HEARING LOSS

The Otolaryngologist's Guide to Amplification

HEARING LOSS

The Otolaryngologist's Guide to Amplification

M. Jennifer Derebery, M.D. and William M. Luxford, M.D.

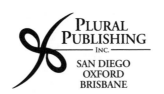

PLURAL
PUBLISHING
INC.

SAN DIEGO
OXFORD
BRISBANE

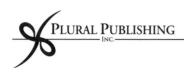

5521 Ruffin Road
San Diego, CA 92123

e-mail: info@pluralpublishing.com
Web site: http://www.pluralpublishing.com

49 Bath Street
Abingdon, Oxfordshire OX14 1EA
United Kingdom

FSC

Mixed Sources
Product group from well-managed
forests and other controlled sources

Cert no. SW-COC-002283
www.fsc.org
© 1996 Forest Stewardship Council

Typeset in 10½/13 Garamond book by Flanagan's Publishing Services, Inc.
Printed in the United States of America by McNaughton & Gunn
Cover design by David Landguth

Library of Congress Cataloging-in-Publication Data

Hearing loss : the otolaryngologist's guide to amplification / [edited by] M. Jennifer
Derebery and William M. Luxford.
        p. ; cm.
  Includes bibliographical references and index.
  ISBN-13: 978-1-59756-188-4 (alk. paper)
  ISBN-10: 1-59756-188-6 (alk. paper)
  1. Hearing aids. I. Derebery, M. Jennifer. II. Luxford, William M.
  [DNLM: 1. Hearing Disorders—therapy. 2. Amplifiers, Electronic. 3. Hearing Aids.
WV 270 H4355 2010]
  RF300.H46 2010
  617.8'9—dc22

                                                                    2009030697

Contents

Foreword

Dr. Derebery and Dr. Luxford have assembled a list of Who's Who to write this important text highlighting the importance of treating the hearing impaired through amplification. As surgeons, otolaryngologists sometimes forget that surgery has risks and complications, hence surgery should be the last resort. There are times when medications and surgery will not alleviate the hearing loss. The 21st century generation of hearing aids can do wonders for our hearing-impaired patients. As an otologist for four decades, I am a successful hearing aid user in each ear.

People saw better with a monocle; however, that was in the 18th century—we now wear a pair of glasses. Hence, binaural hearing is crucial to enjoying life in this fast-paced technologic age. Yet many of us still prescribe only one hearing aid for a patient with bilateral hearing loss.

The editors and the authors of the chapters in this book have contributed greatly in helping us to help our hearing-impaired patients. They are to be congratulated. Our heartfelt thanks.

K. J. Lee, M.D., FACS
Past President, American
Academy of Otolaryngology-
Head and Neck Surgery

Introduction

Hearing loss is the third most common health problem in the United States, and affects more than 31 million Americans. Most hearing loss is sensorineural, which, at the time of this writing, is not "curable" with medical or surgical means. For most patients with clinically significant hearing loss, hearing aids are the best treatment option available.

No patient is happy with the recommendation that they should seek amplification for hearing loss. We are all familiar with the denial that commonly accompanies the recommendation that hearing aids would be of benefit. Yet, most patients will obtain a hearing aid only after a physician, rather than a family member, both confirms that a hearing loss exists, and recommends that amplification is the best treatment available to treat it.

The otolaryngologist is uniquely trained in the ability to diagnose, as well as treat, hearing loss by medical or surgical means. With the aging of the baby boomer population, the significant noise exposure in modern life, as well as the greater comfort the population at large is getting in wearing "ear level" devices for communication, we can expect that the need for professional recommendation for the treatment of hearing loss with hearing aids will continue to increase in the future.

Diagnostic tests for hearing loss and hearing aid dispensing are taught as a core component of otolaryngology residency programs. Questions regarding the treatment of hearing loss with hearing aids are mandated by the American Board of Otolaryngology in both the oral and written examinations taken upon matriculation. The authors intend this book to enhance the training that is already being given in residency programs. The chapters discuss in detail not only technical aspects of hearing aid fitting useful to the physician, but also address specific areas of challenge, such as fitting the pediatric patient with hearing loss, or the patient with hydropic hearing loss with a changing baseline audiogram. We have included research trends in hearing aids, as well as potential nutriceutical interventions to protect hearing health. The related problem of tinnitus management in this population is also of great concern to our patients. Practical solutions for the hearing impaired are at times best addressed by the use of assistive listening devices; to read about them is to begin to think about coping in everyday life from the perspective of the hearing impaired. Bone-anchored hearing aids and other surgically implantable devices are growing in both sophistication and popularity, and also are discussed.

In addition to clinical issues, the well-trained graduating resident or practitioner is faced with the very unfamiliar task of trying to establish both a financial model of how to develop hearing aid dispensing within his or her practice, as well as what they should be looking for in hiring nonphysician professional personnel to join them in practice. Marketing and advertising, foreign concepts to most physicians, can be done both professionally and tastefully to enhance both the hearing aid dispensing as well as the medical and surgical components of practice.

This book would not have been possible without the collegiality and professionalism shown by the many contributors. No one profession or group has a monopoly on providing patient care to the hearing impaired. The knowledge shared here is given by top professionals in the audiology, hearing instrument, business, and medical professions, and we editors genuinely have learned by working with them in preparation for this book. It is our hope that in the future, we professionals in varied fields can put aside "turf battles" to work more closely together to better serve the needs of the growing population of the hearing impaired.

William M. Luxford
M. Jennifer Derebery

Contributors

David M. Barrs, M.D.
Department of Audiology
Mayo Clinic Arizona
Phoenix, Arizona
Chapter 3

John R. Coleman, Au.D., FAAA
Orange County Physician's Hearing
   Services
Mission Viejo, California
Chapter 4

M. Jennifer Derebery, M.D.
Associate, House Clinic and Ear
   Institute
Clinical Professor of Otolaryngology
USC Keck School of Medicine
Los Angeles, California
Chapter 8

Randall R. Drullinger
President of the Aegis Group
Portland, Oregon
Chapter 13

Brent Edwards, Ph.D.
Vice President of Research
Starkey Laboratories
Berkeley, California
Chapter 17

David Fabry, Ph.D.
Chief of Audiology
Miller School of Medicine
University of Miami
Miami, Florida
Chapter 6

Neil A. Giddings, M.D.
Spokane Ear Nose and Throat
Spokane, Washington
Chapter 14

Michelle L. Hicks, Ph.D.
Senior Research Audiologist
Center for Amplification and Hearing
   Research
Sonic Innovations
Salt Lake City, Utah
Chapter 2

John W. House, M.D.
House Clinic
Clinical Professor,
Department of ORL-HNS
Keck School of Medicine
University of Southern California
President,
House Ear Institute
Los Angeles, California
Chapter 9

Margaret M. Jastreboff, Ph.D.
Jastreboff Hearing Disorders
   Foundation, Inc.
Adjunct Professor
School of Audiology
Salus University
Philadelphia, Pennsylvania
Chapter 10

**Pawel J. Jastreboff, Ph.D., Sc.D.,
M.B.A.**
Professor
Department of Otolaryngology
Emory University School of
   Medicine
Atlanta, Georgia
Chapter 10

Sergei Kochkin, Ph.D.
Executive Director
Better Hearing Institute
Washington, DC
Chapter 1

William M. Luxford, M.D.
Associate, House Clinic and Ear
    Institute
Clinical Professor of Otolaryngology
USC Keck School of Medicine
Los Angeles, California
Chapter 1

Michael J. Nilsson, Ph.D.
Director,
Center for Amplification and Hearing
    Research
Sonic Innovations
Salt Lake City, Utah
Chapter 2

Marcia Raggio, Ph.D.
Professor
San Francisco State University
San Francisco, California
Chapter 5

Michael J. A. Robb, M.D.
Private Practice
Neurology, Oto-Neurology and
    Medical Neurotology
Robb Oto-Neurology Clinic
Phoenix, Arizona
Chapter 11

Stephen J. Sanders, Au.D., FAAA
Orange County Physician's Hearing
    Services
Mission Viejo, California
Chapter 4

Michael D. Seidman, M.D., FACS
Medical Director,
Division of Otologic/Neurotologic
    Surgery

Department of Otolaryngology-Head
    and Neck Surgery
Medical Director,
Center for Integrative Medicine
    Program
Henry Ford Health System
Clinical Associate Professor
Department of Otolaryngology
Wayne State University
Detroit, Michigan
Chapter 11

William H. Slattery, III, M.D.
Director, Clinical Studies; House Ear
    Institute
Associate, House Ear Clinic
Clinical Professor, University of
    Southern California
Los Angeles, California
Chapter 12

Michael Valente, Ph.D.
Director of Adult Audiology
Professor of Clinical Otolaryngology
Washington University School of
    Medicine
St. Louis, Missouri
Chapter 16

Brad Volkmer, M.B.A.
President/CEO
Ear Professionals International
    Corporation
City of Industry, California
Chapter 15

Margaret E. Winter, M.S., CCC-A
Board Certified in Audiology
Coordinator of Clinical Services
House Ear Institute
Children's Auditory Research and
    Evaluation (CARE) Center
Los Angeles, California
Chapter 7

Acknowledgments

I would like to both acknowledge and thank the late Aram Glorig, MD, and Alexander Schleuning, MD, both otologists and educators. These gentlemen first taught me to think of hearing aids as an actual treatment for hearing loss, not simply a device.

I would also like to thank my patients, most especially Mr. Richard K. Eamer, who has taught me more than any textbook about the perspective of life from the view of the hearing impaired.

JD

We would like to acknowledge Marian Rush of the House Ear Institute and Brian Hammer of the House Clinic for their help in preparing the manuscript.

WL and JD

This book is dedicated to:

My husband, Gregory Spahr, and daughters Alexandra (A. J.) and Madison Spahr. They have patiently endured the hours I spent working on this book that I could not share with them.
Jennifer Derebery

My wife Margie, my two daughters Lara Logue and Emily Luxford, and my first grandchild Kyla Logue.
William Luxford

1

Why Should I Use Hearing Aids: Talking to the Patient About Hearing Loss

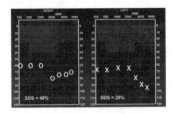

WILLIAM LUXFORD, M.D.
SERGEI KOCHKIN, Ph.D.

Two groups of users are represented by the "I" in the title "Why should I use hearing aids?" The first group consists of hearing professionals: otolaryngologists, audiologists, and hearing aid dispensers who identify and care for patients with hearing loss. The second group consists of the consumers: patients, both adults and children, who would benefit from using hearing aids to treat their hearing loss.

Hearing loss is one of the more common chronic illnesses in the United States. In the year 2000, 28 million Americans, approximately 10% of the population, were hearing impaired. Nine million Americans had mild hearing loss, 10 million had moderate hearing loss, 6 million had moderate to severe hearing loss, and 3 million had severe to profound hearing loss.

In 2004–2005, the population of hearing impaired increased to over 31 million Americans. It is predicted that within the next two decades, the hearing loss population will swell to over 40 million. Approximately 30% of people over the age of 65 are affected by hearing impairment, with the figure rising to 35–40% of those older than 75 years.

Age-related hearing loss (presbycusis) occurs gradually and, although it may go unnoticed by the individual, it is quite apparent to family and friends. Presbycusis is the most common cause of hearing loss in the United States. The aging of the baby boomers is swelling the over 60-year population, increasing the number of elderly adults with hearing loss (Kochkin, 2005b).

Although hearing impairment traditionally has been associated with the elderly, hearing loss has increased markedly across all age groups. Excessive noise is the likely culprit for the increase in the incidence of hearing impairment in the younger age groups. Damaging noise exposure may occur at rock concerts, movies, and aerobic classes. Noise-induced hearing loss may also result from the use of personal music players using in-the-ear buds.

Difficulty in understanding conversation can be secondary to two problems. The first is lack of audibility. If one cannot hear what is said, he or she has nothing to process and, therefore, will not understand what is said. The second is a problem of processing; the inability to discriminate. There are individuals who do not have audibility problem, that is, they are able to hear conversation. However, despite hearing the words, they are not able to clearly process what they hear. Therefore, even though the conversation has been "heard" the conversation is still difficult to understand.

Hearing aids can improve the audibility. They can improve the patient's ability to hear conversation. However, the hearing aids do not improve the processing of what is heard. They do not correct the underlying inability to discriminate.

Hearing-impaired patients can also receive benefit from the use of assistive devices, whether or not they use a hearing aid. Devices are available that can assist with the use of a telephone, television, movies, and in live theaters.

Older adults with hearing loss who do not use amplification are more likely to report feelings of sadness, depression, anxiety, and emotional turmoil. In contrast, for the most part, aided elderly adults experience an overall improvement in quality of life, relationships, and feelings about themselves following acquisition of hearing aids (Kochkin & Rogin, 2000).

Talking to the Patient

The first step in assessing a patient with hearing loss is to define, through a history, physical exam, and audiologic tests, the nature of the patient's hearing loss.

There are several ways to approach the patient who has sensorineural hearing loss. One approach that may discourage the patient from following through with a hearing aid evaluation is one in which the physician states "nothing but the facts."

He says in so many words to the patient: (1) "You have an inner ear or nerve loss," (2) "There is nothing that can be done for your problem," (3) "You need a hearing aid," and (4) "No return appointment is necessary."

What the patient hears is: "There is nothing you want to do to try and help me. You are really not interested in my problem. All you want to do is sell me an expensive hearing aid. You want me to get out of your office and never bother you again."

Another approach, which the author finds may actually encourage the patient to use a hearing aid, provides the same factual information as in the first example, but presents the facts with phrases that provide a better understanding of the problem, increases acceptance of the hearing loss, and encourages the patient that something positive can be done.

Essentially, what is said to the patient is that "You do have a sensorineural or nerve loss that involves your inner ear and, as such, there is no medicine or surgery that will restore your hearing to normal."

A more positive approach is to give the following points of information: "There are some things that can be done to try and make your hearing better. These include (1) being more assertive within your family, social, and work environments to let others know you do have a hearing loss so they will talk more directly to you; (2) providing others with a simple list of do's and don'ts they should use when talking to a person with hearing impairment; (3) consider using speech reading skills to enhance your understanding. Formal speech reading classes are available in many communities; (4) make use of assistive listening devices, including devices to improve telephone communication and listening to television and radio to help with particular areas of difficulty. Adjust the base and treble switches (lower the base and increase the treble) to accentuate the higher frequencies to improve the awareness of consonants sounds that usually create the most difficulty for individuals with hearing impairment; and (5) the possible use of hearing aids.

It is very important for the patient to understand the goals and limits of amplification. Patients need to be aware that their hearing loss cannot be "cured" by simply placing a device on or in the ear. A more reasonable expectation of bene-

fits may include the following points: "Hearing aids will not restore your hearing to normal, but they can provide some increased benefit. It is important to have the appropriate expectation of what hearing aids will provide and, more importantly, what they will not provide, especially in certain situations. Hearing aid use has to be the choice of you, the patient, not that of a family member or physicians. You do have a loss in both ears and, therefore, it is better for you to use aids in both ears. Most likely, over time, you will find hearing aids to be beneficial for you."

Patients need to understand that hearing loss is a medical condition, and that they are not being abandoned in seeking treatment. They also frequently harbor an unvoiced fear that they will "go deaf" ultimately. They should be reassured specifically that this last point is unlikely. An appropriate parting conversation may include the following: "Finally, I am interested in how you are doing, so I feel it is important you return in one year to have your hearing reevaluated to be sure there has been no progression of hearing loss."

The above encouraging approach, taught by Dr. Howard House, is an approach that has proven to be very successful in caring for patients with aidable sensorineural hearing impairment.

Motivation and expectation are the two important parameters for the hearing aid user. It is important for the physician to discuss with the patient his or her motivation to use a hearing aid and expectations of what the hearing aid will provide. Individuals who seek hearing aid use on their own are more likely to be successful users when compared to individuals who purchase the hearing aid to please their spouse or other family members. Individuals who expect to hear "normally" while wearing a hearing aid inevitably will be disappointed. The physician should educate the potential hearing aid user and all family members regarding appropriate expectations for hearing aid use.

The Food and Drug Administration (FDA) has exempted hearing aid manufacturers from premarket notification requirements. Therefore, as opposed to pharmaceuticals, marketing claims for new products may be advertised without FDA clearance. The advertisements may mislead the reader into thinking the more sophisticated more expensive digital hearing aids can restore normal hearing.

Hearing aids are mechanical devices which, although they may improve one's hearing, are unable to restore hearing that is perfect in every setting. Patients must be reminded that good hearing depends on factors other than just the ear and how the ear functions with the use of a hearing aid.

Like a radio or television signal, hearing is dependent on the sound source, a transmitter, as well as the distance the sound must travel from the source to the ear, the receiver. The ear must first receive the signal, that is, hear it, so that the ear can send the information along to the central auditory system where that signal is processed.

A poor transmission from a person who is mumbling or not projecting his or her voice will affect hearing adversely. A large separation between the transmitter and the receiver, such as from upstairs to downstairs or down a long hall, or from one room to another, or an interference in the clarity of the signal by background sound, at large family gatherings, cocktail parties, or restaurant settings, will affect hearing adversely. A receiver that is not tuned in, as for example; may occur when the hearing aid wearer is tired or concentrating on another activity, also will impair hearing.

It is essential to review these situations with the patient who will be using a hearing aid, emphasizing that it is unreasonable to expect perfect hearing in settings where there is a poor transmitter, significant noise interfering with the signal, or even when the user may be tired or under a great deal of stress (Ross, 2008). Explain to the patient that noise may have an impact on auditory function to a greater degree in aided individuals than in matched counterparts with normal hearing.

There are some patients who feel that they have a great deal of difficulty hearing in settings with background sound. Yet, a thorough audiologic assessment shows that they have hearing within the normal range with excellent speech discrimination scores. Occasionally, further testing is ordered, which may include an ABR or even an MRI scan with gadolinium. These tests are almost always normal. In our office, we feel the appropriate diagnosis for these patients is "Discrimination hearing loss, cause unknown."

The majority of patients who have difficulty understanding speech (either recognized by themselves or by a family member) will be found to have some objective hearing loss on the audiometric testing. Patients with mild to moderate hearing loss, as opposed to more moderate to severe, are more likely not to recognize the loss that is present.

Speech is a combination of vowels and consonants. The vowels are primarily lower frequency sounds, whereas consonants are primarily in the mid to high frequencies of the speech range, which is almost completely contained within 500 to 3000 cycles. Most hearing losses that occur either through presbycusis or noise exposure involve the high frequencies, which adversely affect the patient's ability to hear consonants, especially in settings with background sound. It is not unusual for the patient sitting in the professional's office not to recognize a mild or moderate high-frequency loss in a quiet setting while the professional is speaking directly to the patient in a well-lighted room and the professional projects his or her voice using an enunciated speech pattern.

The response from the patient, usually a man to his spouse is, "See, honey, I told you I didn't have a hearing problem. Our difficulty in communicating must be your fault." It is important for the professional, now acting as a marriage counselor, to educate the patient, that yes, he has done well in the quiet office environment, but in the typical home and work environment that represents his real, more noisy, world, his hearing loss most likely will affect his ability to communicate with others.

Within the quiet environment, one to one, the patient is able to hear and see the speaker and, therefore, uses hearing and speech reading to pick up vowels and consonants. In the real world, the chips are stacked against him. His mild to moderate sloping, high-frequency sensorineural hearing loss makes it more difficult for him to understand the higher pitched voice of a female or young child compared to the lower pitched voice of a male adult speaker.

In the typical family setting, in the den watching television, or in the kitchen where he is sitting at the table while his wife is moving around preparing or cleaning up after a meal, he probably will hear the lower pitched vowel components of his wife's speech but not hear the higher

pitched consonants. Unfortunately, it is usually these consonants that give distinct meaning to a word.

Several paths are now open to the patient. The first path is the path of non-response. The patient does not acknowledge that his wife has spoken, which results in her saying: "Sweetheart, don't you hear me?" The second path is the path of indifference. His response is to slowly lift his head and say: "What?" Her response is to say: "Sweetheart, focus. Pay attention. You have to listen to me." The third path is the path of action. He feels he has heard his wife's explicit instructions. At the next commercial break, he pulls himself out of his favorite rocking chair, exits the den, returning a few minutes later kissing his wife on the forehead saying, as he sits back in his favorite rocker to continue watching his basketball game: "I'm surprised you asked me to empty the bucket. There wasn't much there." At that point, the wife slowly turns to her husband to ask: "What did I ask you to do?" and his response: "You asked me to take out the trash." The wife replies: "No, I did not. I asked you to turn on Johnny Cash."

Not only can the hearing-impaired patient misinterpret what is said, but also those around him can misinterpret his responses and actions. As noted above, the patient with the mild to moderate high-frequency hearing loss will have less difficulty hearing and understanding a low-pitched male speaker.

This improved ability to hear the male voice over the female's may result in problems within the family setting after, for example, the husband and wife have returned home from seeing the relatives. The wife states: "You spent all night talking and laughing with my brother and Uncle Dan. All I got out of you was an occasional 'What.' Don't you love me anymore?"

Misinterpretation may also affect the patient's work environment. For example, after a business meeting, one of my patients was called aside by a female employee who told him: "I am glad to see you are getting along with John and Derald, but it is essential that you also acknowledge and listen to me, since I am your boss." Because hearing loss is rarely obvious, it is important for the patient to realize for himself and to explain to others, including his spouse, family, friends, coworkers, and boss, that there are two aspects to hearing: awareness and understanding. Even though he is aware something is said, he may not always understand what is said.

In the Howard House approach to hearing loss, there are many options the patient has to improve his hearing, that is, to improve not only his awareness but, and also more importantly, his understanding. The use of hearing aids is an integral component in improving the hearing impaired patient's awareness of all the speech frequencies, including vowels and consonants.

Effect of Hearing Loss on Adults and Children

Hearing loss is not confined only to the elderly Of the more than 31 million Americans suffering from some degree of hearing loss, over 1 million are children (0–18 years). Additionally 18.4 million are grouped as working adults (18–64 years), and 11.6 million are over 65 years of age.

There are two types of hearing loss; conductive and sensorineural. Conductive hearing loss often can be improved through medicine or surgery, whereas most individuals with sensorineural hearing loss, the more common type of loss, can benefit from the use of appropriately fitted hearing aids, or other assistive devices.

Essentially all hearing aids prescribed today are digital products. Digital hearing aids are reported to provide significantly higher overall satisfaction and benefit, improved sound quality, reduction in feedback and improved performance in noisy situations (Kochkin, 2005a).

Despite changes in technology, acceptance of hearing aids remains poor. Only 23% of those individuals with losses that can benefit from hearing aids own hearing aids. Many of these patients do not actually use their hearing instrument(s). Approximately half of the owners are satisfied or very satisfied with their hearing aids, whereas about 10% are dissatisfied or very dissatisfied (Kochkin, 2005a).

Customer adoption of hearing aids has not improved appreciably since the initial tracking in 1991. The largest percentage of nonusers is in the age range of 45 to 54 years. Problems with conventional amplification cited as reasons for not using hearing aids include: benefit, acoustic feedback, poor fidelity, difficulty listening in noise, cosmetics, cost, and a perceived stigma (Kochkin, 2007).

Patients who do use hearing aids usually have more severe hearing loss than those who do not purchase or use hearing aids and are also more likely to be older. The percentage of "retired" adults (older than 65 years) using hearing aids is 42%, whereas the percentage of "working" adults (18–64 years) using hearing aids is 12.5%. Hearing aid use in children is also around 12%.

Hearing loss definitely impacts quality of life for the patient and the family. It has a negative impact, not only on physical, emotional, and mental health but also on work and school performance.

In most work settings, hearing is necessary for effective communication to create an efficient and safe environment. Compared to normal hearing individuals, not only workers with severe to profound hearing loss but also workers with mild to moderate hearing loss are more likely to be unemployed or under employed, leading to significant personal and social adverse effects. Treating the hearing loss, whether it is mild, moderate, or severe, with hearing aids when appropriate can improve the earning power of the worker. Not treating the loss can lead to lost wages, lost promotions, lost opportunities, and, as a result, lower income in retirement (Kochkin, 2007b).

Hearing loss also can markedly affect the life of a child. Identification of treatable hearing loss is still a problem. Although states now mandate newborn hearing screening, only about two-thirds of those who fail the screening procedure receive appropriate follow-up (White, 2007).

Children with severe to profound hearing loss are more likely to receive further testing and treatment, while children with milder losses are often not identified or treated. However, even a "mild" hearing loss can have a significant negative effect on speech development, educational achievement, and formation of social skills. The lack of follow-up or treatment of children with loss can often be attributed to minimization of the effect of hearing loss by the family doctor, pediatrician, educator, or parent. Two other reasons for nontreatment with aidable hearing loss are the stigma associated with the use of hearing aids and the financial burden on the family with the purchase of hearing aids (Kochkin et al., 2007).

Auditory deprivation can lead to further deterioration of the auditory system and clearly occurs in infants, children, and young and older adults who are fitted with a hearing aid in only one ear. It occurs in patients with binaural sensorineural hearing loss who are fitted with a single hearing aid, and patients with unilateral sensorineural hearing loss who are unaided, and in the unaided poorer ear in patients with asymmetric sensorineural hearing loss, where the better ear is close to normal. It is also present in patients with bilateral conductive hearing loss using only one hearing aid.

The effects of auditory deprivation are more pronounced in patients with unilateral and asymmetrical losses and occur more often with a moderate to severe sensorineural hearing loss than with a loss that is mild to moderate.

To prevent auditory deprivation, it is suggested that binaural amplification be provided for patients with bilateral sensorineural hearing loss and for patients with bilateral conductive hearing loss who are able to wear hearing aids. Patients who have asymmetric hearing loss should be fitted binaurally in an attempt to maintain the worst ear. It is especially important that patients with moderate or severe bilateral sensorineural hearing loss use bilateral aids. A hearing aid should always be recommended for unilateral hearing loss when the affected ear has measurable and usable speech perception.

Late onset auditory deprivation is used to explain reduced word recognition scores in the unaided ear following a period of monaural hearing aid use in a person with bilateral hearing loss. It is a concern for any individual fitted monaurally who has two aidable ears and does not have a general reduction of speech understanding that occurs as part of a normal aging process. The mechanism for auditory deprivation is unknown.

Patients with bilateral sensorineural hearing loss should receive binaural amplification unless there is a medical (draining ear) and/or audiologic (unaidable ear due to profound hearing loss) reason not to do so (Emmer, 1999).

What Can the Physician Do?

The marketing portrayal of digital hearing aids and their increased retail cost leads to higher, often unrealistic, expectations. Aural rehabilitation and counseling leading to more appropriate expectations can improve patient satisfaction, reducing the hearing aid return for credit rate. (Huch, 1999).

The rehabilitation strategies help the patient to learn to listen better. Involving the family in the rehabilitation is helpful (Northern & Beyer, 1999).

Increasing the percentage of aidable adults and children who actually use hearing aids (improving market penetration) will depend on educating both consumers and primary caregivers, of the benefits hearing aids offer for those who are hearing impaired. The Better Hearing Institute (BHI www.betterhearing.org) promotes public awareness of the importance of hearing and hearing care (Kirkwood, 2007). Consumer education also is an important goal of AARP. Their published brochure, titled "Consumer Guide to Hearing Aids," provides accurate information about hearing aids.

Otolaryngologists are an integral component of the hearing health care team. The patient is most likely to treat his or her hearing impairment with hearing aids when the physician has suggested to him or her that it is appropriate, and that help is available. The otolaryngologist should lead the education of the consumers and their primary care physicians on the impact of hearing loss, even a mild impairment, on the quality of life of the patient. Medical management, including the use of hearing aids, can significantly improve the life of a hearing-impaired adult or child.

References

Emmer, M. B. (1999). Review of the late onset auditory deprivation and clinical implications. *Hearing Journal, 52*(11), 26-32.

Huch, J. (1999). In documenting user benefit/satisfaction, there are many tools to choose among. *Hearing Journal, 52*(4), 60-70.

Kirkwood, D. (2007). Ducking bad economic news, hearing aid sales rise by 5.4% on way to record year. *Hearing Journal, 60*, 11-16.

Kochkin, S., & Rogin, C. M. (2000) Quantifying the obvious: The impact of hearing instruments on quality of life. *Hearing Review, 7*(1), 6-34.

Kochkin, S. (2005a). Customer satisfaction with hearing aids in the digital age. *Hearing Journal, 58*(9), 30-39.

Kochkin, S. (2005b). MarkeTrak VII: Hearing loss population tops thirty-one million people. *Hearing Review, 12*(7), 16-29.

Kochkin, S. (2007a). MarkeTrak VII: Obstacles to adult non-user adoption of hearing aids. *Hearing Journal, 60*(4), 24-50.

Kochkin, S. (2007b). The impact of untreated hearing loss on household income. Better Hearing Institute: Washington, DC. http://www.betterhearing.org/pdfs/marketrak_income.pdf

Kochkin, S., Luxford, W., Northern, J. L., Mason, P., & Tharpe, A. M. (2007). MarkeTrak VII: Are one million dependents with hearing loss in America being left behind? *Hearing Review, 14*, 10-36.

Northern, J., & Beyer, C. M. (1999). Reducing hearing aid returns through patient education. *Audiology Today*, *11*(2), 10-11.

Ross, M. (2008, Jan/Feb). *Hearing Loss Magazine*, *29*(1), 2-24. Bethesda, MD: Hearing Loss Association of America.

White, K. R. (2007). Early identification of hearing loss: The best of times . . . the worst of times. *Hearing Health*, *23*(3), 16-18.

2

Review of Audiometry

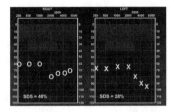

MICHAEL J. NILSSON, Pн.D.
MICHELLE L. HICKS, Pн.D.

The Purpose of Audiometric Testing

The purpose of audiometric testing is to determine the presence and degree of hearing loss and the site of lesion. Hearing loss is defined as a frequency-dependent loss of sensitivity to soft sounds (typically tones) relative to expected normal sensitivity as reported by the audiogram. Normal hearing sensitivity across frequency is defined for young adults by the American National Standards Institute (ANSI) standards (ANSI S3.21-2004). Functional ability beyond pure-tone sensitivity is included in typical clinical testing of hearing mainly as a tool to locate the site of lesion if elevated thresholds are found. That is to say, the presence or absence of a hearing loss is not defined by functional testing, but this testing is specifically intended for site-of-lesion identification. Specific protocols are available describing the measurement of the audiogram (which transducers should be used, preferred and optional presentation methods and strategies, specifics on recording results for uniformity and ease of interpretation, interpretation of results, etc.) and are published by the American Speech-Language-Hearing Association (ASHA). ANSI and ASHA have historical precedence with regulations and recommendations to control/limit/protect the assessment of hearing loss.

Hearing loss can be attributed to a number of different causes. These include conductive components (physical or mechanical obstructions in the outer or middle ear that prevent signals from entering the cochlea) and sensorineural components (typically, some form of damage in the cochlea be it genetic/hereditary, noise-induced, or age-related). Additional, but less frequent causes are central components (pressure on the auditory pathways from tumors, degenerative diseases, processing disorders), or mixed causes (with components from more than one area).

Audiometric testing was designed for diagnostic purposes, but also is the primary method to assess hearing aid candidacy. In these venues, these tests often are used to determine the need for further testing and/or medical treatment versus rehabilitation with amplification. It is the responsibility of any clinician screening hearing to make a referral for medical evaluation when specific indicators are found (such as sudden hearing loss, asymmetric hearing loss, poor speech discrimination, etc.). Success with amplification can be associated with the type of hearing loss, the degree of hearing, and the motivation or communication needs of the patient. A significant hearing loss that impacts enough listening situations to impede normal functioning will respond better to amplification than very mild losses with little or no communication handicap. Patients with high-frequency, sensorineural losses with good discrimination ability will respond better to amplification than patients with poor discrimination or atypical hearing loss configurations.[1] An unmotivated patient

unwilling to learn to listen with amplification often will give up before giving their auditory system time to make use of the newly audible information. Limitations in current amplification systems that distort some of the sounds that were still audible without amplification create cost/benefit tradeoffs between unaided and aided hearing. Internally generated sounds (such as the patient's own voice or other noises generated in the mouth) are often changed, making the familiar action of speaking or eating more difficult than it would be without amplification. If amplification does not provide sufficient improvements to outweigh these difficulties, hearing aid acceptance will be difficult.

Who Can Perform Audiometric Testing?

Audiometric testing can be completed by a number of qualified professionals, including otolaryngologists, audiologists, audiometric technicians, and hearing instrument specialists. Most states require these individuals to be licensed to practice their profession, abide by a code of conduct, and complete continuing education and training in order to maintain their license. Otolaryngologists are medical doctors that specialize in the diagnosis and treatment of diseases of the ear, nose, and throat. They can determine the nature and extent of a hearing disorder, and prescribe and administer medical or surgical intervention as appropriate.

[1]Patients with poor discrimination cannot make good use of speech information even when it is made loud enough to be audible. Therefore, poor discrimination scores denote individuals who will have speech understanding problems even when amplification compensates for their loss of sensitivity.

Whereas otolaryngologists rarely complete audiometric testing themselves, they typically work with or refer to an audiologist or technician for evaluation.

Audiologists are professionals with advanced graduate training in the identification, evaluation, and treatment of hearing and balance function. Audiologists administer and interpret basic and advanced audiometric tests to determine the degree of impairment, site of lesion, the impact on communication, and the need for medical referral. Audiologists receive specialized training in the evaluation of patients across the life span, and in habilitation and rehabilitation services, such as the selection and fit of hearing aids and assistive listening devices.

Audiometric technicians typically work under the supervision of otolaryngologists or audiologists and are trained to conduct audiometric screening and a basic audiometric test battery. They refer to an audiologist for test interpretation or more advanced diagnostic testing, or to an otolaryngologist for medical evaluation.

Hearing instrument specialists receive specialized training in administering the basic audiometric test battery for the purpose of selecting and fitting hearing aids. As with audiometric technicians, they should refer to an audiologist for more advanced diagnostic testing or to an otolaryngologist for medical evaluation if needed.

Test Environments and Equipment

Audiometric testing is intended to measure the limits (softest to loudest) of hearing across frequencies. The ability to detect soft sounds can be impaired either by damage or limitations in the auditory system, or because of other signals that are louder than the test signal and therefore mask it. If the auditory system is already occupied with a louder signal, the softer signal will not be detected. Therefore, controls are necessary to guarantee that elevated thresholds are not due to environmental factors.

The primary environmental control is provided by the audiometric test room. This is a sound-controlled room that prevents extraneous sounds from interfering with testing at the lower limits of human hearing. It is designed to establish a fair and comfortable testing environment that will work with the necessary equipment to evaluate hearing. This involves atmospheric (temperature) and luminosity controls (lighting) that have minimal impact on ambient noise. When installed, an audiometric test room should meet ANSI standards (ANSI S3.1-1999 [R2008]) for noise attenuation and ambient noise within the room while the air circulation fans are turned on. Problems are not uncommon with respect to doors sealing properly, and air circulation fans being too noisy.

Once the test environment is created, test signals must be generated with an audiometer and presented via headphones or insert earphones. The advantages of insert earphones are related to interaural attenuation and collapsing ear canals. The pressure exerted by headphones in order to create a seal can cause ear canals to "collapse" and prevent sound from reaching the tympanic membrane. Insert earphones, which have foam tips with sound tubes in the middle, avoid this problem and prevent sound from leaking out of the ear, stimulating the opposite ear. An audiometer is used to generate the sounds that are played through the transducers, and comes in a wide range of models (ANSI S3.6-2004). Testing flexibility and independence of controls between ears are associated with various prices. The most sophisticated audiometers will have completely independent signal generation and control for the two ears. Simpler, less expensive audiometers will have only one channel to test both ears (only test one ear at a time without "bilateral" test signals). The complexity of testing and goal of testing will help clinics decide which type of audiometer is necessary. All clinical equipment should be calibrated annually.

Audiometric testing often includes evaluation with speech (for speech recognition and discrimination testing). Speech materials have been standardized, but presentation method has not. Clinicians can use recorded materials or use "monitored live voice," where the clinician performing the test reads the materials in a steady voice, while monitoring the level meter for the desired levels. Recorded materials have several advantages and should be used rather than monitored live voice. Recorded materials improve test-retest reliability, reduce the chances of generating feedback in the test room, and guarantee uniform and controlled presentation levels. The hesitation with using recorded materials typically is associated with extra physical steps in controlling the equipment, but modern equipment makes the process simple and fast, once the clinician is familiar with the process.

The Basic Audiometric Test Battery

The basic audiometric evaluation answers several questions. First, is a hearing impairment present? Second, what is the severity of the hearing loss? And, third, is the hearing impairment conductive, sensorineural, or mixed? Additional advanced testing can supplement the basic audiometric test battery to identify the probable site of lesion and to evaluate the communication ability or hearing handicap. The purpose of this section is to describe the principles necessary for understanding how to administer and to interpret the results from a basic audiometric test battery, which includes puretone air and bone conduction audiometry and speech audiometry.

Tuning Fork Tests

Pure-tone audiometry evolved from tuning fork tests, a staple of the otologic test battery used in the differential diagnosis of conductive and sensorineural hearing losses. The principles behind tuning fork tests are the same as those for pure-tone air- and bone-conduction audiometry, and thus should corroborate each other. Tuning forks resonate at a single frequency when struck with a hard or firm surface. The frequency is dependent on the physical properties of the tuning fork, and typically ranges in octave steps from 128 to 4096 Hz. The most common tuning forks used in the otologic test battery resonate at 512 and 1024 Hz.

The Weber test relies on bone conduction to determine if a unilateral or asymmetric hearing loss is conductive or sensorineural. The stem of the tuning fork typically is placed midline on the frontal sinus of the forehead. The patient indicates whether the tone is heard louder in one ear than the other. If the tone is heard equally in the two ears (i.e., no lateralization), hearing is considered symmetric in the two ears. If the tone lateralizes to the better hearing ear, a sensorineural hearing loss is indicated. If the tone lateralizes to the poorer hearing ear, a conductive loss is indicated.

The Bing test is another bone-conduction test used to determine if there is a conductive component to the hearing loss. The stem of the tuning fork is again placed midline on the forehead as the examiner occludes the patient's ear by closing the tragus over the external auditory canal. If the patient reports that the tone becomes louder in the occluded ear, no conductive component is indicated. If there is no noticeable change in loudness, there is likely to be at least a 5- to 10-dB conductive component to the hearing loss.

The Rinne test relies on both air and bone conduction to determine the nature of a hearing loss. The tuning fork is held approximately 2 inches from the opening of the ear canal, and the patient is asked to indicate when he or she no longer hears the tone. The tuning fork is then quickly placed on the prominence of the mastoid without touching the pinna. A conductive hearing loss is indicated if the patient reports that the tone returned. If a tone did not return, a sensorineural loss is likely.

The Swabach test can be completed by air or bone conduction and requires an examiner with normal hearing. The tuning fork is placed by the ear canal or on the mastoid of the patient. When the patient indicates that he or she no longer hears the tone, the examiner quickly places the tuning fork to their own ear. If the examiner hears the tone, a hearing loss is indicated. To quantify the hearing loss, the length of time that the examiner hears the tone is recorded, and a threshold is estimated using the decay rate for a particular tuning fork (Chartrand, 2007).

Pure-Tone Air-Conduction Audiometry

In audiometry, the threshold of hearing is defined as the minimum sound pressure level of a given signal that is capable of producing an audible sensation at least 50% of the time. The most common signal used for audiometry is a pure tone, which results from a simple sinusoidal sound wave. Pure tones have the majority of their energy concentrated at a single frequency, which allows for testing multiple discrete frequencies across the bandwidth of hearing. Thresholds are typically reported in decibel hearing level (dB HL), where 0 dB HL represents the average threshold of young, normal hearing individuals. Thus, positive numbers greater than 0 dB HL indicate thresholds that are worse than the average.

Audiometry is completed using air- and bone-conducted stimuli. Air-conduction audiometry is completed using circum- or supra-aural earphones that rest on or around the pinna, respectively, or insert earphones, in which foam tips are placed into the external auditory canal. In some circumstances soundfield loudspeakers may be used, for example, for children who are unable or unwilling to wear earphones. Earphones have the obvious advantage that they allow independent testing of each ear separately, and insert earphones specifically have the added advantages of preventing collapsed canals, reducing ambient noise, and reducing the chance of crossover hearing to the other ear (see section on masking below).

The evaluation begins by seating the patient comfortably in the audiometric test room, facing toward or in profile to the examiner. Care should be taken not to provide inadvertent visual cues, such as arm movements or facial expressions, as to when a sound will be presented. Although it is preferable to have the patient and examiner in separate rooms with a window that allows for observation of the patient, testing in the same room is possible. The patient is then instructed to listen for a series of tones presented to each ear and to respond to those tones even if they are very faint. Patients typically respond by raising a hand, pressing a response button, or giving a verbal response. After the examiner is confident that the patient understands the instructions, the earphones are carefully centered over the pinna, or, for insert earphones, the foam tips are placed securely into the ear canals. Prior to placing the earphones, a thorough otoscopic examination should be completed to look for signs of pathology, cerumen, or the possibility of collapsed ear canals.

Numerous procedures have been described for finding thresholds, although the most common is a modification of the methods proposed by Hughson and Westlake (1944) and Carhart and Jerger (1959). The procedure is described in detail in guidelines published by the American Speech-Language-Hearing Association (ASHA) on manual pure-tone audiometry (2005). To familiarize the patient with the task, the examiner presents a 1000-Hz tone to the better hearing ear (if an asymmetry exists) at a level that should be clearly audible to the patient. ASHA recommends starting at 30 dB HL. If the patient does not respond, the level is increased to 50 dB HL and then in 10-dB increments until a response occurs. Once a definitive response occurs, threshold testing begins. Using tones of approximately 1 to 2 seconds in duration, the first tone is presented at a level below the expected threshold. If the patient does not respond that he or she heard the tone, the level is increased in 5-dB steps until a response occurs. Once a response occurs, the tone level is decreased in 10-dB steps until the patient stops responding. This "down 10, up 5," descending-ascending approach continues until the examiner has identified the lowest level at which the patient responds to at least half, or two out of three, of the presentations on an ascending series. This level is the patient's *threshold*. After threshold is found for the 1000-Hz tone, the procedure is repeated for the octave frequencies of 2000, 4000, 8000, 1000 (retest for response reliability), 500, and 250 Hz. Occasionally, 3000 and 6000 Hz are added, as well as other interoctave frequencies if there is more than a 20-dB threshold difference between the octave frequencies. Once testing is completed in the better ear, the process is repeated for the poorer ear.

Pure-Tone Bone-Conduction Audiometry

Whereas air-conduction thresholds can be affected by pathology in the outer, middle, or inner ear, and thus provide an overview of the entire auditory system, bone-conduction testing bypasses the outer and middle ear and primarily reflects the functioning of the inner ear. Testing proceeds with essentially the same process as air-conduction testing, but with a bone vibrator placed on the mastoid or forehead. It is critical that the bone vibrator be held in place with the headband with sufficient tension to produce correctly calibrated signal levels and to avoid dislodging the transducer. As bone-conducted stimuli will vibrate the skull and stimulate both inner ears equally, it is not possible to test each ear independently without the use of masking in the nontest ear (see later section on masking). Otherwise, the test procedure and stimuli are as described for air-conduction testing, with the exception that testing may not be possible at 250 Hz or above 4000 Hz, due to vibrotactile sensations or limitations in the frequency response of the transducer.

Masking

Masking is the *process* or the *amount* by which the audibility of one sound is raised by the presence of another sound (ANSI, 1989). In audiometry, masking is used when it becomes necessary to occupy, or mask, the nontest ear to eliminate its participation during assessment of the test ear. This may occur, for example, when there is an asymmetric hearing loss, and the thresholds in the test ear are significantly worse than the nontest ear. When the level in the test ear reaches an intensity level sufficient for it to "cross over" to the other ear via bone conduction of the skull, masking noise should be presented to the nontest ear to prevent the patient from hearing the tone in that ear and only respond when the tone is heard in the test ear. In pure-tone audiometry, the most effective masking noise is a narrowband of noise centered at the signal frequency. For speech audiometry (see later section), the most effective masker is broadband, or speech-spectrum, noise.

The rules for when to mask rely on the amount of *interaural attenuation*. Interaural attenuation is the reduction in sound energy that occurs when the sig-

nal crosses over via bone conduction from one side of the head to the cochlea on the other side. The amount of interaural attenuation is dependent on the signal frequency and the mode of presentation. For air-conducted signals presented via supra-aural headphones, the minimum interaural attenuation is assumed to be 40 dB (Martin & Clark, 2003), whereas for insert earphones, it is 50 dB. This suggests that, whenever an air-conducted signal presented to the test ear exceeds the bone-conducted threshold of the contest ear by 40 (or 50) dB or more, it is possible that the patient may hear the signal in the nontest ear. Thus, masking noise should be presented to the nontest ear to isolate that ear from the test situation.

For bone-conduction testing, interaural attenuation is 0 dB because signals presented via a bone vibrator will reach each cochlea at approximately the same level, regardless of placement of the vibrator. The patient's response will originate from the better, or more sensitive, cochlea. Thus, whenever there is the potential for more than a 10 dB air-bone gap in the test ear, it is necessary to present masking (via air conduction) to the nontest ear, while completing bone-conduction testing in the test ear.

Although the rules for when to mask are generally simple, the procedures for how to mask, and the knowledge of when sufficient masking has been applied are more involved. A thorough understanding of the principles of masking and proper masking techniques is critical for accurate threshold measurement. Several methods for determining effective masking levels and measuring masked thresholds have been proposed, although the most widely cited is the plateau method. The plateau method, also referred to as the Hood technique (Hood, 1960), is a time-consuming procedure, but generally ensures that neither undermasking nor overmasking occurs.

The procedure begins by first establishing unmasked thresholds and determining which thresholds may be influenced by cross hearing. A continuous masking noise is introduced via air conduction to the non-test ear at 10 dB above its air-conduction threshold. Threshold is reestablished in the test ear. The level of the masking noise is increased in 10-dB steps, each time rechecking the threshold in the test ear. If the threshold increases as the masking level increases, cross hearing is occurring and the nontest ear is undermasked. If there is no increase in threshold as the masker level increases over at least a 20 to 30-dB range, the nontest ear is adequately masked and an accurate threshold has been obtained for the test ear. The range over which the threshold stays constant is known as the plateau. Overmasking occurs if additional increases in masker level further elevate the threshold in the test ear. In this case, it is the masking noise that is crossing over to the test ear and interfering with the threshold measurement. The region of undermasking, the plateau, and overmasking are illustrated in Figure 2–1.

Masking for bone-conduction thresholds follows essentially the same procedure. However, the initial masking level usually is increased by an amount equal to the *occlusion effect* for a particular frequency. The occlusion effect is observed as an improvement in the bone-conduction threshold in the nontest ear that occurs when that ear is occluded by an earphone. The improvement does not represent a true increase in sensitivity; rather, it reflects the added energy introduced into the ear canal when the ear is occluded. The size of the occlusion effect differs by

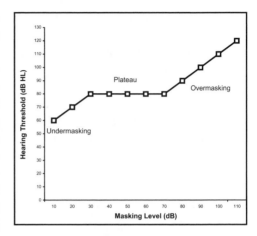

Figure 2–1. Masking levels showing undermasking, the plateau, and overmasking.

frequency and is largest at low frequencies. Additional details on the occlusion effect, the plateau method, and other masking procedures can be found in Yacullo (1996) or Katz (2009).

Audiogram Interpretation

An audiogram is a graphical representation of a patient's hearing thresholds, with frequency (in Hz) along the abscissa and hearing threshold (in dB HL) along the ordinate. Frequency is shown in ascending order from left to right on a logarithmic scale, and hearing level is shown in ascending order from top to bottom on a linear scale. Thresholds for right and left ears can be recorded on the same or separate audiograms, although unique symbols are typically used for each ear, as well as for air- and bone-conduction thresholds, and for masked and unmasked thresholds (ASHA, 1990). The audiometric symbols can be seen in Figures 2–2 through 2–4.

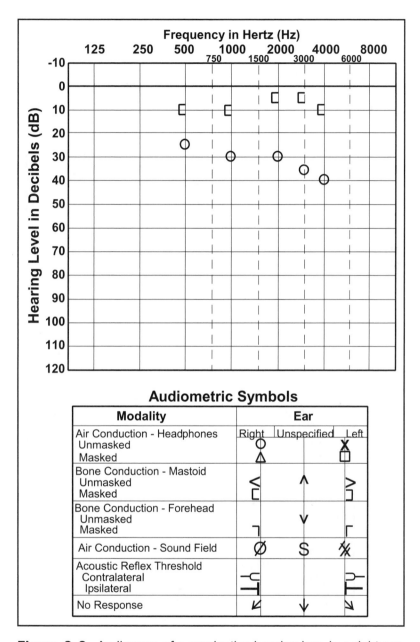

Figure 2–2. Audiogram of a conductive hearing loss in a right ear.

Air-conducted thresholds provide information about the degree of hearing sensitivity, which ranges from normal to profound hearing loss. It is common to divide the audiometric range into cate- gories when describing the hearing loss. One convention, shown below, identifies six categories of hearing sensitivity, based on the level, in dB HL, of the air-conduction thresholds (Bess & Humes, 1995):

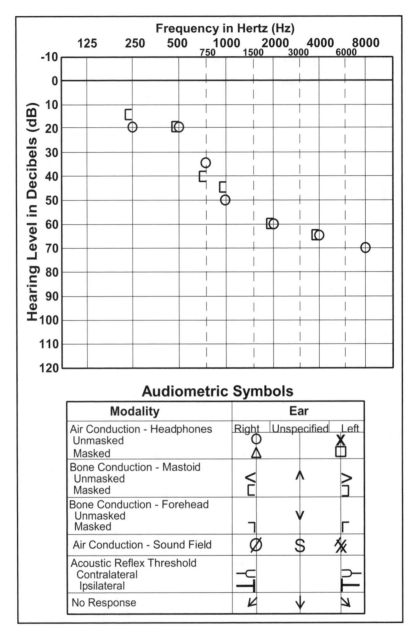

Figure 2–3. Audiogram of a sensorineural hearing loss in a right ear.

Threshold in dB HL	Hearing Sensitivity	Threshold in dB HL	Hearing Sensitivity
10 to 25	normal	56 to 70	moderately severe
26 to 40	mild	71 to 90	severe
41 to 55	moderate	91 or greater	profound

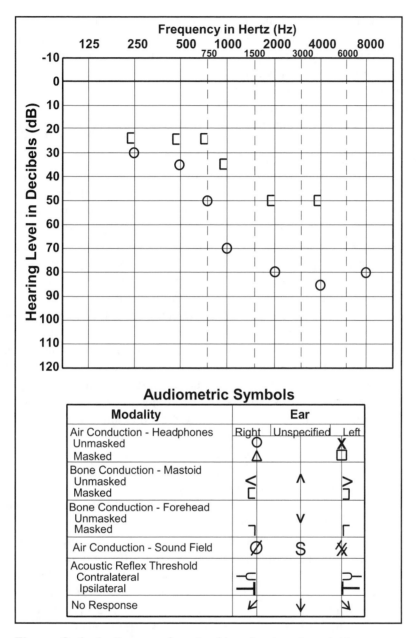

Figure 2–4. Audiogram of a mixed hearing loss in a right ear.

Whereas air-conduction thresholds define the degree of hearing loss, a comparison of air- and bone-conduction thresholds determines the type of hearing loss. Results typically are classified as normal, conductive, sensorineural, or mixed. An ear with normal hearing will have both air- and bone-conduction thresholds within the range of normal sensitivity. An ear with conductive hearing loss will demonstrate bone-conduction thresholds within the range of normal, but abnormal air-conduction thresholds as shown by the audiogram in Figure 2–2. The difference, in dB, between the air- and bone-conduction thresholds is known as the air-bone gap. The poorer air-conduction thresholds reflect reduced transmission of sound energy through the outer or middle ear, suggestive of pathology in one or both of those areas of the auditory system. An ear with sensorineural hearing loss will reveal air- and bone-conduction thresholds that are both outside the range of normal sensitivity, but within 10 dB of each other (i.e., no air-bone gap). A sensorineural hearing loss as seen in Figure 2–3 is suggestive of pathology in the inner ear or auditory nerve. An ear with mixed hearing loss demonstrates air- and bone-conduction thresholds that are also outside the range of normal, but with an air-bone gap that is greater than 10 dB. This result is shown in the audiogram in Figure 2–4. A mixed loss suggests pathology in the outer or middle ear, as well as the inner ear with the size of the air-bone gap reflecting the degree of outer or middle ear involvement. It is important to note that a given ear may exhibit more than one type of hearing loss. For example, a patient may have a mild, conductive hearing loss in the low frequencies, due to possible middle ear dysfunction, but a moderate sensorineural hearing loss in the higher frequencies due to inner ear damage.

Following completion of pure-tone audiometry, one can calculate the pure-tone average (PTA) as a means of summarizing the hearing thresholds. The PTA is an average of the air-conduction thresholds at 500, 1000, and 2000 Hz. In instances of sharply sloping or rising audiograms, where the threshold at one frequency is significantly better or poorer than the other two, the traditional PTA may not accurately reflect the hearing loss. Thus, it is acceptable to calculate a two-frequency PTA, as long as the specific frequencies in the calculation are reported.

Speech Audiometry

Two common speech audiometry tests are speech recognition threshold (SRT) and word recognition ability. The SRT is a cross-check against the reliability and accuracy of the pure-tone audiogram, whereas word recognition testing can help determine site of lesion as well as quantify maximum speech understanding. Although it is possible to administer these tests using monitored live voice by speaking into a microphone, the difficulty in maintaining a consistent intensity level during testing makes using tape or CD recordings preferable. Most of the well-known, common word lists are available for purchase on CD, and in some cases, in multiple languages.

Speech Recognition Thresholds

The speech recognition threshold (SRT) is defined as the "minimum hearing level for speech at which an individual can recognize 50% of the speech material" (ASHA, 1988). The SRT, although measuring the softest level at which an individual can recognize speech, can provide an estimate of the reliability of the test measurements or of the patient's responses. In general, the SRT should agree within ±6 dB of the PTA, otherwise one should suspect that one or both of the test results are questionable, or that the patient's responses are unreliable. Indeed, a large PTA-SRT discrepancy could indicate a nonorganic or exaggerated hearing loss. However, in cases of steeply sloping or rising hearing loss, the SRT may more closely match the best one or two frequencies in the PTA, rather than an average of the three frequencies.

SRT testing begins by familiarizing the patient with a list of common two-syllable words, known as *spondees*. Spondees are words with equal stress on each of the syllables, such as hotdog, cowboy, or toothbrush. The words should be presented at a comfortable listening level, and once the patient is familiar with the list of words, testing can begin. Patients are instructed to repeat back the words that they hear even when the words become very soft. The words can be presented using an ascending, descending, or a combination of ascending and descending methods. The most recent guidelines published by ASHA (1988) recommend using a descending approach, where three to six words are presented at each level, and the intensity level is continually decreased by 5 dB until the patient is unable to correctly identify at least three of the six words at that level. The lowest level at which the patient could correctly identifies at least three of the words is the SRT.

Word Recognition

The purpose of word recognition testing is to evaluate a patient's ability to understand single-syllable words presented at a level above their threshold. The scores can be used to determine a patient's maximum speech understanding ability or to identify a site-of-lesion beyond the cochlea. Most common monosyllabic word lists are constructed of phonetically balanced (PB) words that use sounds that occur in proportion to their frequency of use in spoken English. Well-known lists include the Northwestern University Auditory Test No. 6 (NU-6) (Tillman & Carhart, 1966) and the Central Institute for the Deaf Auditory Tests (CID W-22) (Hirsch et al., 1952). The NU-6 word lists are generally judged to be more difficult and appropriate for adult patients, whereas the CID W-22 words are somewhat easier, and would work well for younger populations. Each list is presented at a single, suprathreshold level and scored as a percentage of words correctly identified. Unlike with the SRT, patients are not familiarized with the word lists prior to testing and a carrier phrase, such as "Say the word _____" is presented before each of the words in the list.

To determine maximum performance, multiple lists should be presented at varying levels, starting near threshold and continuing until performance plateaus. A performance-intensity (PI) function, showing percent correct as a function of presentation level (in dB HL) will identify maximum performance, or *PB Max*. In addition, the PI function can be used to identify possible lesions in the auditory system past the cochlea. When performance significantly declines after reaching PB Max (i.e., performance gets worse as intensity level increases), this suggests a possible retrocochlear, or neural, lesion. This phenomenon, known as *rollover*, is not a definitive diagnosis of retrocochlear pathology and further testing is suggested.

Measuring word recognition at three or four levels to complete a PI function is time consuming, and not the most efficient use of the time available for diagnostic testing. Thus, testing is frequently completed at a single level, approximately 30 to 40 dB above the SRT. This suprathreshold score may not reveal the patient's true maximum performance and does not permit testing for rollover. However, it does provide, in very general terms, an estimate of how well, or how poorly, a patient might perform when listening at levels well above their threshold.

Other Procedures

Additional clinical procedures are common in an audiometric test battery, but are diagnostic in nature, with little or no impact on hearing aid fittings. These include the immittance test battery, such as tympanometry and acoustic reflex thresholds, auditory evoked potentials, and otoacoustic emissions. Detailed information on these tests can be found in Katz (2002).

Speech in Noise Testing

A move toward clinical testing with increased validity has begun to revive the interest in speech testing with more than just word lists. This testing is typically done with sentence-length (or longer) materials, and is often measured with some form of background noise present during testing. The common application of this testing is as an outcome measure for hearing aid fittings, but there is increasing evidence that the ability to understand speech in noise is poorly related to the audiogram. The ability to understand speech in noise must be measured rather than inferred, but can be used to monitor patient complaints as well as validate aided performance. The two sets of materials currently most pop-

ular are the Hearing in Noise Test (HINT, Nilsson et al., 1994) and the Quick Speech in Noise Test (Quick SIN, Killion et al., 2004). Both of these tests measure signal-to-noise ratio loss (SNR loss), or the decrement in ability to repeat speech in noise relative to normal hearing listeners.

Results from these measures help quantify difficulties in noise that are often reported in the clinic, but are not always associated with abnormal audiograms. The data also can identify patients with unusual difficulties in noise, who are unlikely to be satisfied with amplification not including technologies that can improve the signal-to-noise ratio.

Alternative Test Methods

Various additional methods are available for identifying hearing loss, including: screening audiometry and automated audiometry. These variations on standard clinical protocols serve various purposes, but can also be used for hearing aid screenings.

Screening Audiometry

Screening audiometry often will only identify above normal thresholds without quantifying thresholds or bone-conduction data. Unless audiometric thresholds are measured, screening audiometry will only identify a potential hearing loss, but will require additional testing for a diagnosis or to fit a hearing aid. In addition, no information as to the locus of a hearing loss is given without bone-conduction thresholds, which are rarely, if ever, measured with screening audiometry.

Automated Audiometry

Automated audiometry uses computerized systems to go through the well-defined steps in audiometric testing. These systems will measure the complete audiometric test battery by following standardized protocols with many checks in the process to prevent errors in the measurement process. A battery of air- and bone-conduction audiometry, as well as speech testing, can be completed by having the patient interact with a touch screen or similar system. These measurements are most reliable and useful when carefully monitored, but allow complete evaluations without the physical presence of the clinician. However, interpretation of the test results still requires the knowledge of a skilled clinician.

Interpretation— Who Is a Candidate for Amplification?

Amplification is the treatment of choice for any hearing loss that does not have a medically treatable underlying condition. By amplifying the soft sounds not adequately transmitted through the impaired auditory system to levels that can be detected, the patient is given the opportunity to make use of this information and improve hearing in the real world. This treatment does not repair the damaged system, but attempts to optimize the hearing that is still available. An auditory system that is so distorted that even simple speech that is fully audible cannot be understood will still have intelligibility problems with amplification. The capabilities of the auditory system are still a limiting factor. Hearing aid technology is designed to compensate for damage to the sensory organ itself (the ear and cochlea), but not to compensate for more central issues, though any improvement in signal to noise ratio has the potential to increase understanding.

To make treatment with amplification more difficult, the initial symptom of hearing loss is not the loss of soft sounds, but difficulty with speech understanding in noise. Patients first notice difficulty in group settings or noisy environments. This complaint is not associated with a complete loss of understanding, but instead the increased effort required to converse. Eventually, when it becomes hard enough, patients will stop trying to understand because there is insufficient benefit from the effort.

Of the many individuals with hearing loss who are candidates for amplification, not all will be successful users, nor will all be satisfied. Many attempts to predict hearing aid success have been attempted, but no universal prediction has been identified. Current work out of Anna Nabelek's laboratory (Nabelek, 2006) has shown some promise with the ANL measure (acceptable noise level). Individuals who cannot deal with even limited levels of noise appear to be poor candidates for amplification. Other predictors for success have included amount of hearing loss (enough hearing loss is necessary for amplification to provide a noticeable improvement that compensates for negative side effects associated with hearing aids), speech discrimination scores, lifestyle, motivation, age, and ear canal characteristics. Hearing aid success also is strongly associated with familial support, with interactions and efforts from family increasing the likelihood of acceptance.

References

American National Standards Institute. (1999). *Maximum permissible ambient noise levels for audiometric test rooms* (ANSI S3.1-1999 [R2008]). New York: Author.

American National Standards Institute. (2004a). *Methods for manual pure-tone threshold audiometry* (ANSI S3.21-2004). New York: Author.

American National Standards Institute. (2004b). *Specifications for audiometers* (ANSI S3.6- 2004). New York: Author.

American Speech-Language-Hearing Association. (1988). *Determining threshold level for speech* [Guidelines]. Available from http://www.asha.org/policy

American Speech-Language-Hearing Association. (1990). *Audiometric symbols* [Guidelines]. Available from http://www.asha.org/policy

American Speech-Language-Hearing Association. (2005). *Guidelines for manual pure-tone threshold audiometry* [Guidelines]. Available from http://www.asha.org/policy

Bess, F., & Humes, L. (1995). *Audiology: The fundamentals.* Baltimore: Williams & Wilkins.

Carhart, R., & Jerger, J. (1959). Preferred method for clinical determination of pure-tone thresholds. *Journal of Speech and Hearing Disorders, 16,* 340–345.

Chartrand, M. (September 2007). Indiana Jones and the lost art of tuning fork testing. *Audiology Online,* Retrieved November 30, 2007, from http://www.audiologyonline.com/articles/article_detail.asp?article_id=1871

Hirsch, I., Davis, H., Silverman, S., Reynolds, E., Eldert, E., & Bensen, R. (1952). Development of materials for speech audiometry. *Journal of Speech and Hearing Disorders, 17,* 321–337.

Hood, J. (1960). Principles and practices of bone conduction audiometry. *Laryngoscope, 70,* 1211–1228.

Hughson, W., & Westlake, H. (1944). Manual for program outline for rehabilitation of aural casualties both military and civilian. *Transactions of the American Academy of Ophthalmology and Otolaryngology, 48,* (Suppl.), 1–15.

Katz, J. (2002). *Handbook of clinical audiology* (5th ed.). New York: Lippincott Williams & Wilkins.

Killion, M. C., Niquette, P. A., Gudmundsen, G. I., Revit, L. J., & Banerjee, S. (2004). Development of a quick speech-in-noise test for measuring signal-to-noise ratio loss in normal-hearing and hearing-impaired listeners. *Journal of the Acoustical Society of America, 116*(4 Pt. 1), 2395–2405.

Martin, F., & Clark, J. (2003). *Introduction to audiology* (8th ed.). Boston: Allyn & Bacon.

Nabelek, A. K. (2006). Acceptable noise level: A clinical measure for predicting hearing aid outcome. *Journal of the American Academy of Audiology, 17*(9), 624–625.

Nilsson, M., Soli, S., & Sullivan, J. (1994). Development of the Hearing in Noise Test for the measurement of speech reception thresholds in quiet and in noise. *Journal of the Acoustical Society of America, 95,* 1085–1099.

Tillman, T., & Carhart, R. (1966). An expanded test for speech discrimination utilizing CNC monosyllabic words: Northwestern University test No. 4. *Technical report no. SAM-TDR- 62-135.* San Antonio, TX: USAF School of Aerospace Medicine, Brooks Air Force Base.

Yacullo, W. S. (1996). *Clinical masking procedures.* Boston: Allyn & Bacon.

3

Hearing Aid Types

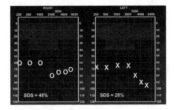

DAVID M. BARRS, M.D.

Hearing Aids

The otolaryngologist is often the initial contact for a patient who has questions about hearing aids. It is important, therefore, that the physician be familiar with the types of hearing aids and current hearing aid technology. The potential hearing aid market in the United States is at least 30 million individuals (Kochkin, 2001; National Institute on Deafness and Other Communication Disorders, 2008). Of this group, only approximately 20% of hearing-impaired individuals obtain a hearing aid, and, of those, one-quarter to one-third do not wear their hearing aids on a regular basis due to problems, such as hearing in background noise (Kochkin, 2001, 2002; The National Council on the Aging, 1999). Patients with hearing impairment are more likely to have communication difficulties and feel depressed and isolated than patients with normal hearing (Kochkin, 2002; Mulrow, Aguilar, & Endicott, 1990). As only a small percentage of the population of patients who could benefit from hearing aids actually do so, the otolaryngologist can perform a significant service to promote hearing aid usage by proper counseling. This chapter reviews the basic types of hearing aids and some of the newer technologies incorporated into contemporary hearing aids.

Hearing Loss Evaluation

The details of a hearing aid evaluation are covered in other chapters. However, portions of the hearing aid evaluation are important in a discussion of hearing aid indications. After the basic audiometric and medical evaluation, the patient is counseled relative to types of hearing aids. Unlike a conductive loss, which requires only an increase in intensity of sound, fitting a patient with sensorineural loss (SNHL) is much more complex (Dillon, 2001). A brief review of the problems associated with this type hearing loss is important in order to understand how new technology in hearing aids tries to correct the loss. The audiometric pattern is down-sloping in 95% of adults and 75% of children, which means that important high-frequency information is missing but the low-frequency power sounds are relatively preserved (Macrae & Dillon, 1996). Sounds are loud enough, but the high frequencies, which give definition to speech, are missing. This leads to the common complaint that sound is loud enough (or too loud!), but comprehension is poor. The steeper the audiometric curve, the more disparity in loss of information, and the harder it is to amplify the high frequencies and preserve the low-frequency sounds. Additionally, loss of cochlear hair cells means that the cochlea loses its ability to fine tune sounds to a specific frequency, also resulting in a loss of clarity. The effect of both the high-frequency loss and the loss of sharply tuned cochlear cells is worsened in noise. Hearing-impaired patients need more information in noise, or, in audiometric terms, they need more signal (speech)-to-noise ratio. Signal-to-noise ratio (SNR) for speech is the sound level of speech compared to background noise. For example, a speech level of 70 decibels (dB) in 60 dB of background noise would have a 10 dB signal-to-noise ratio (Palmer & Ortmann, 2005). Lastly, many patients with SNHL have a narrowed dynamic range (Cook & Hawkins, 2006). Dynamic range is the difference between the threshold of audibility and the loudness discomfort level. With a hearing loss, the hearing level is increased and the loudness discomfort level remains the same, yielding a narrowed dynamic range. Amplification cannot be linear: soft sounds can be amplified the most, but loud sounds need to be amplified less. The hearing aid must be adjusted to amplify sounds above threshold, but below the loudness discomfort level.

Types of Hearing Aids

Although hearing aids can be classified many ways, the simplest way, and the way that patients think about it, is by size. The major trend in hearing aids has been to produce smaller, more cosmetically appealing devices. The four sizes of hearing aids, progressing from largest to smallest, are behind-the-ear (BTE), in-the-ear (ITE), in-the-canal (ITC), and completely in-the-canal (CIC) (Figures 3–1 and 3–2). An increasingly popular BTE is the "mini-BTE," which is a much smaller hearing aid with an open earmold. Which hearing aid is chosen depends on a number of factors: the power requirements needed to correct the hearing loss, the size and shape of the outer ear and ear canal, the electronic features needed to compensate for the hearing loss, and the cosmetic considerations of the patient, which for many patients is the primary concern. Unlike glasses to correct visual problems, a hearing instrument has carried a stigma of aging and most patients initially ask whether a hearing aid will be visible. Obviously, the smaller the aid the greater chance that it will not be noticed.

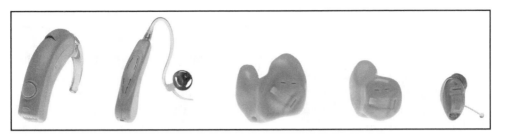

Figure 3–1. Examples of sizes of hearing aids (from right to left): completely in-the canal (CIC), in-the-canal (ITC), in-the-ear (ITE), behind-the-ear (BTE) hearing aid with open mold, and a BTE hearing aid (Courtesy of Starkey Laboratories, Inc., Eden Prairie, Minnesota).

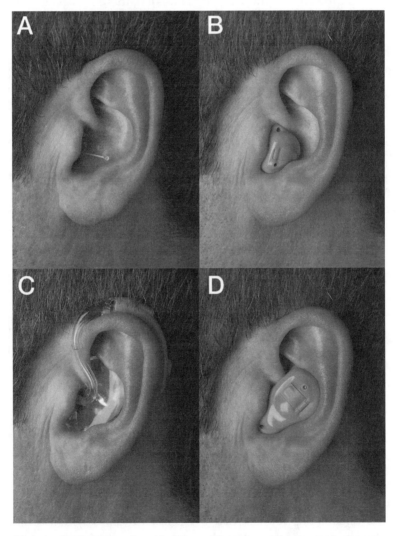

Figure 3–2. Examples of different hearing aids shown in the ear (clockwise from the upper left): completely in-the canal (CIC), in-the-canal (ITC), in-the-ear (ITE), and behind-the-ear (BTE) hearing aids (Courtesy of Starkey Laboratories, Inc., Eden Prairie, Minnesota).

The major benefit of a CIC or ITC type of aid is that it is less noticeable than the other two types. Behind-the-ear hearing aids, however, have become progressively smaller and with thinner tubing; are less noticeable. The BTE fits, as the name implies, behind the ear with a tube running forward over the ear that directs sound into a custom-made mold that fits in the concha and ear canal (Kim & Barrs, 2006). The benefit of the BTE is that it, in general, has the greatest number of features as it has the greatest size for circuitry. They are easy to insert and easy for patients to handle (Kim & Barrs, 2006). In the other three types of hearing aids, the circuitry is in the earmold. The ITE completely fills the concha, includes a large number of features, and is also easy to manage. The ITC is inserted into the ear canal, but protrudes slightly into the concha, so is more visible than the CIC, which is completely in the ear canal. The ITC has a smaller battery, and may contain less circuitry. As the CIC has the fewest features and is the most difficult aid to insert, it is usually recommended for patients who have medium to large ear canals, a mild hearing loss across all frequencies, the dexterity to place the aid in the ear canal, and a significant concern with cosmetic appearance. The patient with bilateral hearing loss also must decide whether to have one aid (monaural fitting) or two aids (binaural fitting). Evidence supports the advantage of binaural fittings for almost everyone with a moderate to severe SNHL, and even in a milder loss in complex listening situations, such as a workplace (Nobel, 2006; Nobel & Gatehouse, 2006; Ross, 1980). In patients with an asymmetric hearing loss, binaural hearing aids are used, with each instrument programmed to attempt to equalize hearing as much as possible (Kim & Barrs, 2006). Binaural hearing also gives the benefit of localization of sound. There are only a few reasons to use a single aid. The main concern is cost, but even then, the possibility exists to use two lesser priced hearing aids as opposed to one more sophisticated aid (Kim & Barrs, 2006). If only one ear is amplified, there is also evidence to suggest an "unaided ear effect," which is characterized by "auditory deprivation," or progressive degradation of function, in the unaided ear.

Clinicians often see patients with single-sided deafness from such conditions as acoustic neuroma, trauma, or sudden idiopathic SNHL. These patients are candidates for crossover type hearing aids. The patient wears two hearing instruments. On the side with the more severe hearing loss, the instrument has a microphone and a transmitter, which sends the signal to the opposite ear's instrument. This usually is performed as a wireless system. If hearing is normal in the opposite ear, no amplification of the sound is needed and the sound is presented to the normal ear at a comfortable level. This system is called a CROS system, which stands for "contralateral routing of signal." If hearing is decreased in the receiving ear, the incoming signal is amplified. In this situation, the system both detects sound on the poorer side and also acts as a traditional hearing on the better side to provide amplification. This is called a BiCROS signal, or "bilateral contralateral routing of sound." The main complaint against the CROS system is that the normal ear can feel plugged as it is necessary to place a hearing aid type earmold in the ear with no hearing loss. The use of open earmolds (discussed below) has helped to reduce the fullness sensation. Also, the patient cannot localize sound because all sound is transferred to the better ear. Despite these drawbacks, a recent review of digital CROS and BiCROS instruments found that approximately three-quarters of patients kept their device, with a satisfaction rating of 3.4, on a scale of 1 (poor) to 5 (excellent) (Hill, Marcus, & Diggs, 2006). Other options include a surgically implanted bone conducting hearing appliance (BAHA). This technology is discussed in Chapter 12.

Special Features

Digital Sound Processing

In the past two decades, advances have been made not only in miniaturization of components to allow smaller hearing aids, but also in circuitry and technology. These advances have allowed the hearing aid manufacturers to make progress with many of the complaints patients have had with sound processing, especially hearing in background noise. Basically, a hearing aid combines several components: a microphone to receive sound and convert it to an electrical signal, an amplifier to increase the strength of the signal, a receiver that is a miniature loudspeaker to convert the electrical signal back to sound, an earmold to couple the sound to the ear, and a power source (Dillon, 2001b; Kim & Barrs, 2006). Previously, hearing aids used analog technology, with acoustic energy transformed into electrical energy. In this

system, electrical voltage is "analogous" to sound intensity, which is where the term "analog" originates (Dillon, 2001b; Kim & Barrs, 2006). Amplification is achieved by manipulation of the signal voltage and then transformed back to a sound.

Digital signal processing (DSP) has, for the most part, replaced analog technology. It is worthwhile briefly reviewing digital technology as it relates to hearing aids. In digital technology, the input signal (sound in this case) is converted to a series of numbers. The signals from the microphone are analog, and are then converted in an analog-to-digital converter and filtered to reduce distortion. This signal is "sampled" at a very high rate; usually at least twice the highest frequency compared to the input signal (Cook & Hawkins, 2006); Dillon, 2001a). For example, if a hearing aid amplifies sound up to 10,000 hertz (Hz), the converter samples at least every 1/20,000 second. This provides a very large amount of information about the input sound signal, which is then processed in an amplifier for such parameters as volume, loudness growth, and frequency response. This signal is then processed in a digital-to-analog converter back to sound for presentation to the earmold.

An intermediate step in the transition from analog to digital hearing aids was the digitally programmable analog hearing aid. In this case, digital technology was used to program the hearing aid, although the sound was still analog. The DSP allowed the hearing aid to be more easily programmed with different output parameters for different listening situations, such as quiet listening versus a noisy background. The user then selected which program fit a given environment.

Digital sound is not necessarily better accepted by a patient than analog sound. A hearing aid user, for example, who has a severe to profound hearing loss, may prefer the more "booming" analog sound, compared to the softer digital amplification. The main advantage of DSP is that it supports a greater number of features, which in turn may improve sound quality as compared with analog processing (Kim & Barrs, 2006). These features include compression, noise reduction, feedback suppression, and directional microphones, among others, and are discussed later. Digital technology allows these complex functions to be performed more efficiently, with less circuitry and power consumption, which translates to smaller hearing aids and reduced battery de-mand. Although some studies show that patients do not necessarily prefer digital hearing aids to analog hearing aids, the ease of programming and lower production costs associated with digital hearing aids have led to the fact that digital hearing aids have almost completely replaced analog hearing aids (Paring, 2003; Strom, 2005; Wood & Lutman, 2004).

Compression

Most patients with hearing loss have a reduced dynamic range. The challenge for the hearing aid is to raise the audible sound to be heard, but not too loud to be uncomfortable. As speech and environmental sounds vary enormously in intensity, this is a significant challenge, especially the control of sudden loud sounds. If sound is visualized as a sine wave, then one traditional method of decreasing uncomfortable sound is a clipping of the tops of the sound peaks. The problem comes if the intensity is clipped at too low a level, then auditory information is lost and the output sound, such as speech, becomes distorted and less intelligible. In other words, the compression circuit limits the output of the sound. Compression is the technology name for DSP circuits that dampen this sudden onset of sound without the loss of auditory information from simple peak clipping. The theory is that soft sounds will be amplified more than loud sounds. To be the most effective, the sound must be split into different frequency widths, and the loudness manipulated for each frequency. With DSP, this can be done across the auditory spectrum for the speech ranges. It is currently termed "wide dynamic range compression," as the compression occurs across a wide range of frequencies, and is the industry norm (Kates, 2005); a side effect of compression technology is that volume is automatically controlled. The hearing aid is set for soft or comfortable sounds, and, if a loud sound occurs, the volume is decreased. For most patients, this technique has taken the place of a volume control. This can present as a potential problem for people with conditions with fluctuating hearing, such as Ménière's disease, as their requirements for amplification may vary. In the future, it may become more difficult to have manual volume control as an option.

Noise Suppression

As one author has stated, noise is simply unwanted sound (Wood & Lutman, 2004). Background noise is mostly in the low-frequency range; so, in the past, reduction of this unwanted noise was accomplished by filtering out low-frequency sounds. Unfortunately, this also removed desired information from speech. Digitally programmable analog hearing aids attenuated low frequencies and enhanced high frequencies with different combinations programmed for different noise levels. Current DSP digital hearing aids attempt to actually recognize noise, which is a constant sound, and differentiate it from speech, which modulates (Kim & Barrs, 2006). This can be done through the same frequency bands as mentioned for compression, so noise and speech can be detected within frequency ranges. The attempt is made not just to filter a set frequency at a set level, but also to detect the temporal characteristics of the sound (Bentler & Chiou, 2006). In other words, measure and react to noise in real time. The hearing aid then can reduce the lower frequency noise levels, while preserving the information in the speech frequencies. The dilemma for manufacturers is where to set the threshold for activation. If the threshold is too low, then suppression will limit audibility, and if it is set too high there will be too much noise. Most manufacturers allow some noise in a trade-off for audibility, and at least one study shows that hearing aid usage is increased if audibility is greater in background noise (Bentler & Chiou, 2006; Souza, Yueh, & Sarubbi, 2000).

A second factor of noise suppression is the speed of onset of the suppression (Kates, 2005; Wood & Lutman, 2004). When noise is presented, the noise suppression circuit detects the sound and, after a given period of time, suppresses the sound. On the one hand, if the onset of suppression is too slow, then the noise interferes with speech detection. On the other hand, fast onset noise suppression is desirable so noise can be reduced, even between words, leading to much clearer

speech understanding (Bentler & Chiou, 2006; Chung, 2004).

Feedback Suppression

Feedback is that unwanted squeal that is heard when a microphone is placed too close to a speaker, and is common in hearing aids when they are placed in the hand or, at times, in the ear canal. Who hasn't heard a spouse say, "Turn off your hearing aids, they're squealing!" Analog processing reduces feedback by reducing gain especially in the high frequencies. Digital signal processing uses a different technique of producing a counterphase signal that cancels the feedback. When feedback is detected, canceling it with a counterphase signal controls feedback without having to reduce gain, again improving the speech signal intensity.

Directional Microphones

A hearing aid with one omnidirectional microphone indiscriminately collects and amplifies speech and noise from all directions. A hearing aid with two (sometimes more) microphones can increase or decrease sounds from different directions. The directional microphone can be two ports on the single microphone, or multiple independent microphones. In most conversational situations, a speaker is directly in front of a listener. Noise that is off to the side, or in the back, is less important to the listener and interferes with the speech signal. With directional microphones, for the most part, there is a microphone that receives sound from the front and one that receives sound from the back. In a conversational setting such as a restaurant, speech detected by

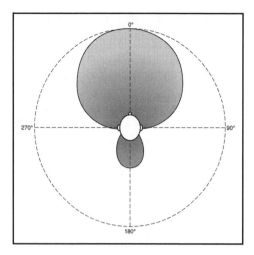

Figure 3–3. Directional microphone field, emphasizing input from the area in front of the listener, and minimizing input from behind the listener.

the frontal microphone can be increased while the noise from other tables to the back and side can be decreased. The obvious benefit is that sound from an object of interest to the listener can be increased and sounds of less interest decreased (Figure 3-3). The resulting increased signal-to-noise ratio hopefully can improve comprehension in noise. In a quieter situation, the microphone outputs can be more equalized. This change can occur either manually or automatically. Also, a technique called adaptive microphone technology can automatically maintain the anterior hemisphere (the hemisphere out in front of the listener) as the most sensitive direction. With continual monitoring of sound input, the aid can determine the direction of sounds with the greatest delay and suppression, change to input from the microphones to maximize SNR. Not all hearing aids can have directional microphones. A CIC is too small, and is buried in the ear

canal, so there is no space for placement of two microphones. Both BTE and ITE hearing aids can be constructed with directional microphones, but it is difficult with an ITC aid.

The amount of benefit gained from noise reduction circuitry and directional microphones is not without controversy. One study compared normal hearing individuals with patients using binaural hearing aids with directional microphones, and showed benefit with the directional microphones, approaching that of the normal group (Bentler, Palmer, & Dittberner, 2004). Two other studies showed 3.4 to 6.6 dB improvements in SNR with directional microphones as compared with omnidirectional microphones (Wouters, Litiere, & van Wieregan, 1999). In real world listening situations, users preferred directional microphones to omnidirectional (Walden, Surr, & Cord, 2004). Relative to adaptive microphone technology, several reports did not find a significant difference from fixed directional microphones (Kak, Kennan, & Lay, 2005), whereas at least one study found improved speech intelligibility with adaptive microphones in the presence of noise introduced laterally. A recent review chronicles the development of directional hearing aids, stating that most hearing aid users will derive some benefit in some listening environments with directional microphones (Ricketts, 2005). The same findings apply to digital noise reduction, with studies showing that noise reduction did not improve speech comprehension in certain noise environments (Smeds, Keidser, & Zakis, 2006a). There also are studies, however, that show there are characteristics of the impaired auditory system that influence these results. Hearing-impaired individuals prefer sound at a lower loudness level than a comparable demographic group with normal hearing (Smeds, Keidser, & Zakis, 2006b). An interesting phenomenon is plasticity of the auditory system after hearing aid usage. Summarized briefly, hearing aid users, either monaural or binaural, developed greater tolerance to loud sounds and increased discrimination performance after hearing aid usage (Gabriel, Veuillet, & Vesson, 2006; Munro & Trotter, 2006). Regardless of the studies, manufacturers increasingly are developing algorithms to sample the sound environment and then "steer" special features such as directional microphones and noise reduction circuitry to provide optimal output (Kates, 2005). These special features are no longer used in isolation, but in combination (Kates, 2005; Nordrum, Erler, & Garstecki, 2006).

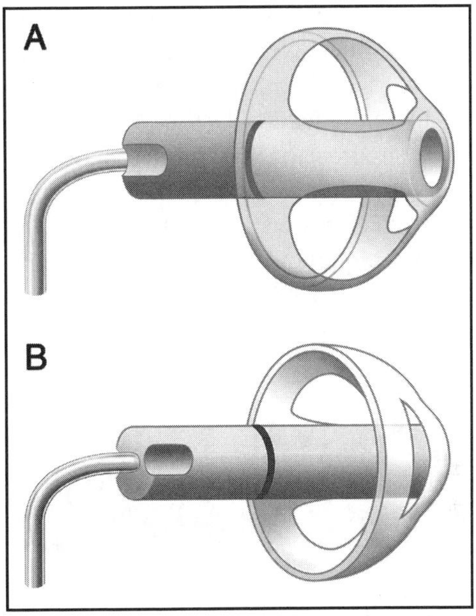

Figure 3–4. An open mold, demonstrating the nonoccluding structure of the earmold, as seen from the front (**A**) and back (**B**).

Open Fitting Hearing Aids

A vented earmold is an earmold that has a hole placed through it to allow air and sound to enter the ear canal. It can accomplish two goals: (1) it allows low-frequency sounds to enter the ear canal in patients who need only amplification for higher frequencies, and (2) it helps relieve the "occlusion effect," which is the feeling that the ear canal is plugged when a solid earmold is placed in the ear canal. An "open mold" attempts to accentuate the vent by making the earmold a shell that only minimally occludes the ear canal (Figure 3–4). This is most useful for a BTE product as the electronics can be placed behind the ear, and a thin tube connected to a minimally occluding open mold (Cook & Hawkins, 2006). This is an especially good choice for mild to

moderately severe high-frequency hearing loss, otherwise known as "Baby Boomer" hearing loss. The second benefit is that the open mold allows the echo or hollow sound from one's own voice to escape. This "occlusion effect" is the second most common reason, after difficulty in noise, for nonusage of a hearing aid. Some mini-BTE hearing aids come premounted with an open earmold, which is not a custom-fit earmold. These are small hearing aids that are specifically designed for mild to moderate high-frequency loss, and usually have three or four different sizes of open earmolds to accommodate different sizes of the ear canal. Like a standard BTE, they are digitally programmable, have directional features, but usually do not have multiple programs. One potential problem of the open earmold is that feedback can limit the amount of gain that can be delivered to the ear canal. In one study, the maximum gain was only 19 dB before feedback (Kuk, 1994). Feedback suppression has helped with this problem, adding an additional 10 to 12 dB gain, which allows minimal amplification of low frequencies and 30 dB of amplification above 1000 Hz (Kuk, Ludvigsen, & Kaulberg, 2002).

Induction Loops (Telecoil and Frequency-Modulated Systems)

Telecoils

These are devices that attempt to minimize the effect of noise by providing a direct connection from the speaker to the listener by induction technology. Induction technology is based on the generation of a magnetic field by an electrical current from the microphone. If the listener is within the magnetic field, an induction device can, in turn, change the magnetic field into an electrical current, which can power a loudspeaker. On a large scale, wires in the walls of auditoriums can detect signals transmitted from a speaker, and then transmit to a hearing impaired person in the audience using a headset. On a smaller scale, the "telecoil" in a hearing aid is an induction device that uses the magnetic field in the telephone to transmit to the hearing aid. In the future, wireless technology may replace the telecoil, which will be more convenient and allow telephone use without having to have proper alignment of the telephone and hearing aid (Levitt, 2007).

Frequency-Modulated (FM) Systems

Assistive listening devices are covered in Chapter 13, but are mentioned here in relation to their connection to hearing aids. With an FM system, a transmitter is used to send a signal from a speaker's microphone directly to a receiver worn by a patient. An FM system can be coupled directly to the hearing aid, by means of a boot, or sometimes incorporated into the hearing aid (Figures 3-5 and 3-6). The use of FM systems significantly improves speech reception, especially in a noisy environment (Chisolm, Noe, & McArdle, 2007). An audio input can be directly attached to the hearing aid by a wire, termed direct audio input.

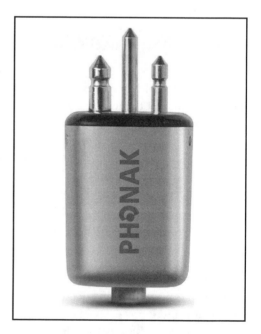

Figure 3–5. An example of a frequency-modulated (FM) attachment for hearing aids (Courtesy of Phonak Instruments, Warrenville, Illinois).

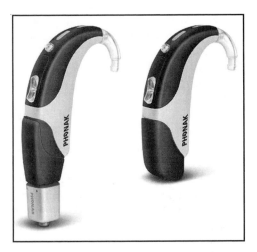

Figure 3–6. A hearing aid with and without the FM attachment (Courtesy of Phonak Instruments, Warrenville, Illinois).

References

Bentler, R., & Chiou, L. K. (2006). Digital noise reduction: An overview. *Trends in Amplification*, *10*(2), 67–82.

Bentler, R. A., Palmer, C., & Dittberner, A. B. (2004). Hearing-in-noise: comparison of listeners with normal and (aided). Impaired hearing. *Journal of the American Academy of Audiology*, *15*, 216–225.

Chisolm, T. H., Noe, C. M., McArdle, R., & Abrams, H. (2007). Evidence for the use of hearing assistive technology by adults: The role of the FM system. *Trends in Amplification*, *11*, 73–89.

Chung, K. (2004). Challenges in recent developments in hearing aids, 1: Speech understanding in noise, microphone technologies and noise reduction algorithms. *Trends in Amplification*, *8*, 83–124.

Cook, J. A., & Hawkins, D. B. (2006). Hearing loss and hearing aid treatment options. *Mayo Clinic Proceedings*, *81*(2), 234–237.

Dillon, H. (2001a). Hearing aid components. In H. Dillon, *Hearing aids* (pp. 18–47). Turramurra, Australia: Boomerang Press.

Dillon (2001b). Introductory concepts. In H. Dillon, *Hearing aids* (pp. 1–17). Turramurra, Australia: Boomerang Press.

Gabriel, D., Veuillet, E., Vesson, J. F., & Collet, L. (2006). Rehabilitation plasticity: Influence of hearing aid fitting on frequency discrimination performance near the hearing-loss cut-off. *Hearing Research*, *213*, 49–57.

Hill, S. L., 3rd, Marcus, A., Digges, E. N., Gillman, N., & Silverstein, H. (2006). Assessment of patient satisfaction with various configurations of digital CROS and BiCROS hearing aids. *Ear, Nose, and Throat Journal*, *85*(7), 427–427, 442.

Kates, J. M. (2005). Principles of digital dynamic-range compression. *Trends in Amplification*, *9*(2), 45–76.

Kim, H. H., & Barrs, D. M. (2006). Hearing aids: A review of what's new. *Otolaryngology-Head and Neck Surgery*, *134*(6), 1043–1050.

Kochkin, S. (2001). The VA and direct mail sales spark growth in hearing aid market. *Hearing Review*, *8*(12), 16–24, 63–65.

Kochkin, S. (2002). MarkeTrak VI: 10-year customer satisfaction trends in the US hearing instrument market. *Hearing Review*, *9*, 14–46.

Kuk, F. (1994). Maximum usable insertion gain with various earmold configurations. *Journal of the American Academy of Audiology*, *5*, 44–51.

Kuk, F., Keenan, D., Lau, C. C., & Ludvigsen, C. (2005). Performance of fully adaptive directional microphones to signals presented in various azimuths. *Journal of the American Academy of Audiology*, *16*, 333–347.

Kuk, F., Ludvigsen, C., & Kaulberg, T. (2002). Understanding feedback and digital feedback cancellation strategies. *Hearing Review*, *9*, 36–41.

Levitt, H. (2007). A historical perspective on digital hearing aids: How digital technology has changed modern hearing aids. *Trends in Amplification*, *11*, 7–24.

Macrae, J. H., & Dillon, H. (1996). Gain, frequency response and maximum output requirements for hearing aids. *Journal of Rehabilitation, Research, and Development, 33*(4), 363-374.

Marcoux, A. M., Yathiraj, A., Côté, I., & Logan, J. (2006). The effect of a hearing aid noise reduction algorithm on the acquisition of novel speech contrasts. *International Journal of Audiology, 45*(12), 707-714.

Mulrow, C. D., Aguilar, C., Endicott, J. E., Velez, R., Tuley, M. R., Charlip, W. S., et al. (1990). Association between hearing impairment and the quality of life of elderly individuals. *Journal of the American Geriatrics Society, 38,* 45-50.

Munro, K. J., & Trotter, J. H. (2006). Preliminary evidence of asymmetry in uncomfortable loudness levels after unilateral hearing aid experience: Evidence of functional plasticity in the adult auditory system. *International Journal of Audiology, 45,* 684-688.

National Council on the Aging. (1999). *The consequences of untreated hearing loss in older persons.* Washington, DC. Available at http://www.ncoa.org/attachments/UntreatedHearingLossReport%2Edoc

National Institute on Deafness and Other Communication Disorders. (2008). *Statistics about hearing, balance, ear infections, and deafness.* Bethesda, MD. Available at http://www.nidcd.nih.gov/health/statistics/hearing.asp

Nobel, W. (2006). Bilateral hearing aids: A review of self-reports of benefit in comparison with unilateral fitting. *International Journal of Audiology, 45*(Suppl.), S63-S71.

Nobel, W., & Gatehouse, S. (2006). Effects of bilateral versus unilateral hearing aid fitting on abilities measured by the Speech, Spatial, and Qualities of Hearing scale (SSQ). *International Journal of Audiology, 45,* 172-181.

Nordrum, S., Erler, S., Garstecki, D., & Dhar, S. (2006). Comparison of performance on the Hearing in Noise Test using directional microphones and digital noise reduction algorithms. *American Journal of Audiology, 6*(15), 81-91.

Palmer, C. V., & Ortmann, A. (2005). Hearing loss and hearing aids. *Neurologic Clinics, 23,* 901-918.

Paring, A. (2003). The hearing aid revolution: Fact or fiction. *Acta Otolaryngologica, 123,* 245-248.

Ricketts, T. A. (2005). Directional hearing aids: Then and now. *Journal of Rehabilitation Research and Development, 42*(4), 133-144.

Ross, M. (1980). Binaural versus monaural hearing aid amplification for hearing impaired individuals. In E. R. Libby (Ed.), *Binaural hearing amplification* (pp. 1-23). Chicago: Zenetron.

Smeds, K., Keidser, G., Zakis, J., Dillon, H., Leijon, A., Grant, F., et al. (2006a). Preferred overall loudness. I: Sound field presentation the laboratory. *International Journal of Audiology, 45,* 2-11.

Smeds, K., Keidser, G., Zakis, J., Dillon, H., Leijon, A., Grant, F., et al. (2006b). Preferred overall loudness. II: Listening through hearing aids in field and laboratory tests. *International Journal of Audiology, 45,* 12-25.

Souza, P. E., Yueh, B., Sarubbi, M., & Loovis, C. F. (2000). Fitting hearing aids with the Articulation Index: Impact on hearing and effectiveness. *Journal of Rehabilitation and Research Development, 37*(4), 1-13.

Strom, K. E. (2005). The HR dispenser survey. *Hearing Review, 12,* 18-36.

Walden, B. E., Surr, R. K., Cord, M. T., & Dyrlund, O. (2004). Predicting hearing aid microphone performance in everyday listening. *Journal of the American Academy of Audiology, 15,* 365-396.

Wood, S. A., & Lutman, M. E. (2004). Relative benefits of linear analogue and advanced digital hearing aids. *International Journal of Audiology, 43,* 144-155.

Wouters, J., Litiere, L., & van Wierengan, A. (1999). Speech intelligibility in noisy environments with one- and two-microphone hearing aids. *Audiology, 38,* 91-98.

Subjective and Objective Measures of Hearing Aid Performance

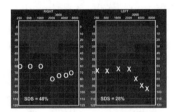

STEPHEN J. SANDERS, Au.D.
JOHN R. COLEMAN, Au.D.

Introduction

Today's hearing instruments are increasingly complex with many programming options available across multiple channels. This chapter reviews the subjective and objective measures used to assess hearing and performance.

Subjective Measurements of Hearing Aid Performance

In the early days of amplification devices for hearing loss, verification of a beneficial or positive outcome was determined by a general subjective assessment from the user. It would be expected that affirmative statements were sought such as, "Yes, I hear better," or, "Yes, I can tell that speech is louder." Whether the device employed was a cow's horn for an ear trumpet, a listening tube with an attached horn on one end and ear tip on the other, or another of the numerous variations on the ear resonator, the acoustic effect was only indirectly assessed by a subjective favorable response.

We now can readily measure the acoustic effects of these devices as typically a resonance at a single central frequency, commonly around 1000 Hz, where energy is collected and focused around a more concentrated, more intense region of tones. Because these devices were not readily tunable, the benefit was a simple yes/no determination. Either the individual could benefit from a constant increase in gain of 10 or 15 dB around the center peak frequency, or not.

The development of electrical amplification of speech for the hearing impaired person provided distinct advantages over previously used ear resonator devices, but did not immediately alter how benefits were verified. The era of biscuit-sized carbon microphones, tube amplifiers, knob-type volume controls, and hand-held speakers enabled the user to vary the overall amount of gain or loudness to a subjective comfort level. This is constrained by the limits of gain provided by the electrical amplification system, but had a distinct advantage of much wider frequency response or wider range of tones that were boosted. These were heavily influenced by the frequency response properties of both the microphone and speaker. Altering the slope or ratio of bass tones to treble tones initially was not an option, but was available in successive generations. The development of smaller components and battery driven systems led to body worn, more portable heading aid assemblages. Verification of favorable impact by devices of this era was still primarily driven by the subjective assessment of the user.

Measurements in a Sound Field

Test procedures that can be used mirror those performed under headphones, but are performed in a calibrated sound field within a sound-treated acoustic booth. An array of speaker placements can be utilized.

Speech understanding at a level that approximates normal conversation level (45 dB–55 dB HL) can be performed for both aided and unaided conditions. Speech stimuli may include single syllable phonetically balanced words; two-syllable spondaic words, sentences, or nonsense sentences. The test condition may include some level of competing noise either mixed into the primary test signal or from another direction in the sound field.

This form of verification can demonstrate hearing aid benefit (if the score is markedly better) and has high face-validity to the user. However significant weaknesses of this approach include poor sensitivity in determining the fine acoustic features of a hearing aid response that are needed for tuning response characteristics (Hawkins & Northern, 1992). High measurement variability is also a problem. Long test times, large numbers of test words, and score differences of 20% or more are often needed.

Another approach that has been used involved measurement of the change in identification of the softest possible sound. This was done in both the unaided and aided condition in the sound field. An advantage of threshold measurements is that they are highly repeatable psychoacoustic measurements, and the testing paradigm is widely used and understood.

Two techniques that have been used are changes in speech reception threshold (SRT) and changes in threshold measurements at discrete tones or frequencies. Measurement of SRT change would identify improvement of the patient's ability to hear soft speech. This is rarely used in hearing aid verification because it is limited to identifying shifts in low- to middle-frequencies of speech, and is of no value in cases of high-frequency hearing loss.

Aided threshold shift in the sound field was the measurement of choice for many audiologists in the time period before the widespread use of ear canal microphone measurement and microprocessor based test systems. A subtraction of the aided from the unaided threshold at a discrete frequency would give the net gain provided by the hearing aid. This is called the functional gain of the hearing aid. By measuring at octave or half-octave frequencies, the actual frequency response of the hearing aid could be derived. This provides information that would allow for more precise tuning of hearing aid frequency response characteristics (Fabry, 2003). This functional gain information was a major source of information that led to the development of amplification targets. Basically, the amount of hearing aid gain per frequency can be correlated to the degree of hearing loss at that frequency. Targets provide a starting place in decision making for hearing aid response characteristics although individual patient's hearing sensitivities contribute to a wide range of variation in determining the best response of the hearing aid.

Objective Measurements of Hearing Aid Performance

There are two principal methods of measuring hearing aid performance available today, electroacoustic analysis, utilizing 2-cc coupler measures, and real-ear probe microphone measures. Other techniques are in widespread use as well, such as visible speech and functional gain measurements (Kuf & Ludvigsen, 2003).

Electroacoustical Analysis

Electroacoustic analysis involves the use of carefully calibrated testing apparatus built to specifications, with standardized (ANSI S3.22) testing protocols allowing for reproducible results concerning the performance of the hearing instrument. This allows for the rapid determination of whether the instrument is performing to manufacturer's specifications (Frye, 2005). Once the hearing instruments are adjusted to the fitter's and wearer's satisfaction, the recording of a frequency response curve and a maximum output curve will serve as a reference for future comparison whenever the performance of the hearing aid may come into question.

The basic physical setup includes an anechoic chamber to conduct the measurements, a loudspeaker to deliver the test stimuli with a control microphone, placed very nearby the hearing aid microphone, which keeps the loudspeaker output at the specified level. The hearing aid is attached to a 2-cc coupler, inside of which a microphone diaphragm comprises one of the boundary walls of the acoustic chamber. This microphone measures the sound pressure level (SPL) in decibels generated by the output of the hearing aid to each controlled stimulus. The difference between the input SPL from the loudspeaker and the output SPL from the hearing aid results in the *gain* for that particular frequency and intensity of the stimulus. The HA-1 coupler typically is the 2-cc coupler in use today and it can be adapted to accept ITE instruments, BTE instruments with the earmold attached, or connect to the tonehook of the BTE instrument directly (Figures 4–1, 4–2, and 4–3).

A consideration when using the acoustic coupler is that its lack of acoustic

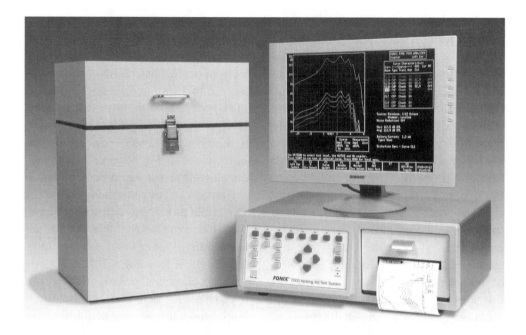

Figure 4–1. Fonix 7000 hearing aid test system. Courtesy of Frye Electronics.

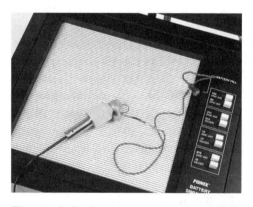

Figure 4–2. 2-cc coupler setup for a BTE instrument. Courtesy of Frye Electronics.

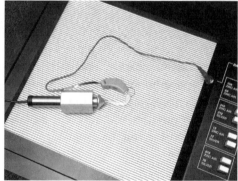

Figure 4–3. 2-cc coupler setup for an ITE instrument. Courtesy of Frye Electronics.

resistance makes it unsuitable for use with vented hearing aids and earmolds unless the vents are closed. The increased popularity of so-called "open fit" hearing instruments utilizing a "slim tube" coupling required a modification of the conventional 2-cc coupler in order to obtain reliable and reproducible results. Although this configuration will not reproduce manufacturer's specifications, it allows for easily measuring and storing a baseline curve for later comparison if the performance of the hearing aid is in question (Figure 4–4).

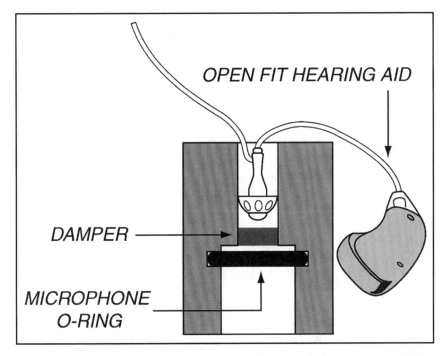

Figure 4–4. Fonix 7000 open fit hearing aid coupler. Courtesy of Frye Electronics.

Electroacoustical Measurements

There are many electroacoustical measurements that can be conducted on hearing instruments, some of which are not feasible or practical in the clinic. The reader is referred to the ANSI S3.22 document for details on all the measurements designed to meet FDA labeling regulations which have been undergoing revision since the initial standard in 1977 to the latest 2003 revision.

Output SPL with a 90 dB Input (OSPL90)

This is a measurement of the SPL developed in the coupler to a 90 dB SPL input stimulus, by frequency, with the hearing aid set to full on. A hearing aid with too low an output will not sound as clear as a more powerful instrument in the case of a more severe hearing impairment requiring louder signals. At the same time, care must be taken that the maximum output doesn't exceed the wearer's loudness discomfort level (LDL), which would lead to poor tolerance of amplification and likely eventual disuse (Kochkin, 2000). The OSPL90 is a curve defining the maximum output of the hearing aid by frequency. To simplify classification of the maximum output, the FDA has defined the HFA-OSPL90 (high-frequency average OSPL90) as the average of the 1000, 1600, and 2500 Hz OSPL90 outputs on the OSPL90 curve. The maximum OSPL90 is simply the maximum value on the OSPL90 curve.

Full-On Gain (FOG)

Acoustic gain is the difference between the output SPL and the input SPL and typically is displayed as a curve as a function of frequency. Full-on gain is measured when the instrument is set to its maximum output settings and the input SPL is at a level below that which could overload the hearing aid. The average gain at three frequencies (1000, 1600, and 2500 Hz) defines the full-on gain of the hearing instrument.

Reference Test Gain (RTG)

Hearing aids are rarely used full-on. A standard was developed to better approximate typical use settings. It is achieved when the gain is reduced so the average SPL values at 1000, 1600, and 2500 Hz, are 17 dB below the HFA-OSPL90. The curve generated at this setting is called the frequency response curve. Several subsequent measurements are made with the instrument set to the reference test gain.

Frequency Range

The frequency response curve is generated with the hearing aid in the reference test gain setting. An average of the SPL is taken at 1000, 1600, and 2500 Hz, and a horizontal line is constructed at a point 20 dB below this. Where this line intersects the hearing instrument's frequency response curve defines its frequency range. It defines the frequency range that the hearing instrument is likely to be effective. The wider the bandwidth of the hearing instrument, the better the audibility of speech cues

Total Harmonic Distortion (THD)

Distortion in hearing aids is expressed by the THD measured at three frequencies (500, 800, and 1600 Hz) at an input level of 70 dB SPL at 500 and 800 Hz, and for a 65 dB SPL input at 1600 Hz with the hearing aid set to the RTG position. This is a representation of the ability of the hearing aid to deliver a clean signal at a realistic output level. It is typical that the distortion in a hearing aid circuit is lower with very soft input levels, but may increase substantially with louder input levels. For this reason, measuring distortion levels at several input levels may allow the detection of undesirable characteristics from an instrument not evident using the ANSI measurement guideline.

Equivalent Input Noise (EIN)

The internal or "circuit noise" of an instrument is quantified by the EIN measurement. This is a measure of the amount of noise that would be required at the input of the hearing aid with its measured gain and frequency response, to account for the output SPL of the hearing aid assuming that it is otherwise noiseless. Most of the noise of a hearing instrument is generated by the microphone. Digital circuitry allows for an expansion kneepoint, below which, the signal receives less gain in order to lessen the effects of microphone noise. This reduces audibility of this noise for wearers with regions of normal hearing.

Input-Output Characteristics

Most modern hearing aids are not linear, meaning, as the level of the input varies, the level of the output is altered by a different amount. Measurements can be made at multiple input levels in different frequency bands to define the behavior of the hearing instrument's compression. Compression is necessary in most fittings to allow enough gain to make soft inputs audible without causing loud inputs to become uncomfortable or saturating the output of the hearing instrument creating potentially unacceptable levels of distortion.

Additionally, most 2-cc test boxes allow for rapid verification of battery current drain, whether or not noise reduction is operating, and telecoil sensitivity. It is also possible to verify the attack and release times, which are the times (in milliseconds) it takes for the instrument to go into and out of compression at various frequencies.

Probe Microphone Measurements

Probe microphone measures, unlike electroacoustic 2-cc coupler measures, are an in situ measurement, taken in the wearer's ear rather than in a standardized test chamber. The probe microphone consists of a microphone with a thin rubber tube attached, which is placed within millimeters of the eardrum while a reference microphone resides above or below the pinna. There are distinct advantages for doing this. In this instance, we no

longer are attempting to replicate a carefully defined set of values that permit quality control assessment and an objective analysis of whether the hearing instrument continues to meet its performance parameters. We now are defining the way the instrument is behaving in the environment for which it is actually intended. To begin with, probe microphone measures are sensitive to individual variability of acoustic impedance at the eardrum (Hellstrom & Axelsson, 1993). Overall gain effects, as a function of the residual volume of the external ear canal, with the hearing instrument in place, are accounted for. This may vary significantly over the continuum from infant to adult and with the insertion depth of the earmold or instrument. The effects of microphone placement, head diffraction, and pinna resonance are accounted for, as are the effects of insertion loss and venting for the individual ear (ANSI 2004 S3.35). Probe microphone measures are typically performed sequentially, comparing aided values to a baseline obtained of the wearer's unaided, unoccluded ear. They are displayed in sound pressure level (SPL) as a function of frequency and generate a curve (Figure 4-5).

Real-Ear Unaided Response (REUR)

REUR is a measurement of the SPL at, or near the tympanic membrane of an open ear (no hearing aid present) (American National Standards Institute, 1997 S3.46). This accounts for resonances of the pinna unique to the individual ear due to volume, shape, and acoustic impedance of the canal walls and at the tympanic membrane.

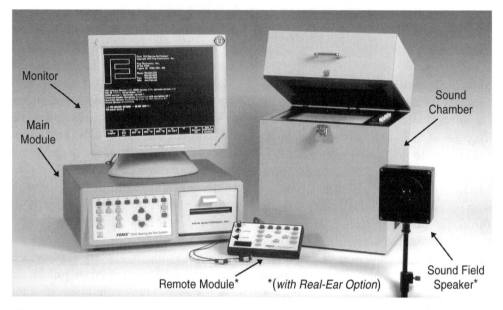

Figure 4–5. Probe microphone test system. Courtesy of Frye Electronics.

Real-Ear Occluded Response (REOR)

A measurement of the SPL at the eardrum with the hearing aid in place, but turned off (American National Standards Institute, 1997 S3.46). This measurement defines the alteration of external ear resonances or *insertion loss* created by the occlusion of the ear by the hearing aid or earmold and its fit or venting characteristics.

Real-Ear Aided Response (REAR)

REAR is a measurement of the SPL at the tympanic membrane with the hearing aid in place and switched on (ANSI, American National Standards Institute, 1997). When compared to the REOR, this generates a curve that displays the hearing aid output for the selected stimulus.

Real-Ear Insertion Response (REIR)

REIR is the difference between the REAR and the REUR. It describes the net effect on the SPL at the eardrum with the hearing aid turned on and in place compared to the open ear canal (American National Standards Institute, 1997 S3.46). It is typically displayed as gain (SPL difference) in decibels as a function of frequency (Figure 4–6).

Real-Ear Saturation Response (RESR)

RESR is a measure of the SPL at the tympanic membrane with the hearing aid in place and turned on, being driven by a stimulus sufficiently loud to ensure that the maximum output of the hearing aid, as it is configured, is achieved (American

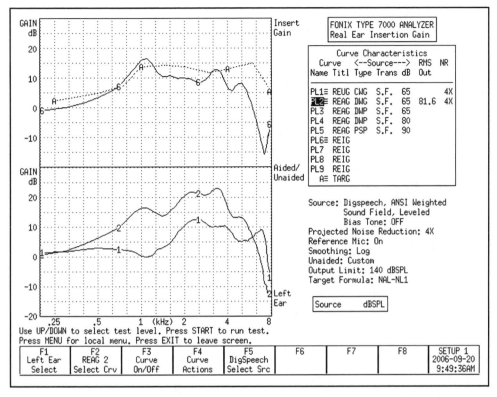

Figure 4–6. Real-ear insertion gain, depicted in the top tracing, is the difference between the REUR and the REAR seen in the bottom tracings. Courtesy of Frye Electronics.

National Standards Institute, 1997 S3.46) This allows for the assessment and adjustment of any peaks in the output which might exceed the wearer's loudness discomfort levels.

The REUR, REAR, and REIR may be performed for various stimulus levels to define the amplification and compression characteristics of the hearing instrument. Newer probe microphone systems will auto adjust the REUR as the level of the stimulus for the REIR is varied, obviating the need to re-measure the REUR each time a new stimulus intensity is chosen. Care must be taken in selecting which hearing instrument signal pro-

cessing features are enabled along with the type of input signal utilized for probe microphone measurements as they may trigger noise reduction or compression effects leading to the underestimation of the instrument's true output (Bray & Nilsson, 2002; Lantz, Jensen, Haastrup, & Olsen, 2007).

Other Applications

Probe microphone measures can be utilized to better predict the performance of the hearing instrument in the wearer's ear when fitting infants and young children, or individuals with limited cooperation (Scollie & Seewald, 2002). Real ear to coupler difference (RECD) is the difference, in SPL, between the REAR and the hearing aid placed in the 2-cc coupler for the same stimulus. Knowing this difference allows for the prediction of the hearing instrument's output at the tympanic membrane when adjustments are being made in the test chamber, significantly reducing the time required for the subject's cooperation.

Another application utilizing probe microphone is visible speech mapping (VSM). VSM utilizes any live voice or recorded signal as the stimulus. The individual's hearing thresholds are plotted on an SPL screen by frequency while the input is displayed relative to the hearing loss. The real-time measurement curve is updated many times a second, which reflects the dynamics of speech, while another curve displays the average output by frequency. The individual and his family can visually understand the degree to which speech is inaudible due to the hearing impairment. The demonstration is repeated with the hearing aid in place showing the benefits of amplification in an easily grasped, visual medium.

Probe microphone measures allow for assessing performance features such as directional microphone response characteristics not possible in conventional electroacoustic test chambers. Polar plots are graphs of the microphone system's sensitivity to a selected stimulus relative to the angle of the stimulus presentation. This can be measured and recorded in two or three dimensions (Preves & Burns, 2007). These measures ascertain that the microphones are wired properly and functioning appropriately.

References

ANSI: American National Standards Institute. (1997). *Methods of measurement of real-ear performance characteristics of hearing aids (S3.46).* New York: Acoustical Society of America.

American National Standards Institute. (2004). *Methods of measurement of performance characteristics of hearing aids under simulated real ear working conditions (S3.35).* New York: Acoustical Society of America.

Bray V., & Nilsson, M. (2002). Assessing hearing aid fittings: An outcome measures battery approach. In M. Valente (Ed.), *Strategies for selecting and verifying hearing aid fittings* (pp. 151–175). New York: Thieme.

Fabry, D. (2003). Nonlinear hearing aids and verification of fitting targets. *Trends in Amplification, 7*(3), 99–115.

Frye, G. (2005). Understanding the ANSI standard as a tool for assessing hearing aid functionality. *Hearing Review, 5,* 22–79.

Hawkins, D., & Northern, J. (1992). Probe-microphone measurements with children. In H. G. Mueller, D. Hawkins, & J. Northern (Eds.), *Probe microphone measurements: Hearing aid selection and measurement* (pp. 159–181). San Diego, CA: Singular.

Hellstrom, P., & Axelsson, A. (1993). Miniature microphone probe tube measurements in the external auditory canal. *Journal of the Acoustical Society of America, 2,* 907–919.

Kochkin, S. (2000). MarkeTrak V: Why my hearing aids are in the drawer: The consumer's perspective. *Hearing Journal, 53*(2), 34–42.

Kuk, F., & Ludvigsen, C. (2003). Reconsidering the concept of the aided threshold for nonlinear hearing aids. *Trends in Amplification, 7*(3), 77–97.

Lantz, J., Jensen, O., Haastrup, A., & Olsen, S. (2007). Real-ear measurement verification for open, non-occluding hearing instruments. *International Journal of Audiology, 46*(1), 11–16.

Preves, D., & Burns, T. (2007). Revised ANSI standard measures hearing aid directionality in 3D. *Hearing Journal*, *60*(1), 36–42.

Scollie, S., & Seewald, R. (2002). A sound foundation through early amplification. *Ear and Hearing*, *16*, 263–273.

5

Hearing Aid
Candidacy in Adults

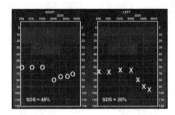

MARCIA RAGGIO, Ph.D.

Adult Hearing Aid Candidacy

With dozens of hearing aid manufacturers, and hundreds of hearing aid possibilities, choosing the best hearing aid for a patient can be a challenging task. On the other hand, nearly all of today's digital hearing aids contain complex integrated circuits that allow for elaborate digital signal processing, while providing great flexibility for fitting essentially any hearing loss. Before any hearing aid choices can be made, however, a combination of other factors must be considered.

The Damaged Cochlea

To best understand how today's hearing aids work, and thus how to best fit them, it is important to know how cochlear function changes with sensorineural hearing loss. That is, modern hearing aids are designed to attempt to compensate for a number of physiological factors that are altered by hearing loss. For example, an audiometric evaluation will reveal how much a patient's pure tone and speech thresholds have shifted from normal with hair cell damage or loss, and thus indicate how much loss of audibility a patient is experiencing. In addition to loss of audibility, the loss of the cochlea's non-linearities or active mechanisms also must be appreciated. The normal cochlea maintains active mechanisms such that it is able to increase the amplification of soft sound, while not amplifying loud sound, since for many cochlear losses, loud sound is still perceived normally (Brownell et al., 2001). On the other hand, some patients experience a deteriorated intensity coding for loud sound. That is, suppressive factors that may have kept loud sound from being perceived as too loud are now compromised, creating uncomfortable loudness perception by the patient (Buus & Florentine, 2001). This means that the patient now experiences a more narrow dynamic range, or the range to which sound can be amplified comfortably for the patient. Lastly, with hair cell damage comes a loss of fine frequency coding necessary for accurate speech discrimination (Oxenham & Bacon, 2003). The consequences of these functional changes are that patients with sensorineural hearing loss process sound with reduced audibility and clarity, both of which causing communicative difficulty particularly in noisy environments. Today's hearing aids have shown promise in attempting to compensate for these functions to some extent.

Degree of Hearing Loss

The degree of hearing loss is a place to start when considering hearing aid choices, but the presence of a loss is not evidence enough to recommend a hearing aid. For adults, pure tone thresholds of 25 dB or greater typically constitute an aidable hearing loss. However, not everyone with a 25 dB loss would consider that loss sufficiently handicapping to warrant wearing a hearing aid. There are those for whom hearing acuity is critical to job performance or lifestyle, and thus will readily consider a hearing aid even with a minimal loss, whereas others with moderate or even severe losses would maintain that a hearing aid is totally unnecessary for their lifestyle. Historically, individuals with hearing losses in the 55–80 dB range were thought to benefit the greatest from wearing amplification. That is, those with mild or profound loss will benefit from using amplification, but the perceptual benefit may not be as great. However, with an increase in the understanding of normal hearing, and thus hearing loss, a better rule of thumb may be that hearing aid benefit is in the ear and mind of the individual hearing aid wearer. Table 5–1 shows a typical categorization of degree of hearing loss, and the associated consequences for speech understanding (Table 5–1).

Type of Hearing Loss

Hearing losses, for which amplification is typically recommended, can be described as sensorineural, conductive, or mixed. Although the majority of hearing aid recommendations are for individuals with sensorineural hearing loss, any type of loss can be suitable for the successful use of amplification. For example, an older individual with a history of otosclerosis or cholesteatoma, both resulting in conductive or mixed hearing loss, may opt to wear amplification to enhance his or her residual hearing, with or without

Table 5–1. Degree of Loss in Relation to Handicap for Speech Understanding

10–25 dB	Normal limits	No significant difficulty with soft speech
26–40 dB	Mild loss	Difficulty hearing soft speech
40–65 dB	Moderate loss	Difficulty hearing normal speech
70–90 dB	Severe loss	Requires loud speech for understanding
90–110 dB+	Profound loss	Cannot understand loud speech

previous surgical intervention. However, individuals with these and other middle ear pathologies should be encouraged to exhaust all medical intervention strategies before amplification is considered. That is, the decision to seek amplification should be made by the physician and the patient together, when no further medical or surgical intervention is advisable.

The majority of all hearing loss is sensorineural (Cruickshank et al., 1996, Gates & Mills, 2005; NIH Fact Sheet, 2007). Thus, little medical or surgical intervention is possible. Exceptions to this finding are cochlear implants for severe to profound hearing loss, brainstem implants for those who have undergone complete VIIIth nerve tumor resection surgery, middle ear implants for various forms of conductive abnormalities, and bone-anchored devices for unilateral or single-sided deafness. Hearing loss due to aging, genetics, excessive noise exposure, ototoxic drugs, vascular disorders, unoperated benign tumors, viruses, skull fracture, Ménière's disease, autoimmune disease, and others are typically successfully fit with amplification.

Pure conductive hearing losses due to pathologies such as otitis media with effusion, typically are not fitted with amplification in adults, as this is a medically treatable condition. However, adult patients with pure conductive losses due to otosclerosis, cholesteatoma, large, dry tympanic membrane perforations, or disarticulation of the ossicular chain due to head trauma are candidates for amplification pursuant to the decision not to apply a surgical remedy. Patients with atresia, and with imaging findings of a fully developed cochlea, may demonstrate a pure conductive hearing loss, thus making those individuals candidates for middle ear or bone-anchored hearing aids.

Age of Onset of Hearing Loss

Hearing loss can occur at any time and at any age. Adults more often have adventitious or acquired hearing loss, but can have congenital hearing loss as well. Acquired hearing loss can be further divided into pre-, peri-, and postlingual hearing loss, although a prelingual hearing loss may actually be an undiagnosed congenital loss. Some adults may have experienced a late onset hearing loss in childhood that allowed for near-complete speech and language development. Adults with acquired or postlingual hearing loss are typically candidates for amplification. The use of amplification by adults with congenital or perilingual loss is variable.

Adults who grew up in an oral/aural environment in which speech was the primary mode of communication may readily wear amplification. Those who were educated in a manual communication environment may or may not choose to wear any form of amplification.

Audiometric Configuration of Hearing Loss

The configuration or shape of an individual's audiometric thresholds will have a bearing on hearing aid candidacy, choosing an appropriate amplification style, as well as deciding on a fitting rationale. Table 5–2 shows the most common hearing loss configurations.

With the flexibility of today's hearing aids, essentially any hearing loss configuration can be fitted with amplification. Hearing aid gain and frequency response schemes are primarily designed for greater high frequency amplification due to the fact that most losses demonstrate a greater loss in the high frequencies than the low frequencies, as well as the importance of high-frequency consonant information for speech understanding. Other patients will demonstrate a flat hearing loss that still requires a high frequency emphasis for better speech understanding. Low-frequency or rising hearing losses can be fitted as well, with a sensitivity for not allowing too much low-frequency gain that can increase background noise, or create upward spreading of masking (powerful low frequencies mask weaker high frequencies).

Word Recognition

Word recognition or speech discrimination is a routine aspect of an audiometric evaluation. This measure, performed under earphones and at a suprathreshold level, is designed to determine the ability of a patient to identify words without benefit of visual cues. From these results, the degree of communicative difficulty

Table 5–2. Hearing Loss Configurations

Flat	Thresholds are within 20 dB of each other across the frequency range
Rising	Low-frequency thresholds at least 20 dB poorer than for high frequencies
Sloping	High-frequency thresholds at least 20 dB poorer than for low frequencies
Low-Frequency	Hearing loss is restricted to the low-frequency region of the audiogram
High-Frequency	Hearing loss is restricted to the high-frequency region of the audiogram
Precipitous	Steeply sloping high-frequency hearing loss of at least 20 dB per octave

a patient may experience, as well as appropriate expectations for successful hearing aid use, can be discussed with a patient. Using monosyllabic word lists of 25 to 50 words, a word recognition score can be determined and categorized with regard to degree of word clarity or the lack of it. A general categorization of word recognition ability and associated communicative difficulty can be seen in Table 5-3.

General word recognition ability can be predicted, to some extent, by the configuration of the hearing loss. This is possible due to the relationship between the frequency and intensity of English speech sounds, and the configuration of a given hearing loss. For counseling purposes, this score provides a way to discuss potential communicative difficulty, as well as the impact of word recognition on successful hearing aid use.

One further aspect of word recognition and hearing aid fitting should be considered. That is, it must be understood that the central auditory nervous system clearly demonstrates plasticity with hearing aid use (Gatehouse, 1992). It has been found that there is a significant decrease in speech recognition in an ear with hearing loss and without amplification rela-

tive to an ear that is aided. Further, it has been demonstrated that speech perception performance can improve over time with hearing aid use. Thus, it seems clear that speech perception ability has a "use it or lose it" aspect that should be appreciated by both those who fit and those who wear amplification.

Impact of Hearing Loss on Communication: "I can hear, but I can't understand."

Hearing health care professionals hear this statement essentially every day, and it is our responsibility to help patients understand why this is the case. The Articulation Index (now more often referred to as the Audibility Index) (AI) provides a way to visually demonstrate the amount of speech signal that is audible to an individual with a given hearing loss. The AI uses a number between 0 and 1.0 to describe the proportion of the average speech signal that would be audible to the patient depending on the hearing loss configuration. The AI divides the speech signal into frequency bands and

Table 5–3. Word Recognition

WR Score in Percent	WR Descriptor	General WR
100–90%	Excellent	Normal
89–80%	Good	Slight difficulty
79–70%	Fair	Moderate difficulty
69–60%	Poor	Marked difficulty
<60%	Very Poor	Visual cues required

assigns various weightings to each band depending on their contribution to an individual's ability to hear and understand the speech signal. For example, the bands whose frequencies represent consonant sounds are given more weight because consonants are more important for speech understanding than vowels. Muller and Killion (1990) developed a simplified way to calculate audibility called a *Count the Dots* method in which 100 dots are used to depict the weighting of English speech sounds. Figure 5–1 shows that the more important the frequency band to speech understanding, the greater the number of dots. In addition, we can see a mild-to-moderate hearing loss superimposed on the Count-the-Dots audiogram. Dots that are found above the black horizontal line can be

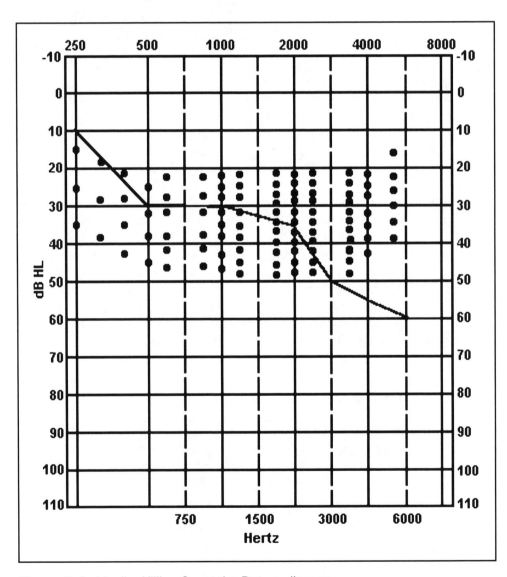

Figure 5–1. Mueller-Killion Count-the-Dots audiogram.

counted as audible to the patient. Those below the red line are counted as inaudible to this patient. Thus, this patient has an AI of 0.44, which means for that this individual, 44% of speech is audible.

In the example above, we can see that this individual is unable to hear a number of important speech sounds spoken at a normal conversational loudness. This information can help determine the degree of difficulty this patient might have hearing normal conversational speech, as well as how to configure the gain and frequency response required of amplification for this patient. However, it should be remembered that for patients with losses in the severe or profound range, normal speech is, for the most part, inaudible, and depending on the amount of damage in a given auditory system, the individual may have little or no word recognition. Another measure, the Speech Intelligibility Index (SII) provides a somewhat more complicated way to predict speech recognition in the presence of noise. That is, the SII can be calculated using a combination of the speech spectrum, the noise spectrum of a given noise source, and the patient's hearing thresholds in discrete frequency bands (ANSI S3.5, 1997).

Most Comfortable Loudness

An additional measure that is important to understanding hearing loss is most comfortable loudness or MCL. A patient's MCL is the level at which he or she prefers to listen to speech. For people with normal hearing, this level is often 40 to 50 dB above the pure tone threshold or speech recognition threshold. However, as the degree of hearing loss

increases, often the MCL gets lower, thus demonstrating a reduced dynamic range. Typically, word recognition is tested at MCL for the best result. MCL can be measured monaurally under earphones, or binaurally in the sound field, with or without hearing aids.

Uncomfortable Loudness Level

Uncomfortable Loudness Level or UCL is a measure of the greatest loudness for speech or tones that a patient can tolerate. For normal hearing people, this level is typically 100 dB HL. In some patients with sensorineural hearing loss, the UCL is much lower, due to recruitment. That is, some sensorineural hearing loss patients will perceive large increases in loudness with only small increases in sound intensity. In cases of recruitment, as the hearing loss increases, the UCL decreases, creating a narrow dynamic range. This can cause a very challenging situation for providing enough gain to amplify speech sounds to a comfortable listening level without causing any sounds to be too loud.

Hearing Aid Evaluations

Those who evaluate a patient for today's hearing aids are faced with many decisions, because so many factors play a part in choosing the most beneficial hearing aid. The patient's degree and type of hearing loss, word recognition ability, loudness tolerance, and perceived handicap are all fundamental pieces of the puzzle. However, understanding the communicative needs of the patient in terms of his or her daily life, the nature of a patient's routine noise environments, dexterity, motivation, cosmetic concerns, expectations for amplification, and financial resources are also some of the primary considerations for choosing a hearing aid or assistive listening devices. Knowledge of the sound and noise processing strategies available in today's hearing aid circuitry is essential, of course, in deciding which product would meet the varied needs of a patient. It is the skill of being able to synthesize all of the above factors, along with important elements of patient counseling and rehabilitation, that makes successful hearing aid fitting an art.

To Wear or Not to Wear

There are two fundamental aspects of successful hearing aid evaluations and fittings, the technical aspects and the psychological aspects. The technical aspects have goals of providing an instrument, or two, that will amplify conversational speech to a comfortable listening level for the patient, while suppressing as much background noise and uncomfortably loud sound as possible. How these goals can be achieved has become much easier with today's sophisticated integrated circuit technology, as well as with the flexibility of today's hearing aid fitting software. However, the psychological or motivational aspects, in some ways, are more difficult to address. For many candidates, there is a kind of resignation that they will become hearing aid wearers when they walk through the door because they and their families have grown tired of their increasing communicative difficulties. Others come in filled with denial, stating that they do not have any com-

municative difficulties, and are wondering why their husbands, wives, or family members have coerced them into having a hearing test. Yet others will attack the problems created by their hearing loss head-on, wanting to minimize communicative concerns as quickly as possible. These are the problem-solvers who are quick to accept any reasonable avenue to restore their hearing as much and as soon as possible. Whichever group the patient falls into, it must be appreciated that there can be a considerable amount of emotion associated with the diagnosis and treatment of hearing loss. Many patients can feel anger, denial, or depression, and it should be understood that it has taken some time, and may take more, for them to accept that they have a loss and to do something about it. In most cases, a physician recommendation for the use of amplification is more likely to be accepted by a patient than one from a spouse or family member.

Self-Assessment of Hearing Aid Goals

Self-assessment scales have proven to be helpful counseling tools for patient who have either accepted the idea of trying amplification, or for those considering it. These scales were developed to assist the patient in determining his or her own areas of perceived communicative difficulty, which can then lead to the development of personal goals for amplification. Two popular scales are the Abbreviated Profile of Hearing Aid Benefit (APHAB; Cox, 1997) and the Client Oriented Scale of Improvement (COSI; Dillon, Birtles, & Lovegrove, 1999). These scales can reflect the patient's subjective perception of his or her communicative difficulty, act as pre- and post-measures of perceived hearing aid benefit, or provide comparisons of communicative function with and without amplification. The APHAB is a multiscenario inventory that places an individual in a number of favorable and unfavorable communicative situations. The patient is then asked to judge his or her perceived functionality in these environments. The COSI asks the patient to prioritize five listening situations in which help with hearing is needed. At some point following the initial hearing aid fitting, or at the conclusion of intervention with amplification, the patient is asked to reassess his or her hearing disability, and the resulting ability to communicate in the original situations is quantified. Thus, both scales provide a means to help direct intervention strategies into areas of greatest perceived need. It is the responsibility of the professional to be ever mindful of the degree to which the patient is adapting to the use of amplification, and make the appropriate accommodations, technically or emotionally, with regard to the patient's needs.

hearing loss. The aids were behind-the-ear models that were worn with a stock earmold. Word recognition testing in quiet and noise, SRT level, and the widest dynamic range with pure tones were performed in a serial fashion in the sound field with each hearing aid. The performance of the patient with each aid was then compared. The aid that provided the best performance was determined to be the one to fit.

Unfortunately, these comparisons are not particularly reliable. Being able to perform well in an artificial environment, like a sound booth, does not always translate to providing the same abilities in real life environments. Also, studies on the statistical treatment of word recognition scores have shown that it takes approximately 250 word administrations per hearing aid to statistically determine that one aid is superior to another (Thornton & Raffin, 1978). Few clinicians have time to administer that many words in this comparative fashion. With these factors known, the comparative method was abandoned.

History: Comparative Analog Hearing Aid Selection

In the past, a hearing aid evaluation (HAE) involved choosing a "best" hearing aid based on a patient's word recognition score, as well as other measures of performance, from a number of hearing aids. That is, the audiologist would choose three or four analog hearing aids that were thought to provide the correct amount of gain, and with the most appropriate frequency response for the patient's

Hearing Aid Signal Processing: Analog Hearing Aids

Until approximately a decade ago, the only hearing aids available used analog signal processing. Analog hearing aids have simple circuits that contain various amplifier stages that increase the intensity, or amplify, incoming sound. Unfortunately, these aids apply a single gain and frequency response to all incoming signals, speech and noise alike. Although the frequency response of these aids is designed to minimally amplify low-frequency sound, they are not particularly effective in reducing significant, low-frequency background noise. Analog aids are able to provide both linear and compression circuits. Thus, in quiet, analog hearing aids work well, but in noise, the wearer is in a constant battle to understand speech by trying to reduce background noise with only the volume control. Trimmer potentiometers offered little resolution to listening in noise for analog wearers. Figure 5-2 shows a typical analog circuit.

Hearing Aid Signal Processing: Digital Hearing Aids

Digital signal processing (DSP) began to be used in hearing aids over ten years ago. In a digital hearing aid, an analog to digital or A/D converter samples the incoming signal many thousands of times per second and converts these samples into positive and negative electrical voltages. The samples are then coded into a series of binary digits that represent the voltages of each positive or negative charge. All of the binary digits are labeled either a 0 or a 1 based on a predetermined value, for example whether a certain frequency is represented. These digits are then fed into the hearing aid's central processing unit, which is able to determine how the signal will be processed, called algorithms. A digital to analog or D/A converter then converts the electrical signal back to an acoustic signal. Generally speaking, the greater the number of samples, the higher the resolution; and thus the better the quality of the amplified sound (see Figure 5-2).

Hearing Aid Fitting

Hearing Aid Gain Decisions

An early fitting principle for choosing a single gain value for an analog hearing aid is referred to as the *half gain rule* suggested by Lybarger (1944, 1963). Lybarger studied the gain preferences of several hundred patients wearing linear hearing aids. He evaluated their pure-tone thresholds and then looked at the gain provided by their hearing aids at their preferred or use volume setting. He discovered that the preferred gain setting of these wearers was essentially half of their hearing loss at a particular frequency. This rule has been modified by a number of the current prescriptive fitting strategies.

Prescriptive Hearing Aid

More recently, target or predictive formulae were developed to help in choosing hearing aid gain and output targets for discrete frequencies. Most prescriptive methods use threshold and suprathreshold data to predict the gain and output needs of the wearer of nonlinear or compression hearing aids, with later formulas allowing for targets for different loudness input levels such as Fig6 (Killion & Fikret-Pasa, 1993), and IHAFF (Cox, 1995). These targets ideally would boost speech to the most comfortable loudness of the hearing aid wearer, or said another way, would boost speech to the same suprathreshold loudness that it is for normal hearing people, while not causing speech or sound to be uncomfortably loud. It should be noted, however, that prescrip-

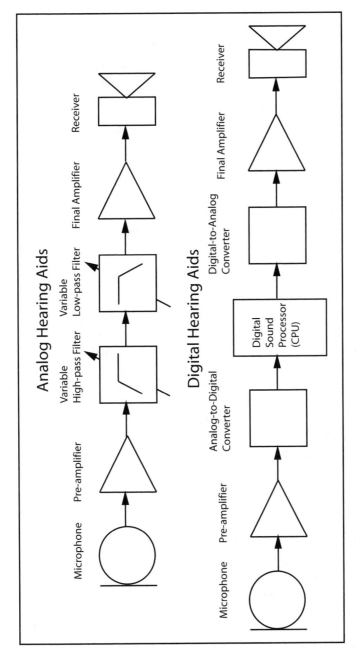

Figure 5–2. Analog and digital hearing aid circuits.

tive methods, based on average data, can have drawbacks as not all patients present with average auditory relationships. Presently, popular prescriptive methods are National Acoustics Laboratory Non-Linear 1 or NAL-NL1 (Dillon et al., 1998) and DSL [i/o] (Seewald, 1992), as well as several others. A variety of these prescriptive methods are available in each manufacturer's hearing aid fitting software.

Long-Term Average

Most prescriptive fitting formulae apply additional principles of speech acoustics for making gain and frequency response decisions, including the long-term average speech spectrum (LTASS), the Audibility Index (AI), and the Speech Intelligibility Index (SII). In fact, these measures provide the foundation for hearing aid sound processing design in terms of meeting gain and frequency response requirements. The LTASS was developed from recordings of the frequency and intensity of speech over time using male and female speakers. The LTASS reveals that there is much greater low-frequency energy present for the average speaker than high-frequency energy. Thus, due to the naturally greater intensity of low-frequency speech sounds, a significant amount of gain for those frequencies is not required. Of course, this must be qualified depending on the configuration of the loss. Alternatively, because high-frequency information is critically important for speech understanding, and contains relatively less natural power, it is necessary to provide relatively greater high-frequency gain. The AI then provides a way to demonstrate the audibility of high frequency, primarily consonant information, for a given hearing loss. Taken together, prescriptive methods use this information, along with patient preference

data for gain and output, to design theoretically appropriate amplification targets.

Nonlinear Sound Processing: Wide Dynamic Range Compression (WDRC)

Most of today's digital hearing aids use a sound processing strategy referred to as wide dynamic range compression or WDRC. The goal of WDRC processing is to provide progressively greater gain as the input signal decreases in intensity. Thus, soft sounds are given greater gain or amplification than loud sounds. This way, the hearing aid is able automatically to maintain a wide range of input sound intensities within a comfortable listening level for the patient. Unlike the "old days" of analog hearing aids when the wearer often had to manipulate the volume control to decrease background noise while trying to hear speech more comfortably, hearing aids using WDRC have reduced this need dramatically. Essentially all digital hearing aids today provide multiband sound processing, and thus may offer differing WDRC ratios, attack and release times, and compression kneepoints in many frequency bands.

Advanced Sound Processing Features

In addition to DSP and the implementation of some form of WDRC, hearing aid manufacturers have developed very sophisticated, high-speed computer chip technology that allows for automatic control of many aspects of speech and noise in a multiband format. In addition, directional microphones are able to adaptively suppress sound from the side or rear of the listener, creating a better signal-to-noise ratio in many circumstances. Thus, modern hearing aids, using timing and loudness input calculations, as well as directionality, are able to determine a voice from a noise, loud from soft, and front from back, essentially all at the same time, creating better speech understanding in the presence of noise. For some high-speed, large memory computer processing units, these many factors can be processed in an integrated fashion with millions of calculations made per second, providing discrete processing in each of many frequency bands. These advances also have increased battery life, while allowing for the development of smaller hearing aids.

A number of other advanced features are available in today's hearing aids. Digital feedback management has made this long-standing problem for hearing aid wearers essentially a thing of the past. Transpositional features have been incorporated into some hearing aids that move inputs from a frequency area for which a wearer has little or no usable hearing to a frequency area where they do. In addition, circuits have been developed that are "trainable" in that they learn the wearer's preferred gain setting or compression needs for different environments and set them automatically. Other hearing aid technology includes the ability of hearing aids to communicate with each other so that, for example, changes in the volume or program of one hearing aid would be changed simultaneously in the other hearing aid. These aids can also share information with regard to the listening environment such that speech and noise processing algorithms can work together. Still others use wireless technology to allow a hearing aid to communicate with a cell phone or television, as well as many other electronic devices.

This growing array of technologically advanced hearing aid features allows the audiologist to use manufacturer software to program hearing aids in a variety of ways. Thus, wearer satisfaction has increased significantly by allowing the audiologist to program the hearing aid to meet the specific needs of the wearer. It can be appreciated that prescriptive methods of hearing fitting are only a place to start, and that complex hearing aid fitting software creates sound treatments that can be individualized and manipulated for greater patient satisfaction. Although hearing aids today are still not perfect, it is unlikely that they ever will be, as the task of replacing the exquisite physiology of the ear is remote. The best hearing aid is only as good as the ear upon which it is fitted, and the brain that is adapting to it. Credit can be given to those who have provided the basic science research on how the ear works, and the hearing aid manufacturers who have tried to incorporate the research findings into their products. Today's hearing aids go a long way to restore audibility and the cochlea's natural compression, as well as appropriate frequency emphasis relative to the loss configuration. These advances have created a remarkably better outcome for most hearing aid wearers than even a decade ago. Aural rehabilitative efforts also have increased the positive aspects of hearing aid fitting.

Binaural Amplification

In many everyday listening situations, wearing two hearing aids is better than one. We know that hearing with two equal ears allows for suppression of background noise (squelch effect), better sound location, and greater loudness. Patients typically note an appreciation for a sense of hearing balance when wearing two hearing aids as well. However, more recent research has demonstrated that binaural amplification in noisy environments, particularly as people age, may have a deleterious effect on speech understanding. In fact, in very noisy environments, it may be helpful to remove one hearing aid for better speech understanding (Walden & Walden, 2005).

Assistive Listening Devices

Patients can opt to compensate for hearing loss using assistive listening devices or ALDs. Room or personal induction loop systems, used in conjunction with the patient's hearing aid telecoil, are growing in popularity. In this way, sound from a speaker's microphone, a music sound source, or any number of acoustic outputs can be received by a wearer's hearing aid, greatly improving the signal to noise ratio. Television devices, which beam the signal directly to a wearer's headset via infrared or FM transmission, as well as television captioning have grown in popularity as well. Bluetooth technology is also quickly being adapted for those with hearing loss. In addition, there are a number of signaling and alerting devices that can be critically important to the hearing impaired. Deciding if an ALD would be helpful to a patient in addition to, or instead of, simply wearing hearing aids, is an important element of the hearing aid evaluation process.

Outcome Measures

Objective and subjective measures of patient satisfaction with hearing aids are essential to a successful hearing aid fitting. Self-assessment scales, electroacoustic analyses of basic hearing aid function, and real-ear measurements, including speech-mapping (Stelmachowicz et al., 1996), are some of the current tools used to verify patient benefit with amplification.

References

ANSI S3.5. (1997). *American National Standard Methods for Calculation of the Speech Intelligibility Index*. New York: American National Standards Institute.

Brownell, W., Spector, A., Raphael, R., & Popel, A. (2001). Micro- and nanomechanics of the cochlear outer hair cell. *Annual Review of Biomedical Engineering*, 3, 169–194.

Buus, S., & Florentine, M. (2001). Growth of loudness in listeners with cochlear hearing losses: Recruitment reconsidered. *Journal of the Association for Research in Otolaryngology*, 3, 120–139.

Cox, R. (1995). Using loudness data for hearing aid selection: The IHAFF approach. *Hearing Journal*, 48(2), 10–44.

Cox, R. (1997). Administration and application of the APHAB. *Hearing Journal*, 50(4), 32–48.

Cruickshank, K., Wiley, T., Tweed, T., Klein, B., Klein, R, Mares-Perlman, J., et al. (1996). Prevalence of hearing loss in older adults in beaver dam, Wisconsin. *American Journal of Epidemiology*, 148(9), 879–886.

Dillon, H., Birtles, G., & Lovegrove, R. (1999). Measuring the outcomes of a national rehabilitation program: Normative data for the Client Oriented Scale of Improvement (COSI) and the Hearing Aid User's Questionnaire (HAUQ). *Journal of the American Academy of Audiology*, *10*, 67–79.

Dillon H., Katsch R., Byrne D., Ching T., Keidser G., & Brewer S. (1998). The NAL-NL1 prescription procedure for non-linear hearing aids. *National Acoustics Laboratories Research and Development, Annual Report 1997/98* (pp. 4–7). Sydney, Australia: National Acoustics Laboratories.

Gatehouse, S. (1992). The time course and magnitude of perceptual acclimatization to frequency responses: evidence from monaural fitting of hearing aids. *Journal of the Acoustical Society of America*, *92*(3), 1258–1268.

Gates, G., & Mills, J. (2005). Presbycusis. *Lancet*, *366*, 1111–1119.

Killion, M., & Fikret-Pasa, S. (1993) The 3 types of sensorineural hearing loss: Loudness and intelligibility considerations. *Hearing Journal*, *46*(11), 1–4.

Lybarger, S. (1944). *U.S. Patent Application SN 543, 278.*

Lybarger, S. (1963). *Simplified fitting system for hearing aids.* Canonsburg, PA: Radio Ear Corp.

Mueller, H., & Killion, M. (1990). An easy method for calculating the articulation index. *Hearing Journal*, *43*(9), 14–17.

National Institutes of Health Fact Sheet. (2007). *Hair cell regeneration and hearing loss.* Available at http://www.nih.gov/about/researchresultsforthepublic/Hair.pdf

Oxenham, A., & Bacon, S., (2003). Cochlear compression: Perceptual measures and implications for normal and impaired hearing. *Ear and Hearing*, *24*(5), 352–366.

Seewald, R. (1992). The desired sensation level method for fitting children: Version 3.0. *Hearing Journal*, *45*(4), 36–41.

Stelmachowicz, P., Kopun, J., Mace, A., & Lewis, D. (1996). Measures of hearing gain for real speech. *Ear and Hearing*, *17*, 520–527.

Thornton, A. R., & Raffin, M. J. (1978). Speech-discrimination scores modeled as a binomial variable. *Journal of Speech and Hearing Research*, *21*, 507–518.

Walden, T., & Walden, B. (2005). Unilateral versus bilateral amplification for adults with impaired hearing. *Journal of the American Academy of Audiology*, *16*, 574–584.

Verification of Hearing Aid Fitting

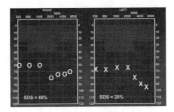

DAVID FABRY, Ph.D.

According to Hearing Industries Association (2008) figures, digital hearing aids represent over 95% of the total hearing aids dispensed in the United States. Although digital technology affords access to unparalleled technology for noise cancellation, multiple-channel compression, adaptive directionality, and adaptive feedback cancellation, the primary advantage compared to analog devices is the sophisticated *control* over these features, enabling optimization to meet individual patient need.

During the past decade, the software used to program hearing aids has improved concomitant to the digital hardware, and many offer both "manual" and "automated" fine-tuning systems to facilitate the verification process. In fact, most manufacturers provide a "simulated" verification in their software, on the basis of the patient's audiometric data and associated prescriptive amplification characteristics. The reality, however, is that the most important component of the fitting—the patient—cannot be automated or simulated in software, and therefore the initial verification requires that the patient be present. Previous studies (Hawkins & Cook, 2003) have shown that *simulated* amplification often overestimates *measured* amplification by 20 to 25 decibels, so it is extremely important to verify hearing aid performance in situ for the best quality of outcome.

Goals of Verification

The most important goals of amplification are to ensure audibility of sound sounds over as broad a frequency range as possible, provide speech intelligibility for quiet and noisy listening environments, and prevent loud sounds from reaching uncomfortable levels.

Verification Methods

A number of measures have been employed for verification of initial hearing aid settings; most involve comparison of unaided and aided performance, in terms of the frequency-specific amplification (gain) provided across the hearing aid bandwidth (typically 200-6000 Hz). Historically, desired gain (also called "target" gain) comprised roughly one-half of the audiometric threshold value at a given frequency (Lybarger, 1944). Although modifications to this "half-gain" prescriptive fitting rule were subsequently developed by Berger (Berger, Hagberg, & Rane, 1977), POGO (McCandless & Lyregaard, 1983), and NAL (Byrne & Dillon, 1986), all are based on an arithmetic computation, based on audiometric thresholds that translate to the "prescribed" gain as a function of frequency. An example of this calculation is shown in Figure 6–1, and illustrates the frequency-specific nature of applied target gain for an individual patient. In turn, verification measures are used to ensure that measured gain values at each frequency approximate target gain within some criterion measure.

Until the past decade, most hearing aids employed "linear" signal processing; that is, once target gain values are applied at a given frequency, they do not change as a function of input until maximum hearing aid output is reached. Figure 6–2 illustrates a sample input-output functions measured in the 2-cc coupler for a linear hearing aid that provides 30 dB gain (output level minus input level) at 2000 Hz, with infinite peak clipping employed to limit maximum output at 115 dB SPL. Note that for all inputs ranging from 20 dB to 95 dB SPL, gain remains the same; when hearing aid output reaches 120 dB SPL, peak clipping restricts any further increase from occurring. The use of an artificial (2-cc) coupler, rather than an actual patient's ear, for some hearing aid measurements dates back to the 1940s (Lybarger, Preves, & Olsen, 1999). Although 2-cc coupler data provide important information regarding hearing aid signal processing, they do not provide sufficient information to predict measured levels in an actual patient's ear when "real-ear" measurements are available.

The reason, of course, that coupler measures do not accurately predict sound pressure levels in individual ears is that the acoustic properties of each ear reflect differences in pinna, concha, ear canal, and eardrum resonances. On average, the sum total of these resonances produces a frequency-dependent "free field to eardrum transformation" (Shaw, 1974) that provides 15 to 20 dB amplification in the frequency region between 2500 to 3500 Hz (Figure 6–3). Slight variations in the size of the pinna, concha, and ear canal will alter this resonance and impact the way that sounds are heard. Furthermore, insertion of a hearing aid or earmold into the patient's ear will alter the acoustic properties of sounds, depending on the type of hearing aid, insertion depth of the shell or earmold, vent size, and hearing aid microphone location.

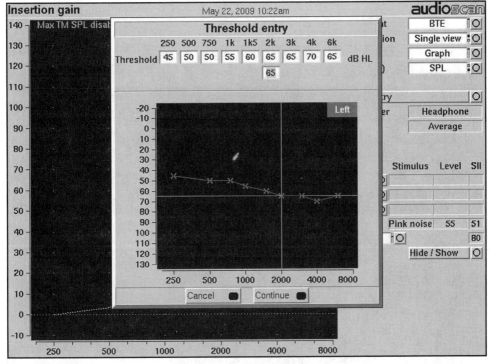

A

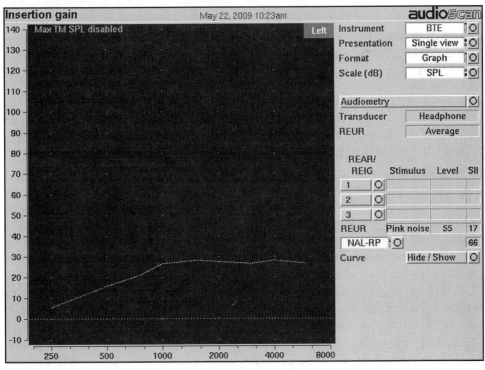

B

Figure 6–1. A. Audiometric thresholds for the left ear of a patient, indicating a moderate, gently sloping hearing loss; **B.** prescriptive gain "target," based on audiometric thresholds displayed in **(A)** according to National Acoustics Laboratories' RP arithmetic formula.

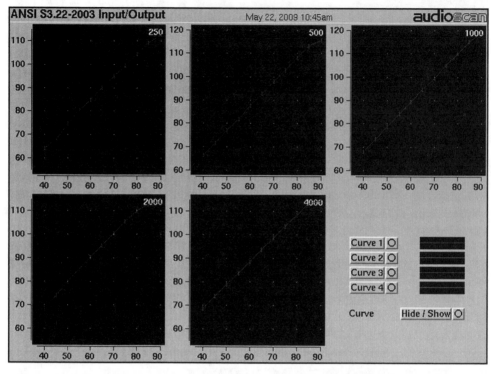

Figure 6–2. Input/output functions, measured according to ANSI S3.22-2003, for 250, 500, 1000, 2000, and 4000 Hz.

As a result, there is no substitute for in situ assessment of hearing aid performance to assess the acoustic interactions between the patient's hearing aid and his or her ear.

For years, "functional gain" measures were the most popular method used by audiologists for verification of initial hearing aid settings. Functional gain measures are obtained using behavioral assessment of aided and unaided sound-field thresholds for frequency-specific stimuli. For a given frequency, functional gain is computed by subtracting aided threshold from unaided threshold. This measure has the advantage of being relatively easy to obtain, and requires minimal specialized equipment, the most important being a calibrated "sound field"

system in an acoustic test chamber or booth (Figure 6–4). Furthermore, because behavioral responses are obtained from the patient, functional gain evaluates the perception of sound, rather than merely the presence of acoustic gain. The disadvantages of functional gain measures, however, outweigh the advantages, especially for modern digital hearing aids that use nonlinear signal processing (compression). These drawbacks include limited frequency resolution (octave or intra-octave frequency resolution at best) and poor test-retest variability (often 10 dB or more). Furthermore, unlike linear hearing aids, gain varies with stimulus level for nonlinear amplification, meaning that more gain typically is present for soft sounds than for loud sounds.

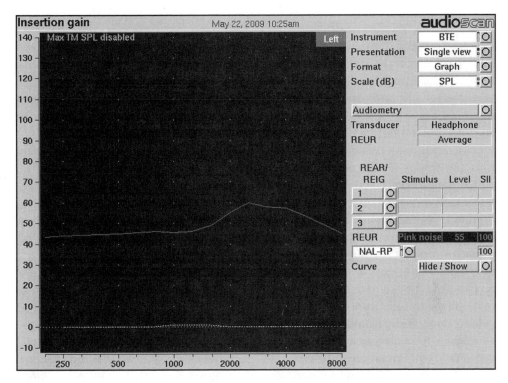

Figure 6–3. Average real-ear unaided response (REUR) for an adult ear, depicting the principal resonance effect (15–20 dB) in the frequency region between 2500 to 3500 Hz.

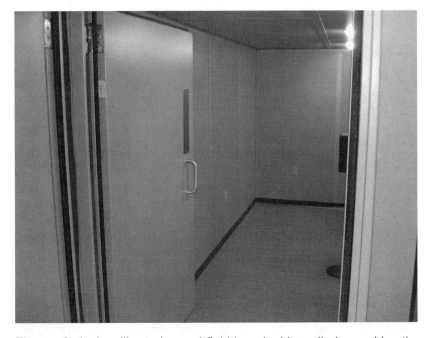

Figure 6–4. A calibrated sound field in a double-walled sound booth.

As a result, varying the presentation level to assess aided functional gain levels will also interact and interfere with accurate threshold levels. Typically, this will result in an overestimation of "actual" gain values for conversational-level speech, which in turn may lead to a poor aided result.

The challenges faced by using functional gain measures to accurately assess nonlinear (compression) hearing aids have led to renewed interest in real-ear probe microphone measurements. Initially developed in the early 1980s (see Mason & Popelka, 1986, for a review), probe microphone techniques assess hearing aid gain by comparing the aided sound pressure levels measured near the tympanic membrane with sound pressure measured at a reference microphone located near the entrance to the ear canal (Figure 6–5). This measure provides an objective estimate of frequency-specific "insertion gain" that offers greater frequency resolution, better test-retest accuracy, and improved face validity than pure-tone functional gain measures when speech stimuli are used. To that end, the choice of test stimulus for use with probe microphone measures is an important one.

Historically, warble tones and swept sinusoidal stimuli were initially used for real-ear measures, but the advent of multiple-channel compression hearing aids required the development of broadband speech-weighted noise (ANSI S3.42-1992). This stimulus reduces the test artifacts that occur when tonal stimuli are used to test compression hearing aids (Preves et al., 1989), but it does not prevent stimulus interference with noise cancellation systems used with digital hearing aids. As a result, the International Collegium for Rehabilitative Audiology (ICRA) developed a collection of noise signals that may be used for hearing aid testing (including real-ear measurements) by using a test stimulus that more closely mimics the temporal and spectral prop-

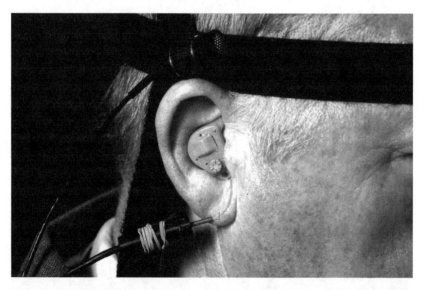

Figure 6–5. Real-ear measurement of an in-the-ear (ITE) hearing aid, with reference microphone (*top*) and probe microphone (*bottom*) inserted into the patient's ear canal.

erties of speech (see Dreschler et al., 2001 for a review). Although used widely in Europe, the ICRA test stimulus has not been used extensively in North America. More recently, the trend in the United States and Canada has been for manufacturers to incorporate "live" or recorded speech for use with probe microphone systems. By using actual speech, rather than pure tones or shaped noise, the measures more closely approximate "real world" use. The primary limitation, however, is that no ANSI standards exist at the present time for the acoustic properties corresponding to "average" speech. As a result, some instrument manufacturers use recorded or live speech samples with male, female, or child talkers, with no consistent method for comparing across devices or clinics. The advantage of recorded speech include improved test-retest accuracy and repeatability, whereas "live" speech testing provides advantages for customizing hearing aid settings for specific voices (think specialized "mother-in-law" or "grandchild" program). At present, the advantages of using actual speech outweigh the disadvantages, but additional information is required to provide a comprehensive evaluation of initial hearing aid settings. Furthermore, as with any prescriptive measure, adjustments may be required from the suggested target values to ensure optimization to meet individual patient need. The following protocol may be used to ensure that modern digital hearing aids achieve the verification goals listed above.

Verification Protocol

The first objective of any verification protocol should be to provide speech audibility over as broad of a frequency range as possible. Probe microphone measures should be completed with the patient seated approximately one meter in front of a loudspeaker positioned at 0 degrees azimuth (directly in front of the patient). The reference microphone/probe microphone assembly should be positioned on the patient's ear, with the reference microphone near the entrance to the ear canal and the probe microphone within 5-10 mm of the tympanic membrane. The patient's audiometric thresholds and loudness discomfort levels provide a graphic depiction of residual auditory area (Figure 6-6). This display format is typically referred to as an "SPL-O-Gram," as opposed to the traditional audiogram format, which is plotted in dB HL.

Initially, the reference microphone must be equalized to ensure that a known SPL is measured at the reference microphone. This equalization measure should be completed for each patient to control for changes in the test environment. Next, recorded or live speech should be delivered through the loudspeaker at 65 to 70 dB SPL, corresponding to the long-term average level for conversational speech. Note that for a constant vocal effort, unaided speech levels at each frequency range over 30 dB from "peak" to "minima" levels, with peak levels roughly 12 dB greater than the long-term average (Figure 6-7). Real-time display of the unaided level provides the audiologist with information regarding speech audibility for "typical" listening situations; some probe microphone test systems calculate and display *expected* speech intelligibility (e.g. the Speech Intelligibility Index) for unaided and aided conditions (see Figure 6-7).

Next, aided measurements of hearing aid performance are made using the same

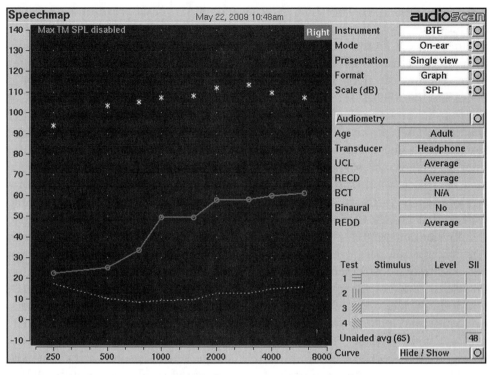

Figure 6–6. SPL-O-Gram, as displayed for dB SPL plotted as a function of frequency. Middle line (*with circles*) depicts unaided thresholds for a patient with sloping mild-to-severe hearing loss; asterisks indicate predicted loudness discomfort levels (LDLs). Residual auditory area is defined as the region bounded by thresholds to LDLs for each audiometric frequency.

speech stimulus (at 65–70 dB SPL) with the hearing aid placed in the patient's ear. The difference between the aided and unaided measurements provides the audiologist with an assessment of frequency-specific insertion gain (Figure 6–8). Additionally, aided speech for conversational speech levels (65–70 dB SPL) should bisect the residual auditory area, midway between the patient's thresholds and loudness discomfort levels (LDLs) to ensure audibility without discomfort. In the past, much attention has been focused on the precision with which prescriptive target is matched, but most modern digital hearing aids use "data logging" of volume control settings to assist with optimization of hearing aid settings based on "real world"

hearing aid use. Consequently, more attention is typically focused on evaluating the dynamic aspects of compression to ensure that soft sounds are audible and loud sounds are not uncomfortable.

Studies of the long-term spectrum of speech as a function of different vocal efforts indicate that 50 dB SPL is a reasonable approximation of "soft" speech for both male and female talkers (Pearsons et al, 1977). As such, this stimulus level is appropriate for use to ensure that compression settings are appropriately set for distant speech and quiet listening environments.

Early compression studies showed that, if ambient sounds were amplified too much, sound quality decreased. Al-

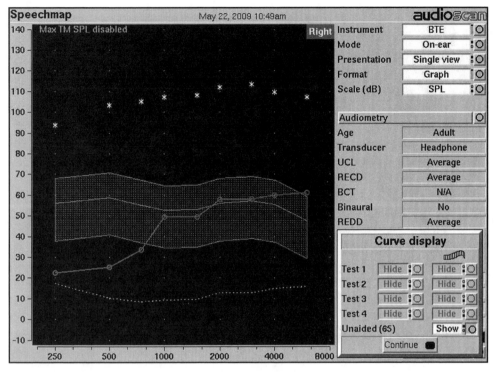

Figure 6–7. Unaided long-term average speech spectrum levels (*hatched region*), plotted on the SPL-O-Gram, with unaided hearing thresholds (*middle line with circles*) and calculated LDLs (*asterisks*).

though extensive review of compression parameters is beyond the scope of this chapter, review of a few basic principles is relevant. Basically, compression systems are governed by the terms compression threshold and compression ratio. Compression threshold, for most systems in use today, is defined by the input level (in dB) at which the system is activated; compression ratio is the change in input divided by the change in output level over a defined intensity range above compression threshold (see Figure 6-8). Most systems today use compression thresholds that activate below 40 dB SPL and compression ratios of less than 2:1, to permit sounds that vary dynamically over a 60- to 80-dB range to fit into the reduced dynamic range that accompanies cochlear hearing loss.

Using the 50 dB SPL speech stimulus, the goal of initial verification is to amplify the average levels and peaks to audibility, but leave the minima below the patient's auditory threshold (Figure 6-9). If the entire speech spectrum is amplified to audibility, it will increase compression ratio to unacceptable levels by acting as an "automatic volume control." In essence, if compression ratio is too high (in excess of 4:1) all amplified sounds will be the same, and the hearing aid user will be unable to distinguish a whisper from a raised voice. It is therefore important to verify that soft sounds are indeed audible—but soft—to the hearing aid user at the time of initial verification.

Loudness recruitment is a frequently observed consequence of sensorineural hearing loss (SNHL). As a result, the

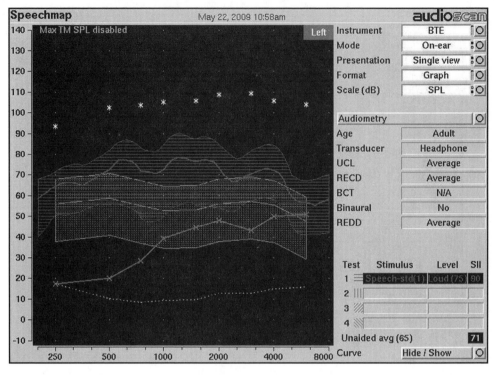

Figure 6–8. Aided speech spectrum (*region with horizontal lines*), displayed within the patient's residual auditory area, with calculated Speech Intelligibility Index (SII) displayed as 0.90, indicating audibility is achieved across nearly all important speech frequencies for speech presented at 75 dB SPL.

growth of loudness from threshold to discomfort occurs over a much narrower range of intensities than for persons with normal hearing. It is therefore extremely important to assess whether hearing aids that provide audibility for soft and average sounds also prevent loudness recruitment from producing discomfort for loud sounds. That is, measurements should be made with frequency-specific high-level inputs (usually 85–90 dB SPL) to ensure that the patient reports that they would be loud, but not uncomfortably loud, if encountered in real-world settings (Figure 6–10). Some audiologists are reticent to use 85 to 90 dB SPL stimuli for fear of causing discomfort for their patients, but it is perhaps one of the most important

checks completed as part of the initial verification battery, as the patient will certainly encounter loud sounds outside the controlled test environment of the audiometric sound suite. This was particularly important in the past, as linear hearing aids required high gain and high output to achieve satisfactory gain, and maximum in situ output levels often exceeded 120 dB SPL for patients with moderate to severe degrees of SNHL. With modern digital hearing aids that use multiple-channel compression, however, maximum power is often set too *low*, which, in turn, reduces the dynamic range by increasing compression ratio. The effect is the same as when soft sounds are amplified too much, in the patient's exposure

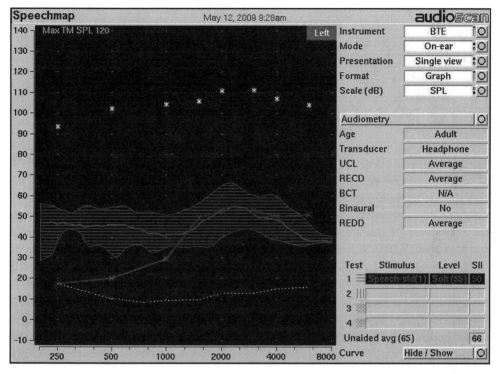

Figure 6–9. Aided speech spectrum (*hatched region*), displayed within the patient's residual auditory area, for speech presented at 55 dB SPL, indicating a calculated SII of 0.50.

to dynamic listening environments is reduced when soft sounds are over-amplified and loud sounds are under-amplified. In summary, the use of multiple input levels (e.g., 50, 65, and 90 dB SPL) with probe-microphone measurements at the initial hearing aid fitting is important to verify that compression thresholds and compression ratios are both set as low as possible to ensure audibility and prevent loudness discomfort. Subsequently, as stated above, the use of data logging of patient-adjusted volume control settings in real-world listening environments will assist with optimization of hearing aid gain for individual patients. It is important to remember that probe microphone measures test gain, not hearing, because they do not typically require a behavioral

response from the patient. For this reason, some clinicians will use speech recognition measures in quiet or in noise to provide additional evidence of a successful fit.

Speech Recognition Testing

The most popular speech measures in use today remain the W-22 (Hirsh et al., 1952) or NU-6 (Tillman & Carhart, 1966) monosyllabic word lists popularized years ago for use with diagnostic audiologic evaluation, but speech-in-noise measures, including the Hearing in Noise Test (Nilsson, Soli, & Sullivan, 1994) and QuickSIN

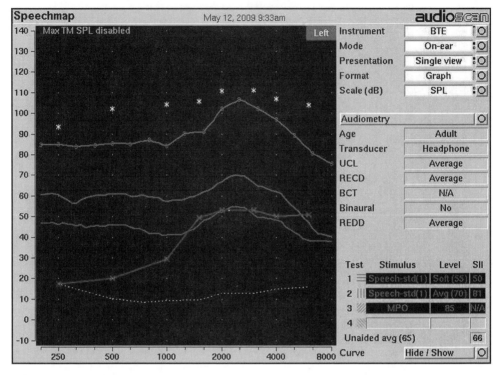

Figure 6–10. Family of measurement curves for speech presented at 55 dB SPL (*third line from top*), 70 dB SPL (*second line from top*), and for a maximum power output (*top line*) swept sinusoidal stimulus presented at 85 dB SPL to ensure that loud sounds do not exceed the patient's LDL.

(Killion et al., 2004) have gained in popularity in recent years because they have demonstrated greater predictive accuracy of benefit from specific hearing aid technology than with the audiogram alone or speech testing in quiet. Furthermore, they provide a behavioral complement to probe microphone measures, because they actually evaluate perception, rather than mere presence of sound in the ear canal, and therefore provide some information regarding expected outcome.

Killion has also suggested that the QuickSIN may be used to predict whether a patient is likely to benefit from specific hearing aid technology, including directional microphones or wireless microphone technology, by comparing indi-

vidual patient performance (aided or unaided) in terms of a "signal-to-noise ratio deficit" relative to normal hearing (Figure 6-11). This type of evaluation has proved very useful both in terms of diagnosis and treatment of hearing loss, and many audiologists have incorporated speech in noise testing into their basic test battery.

Advanced Signal Processing

In recent years, directional microphones have proven to be one of the most important features related to perceived

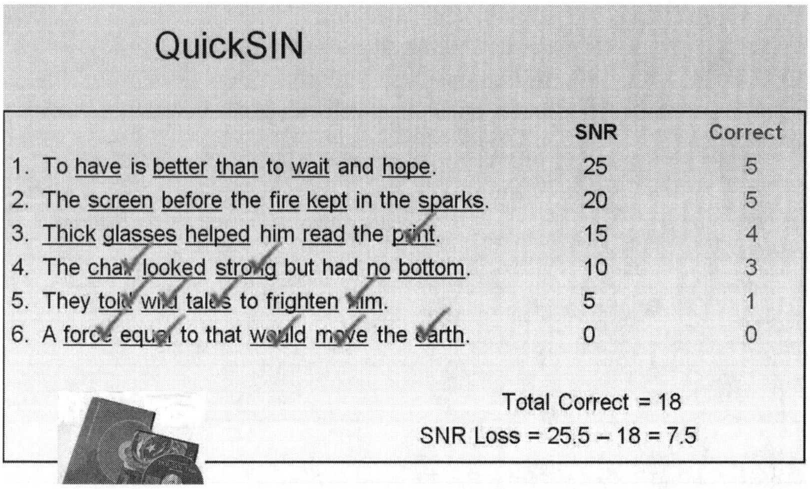

QuickSIN

	SNR	Correct
1. To have is better than to wait and hope.	25	5
2. The screen before the fire kept in the sparks.	20	5
3. Thick glasses helped him read the print.	15	4
4. The chair looked strong but had no bottom.	10	3
5. They told wild tales to frighten him.	5	1
6. A force equal to that would move the earth.	0	0

Total Correct = 18

SNR Loss = 25.5 − 18 = 7.5

Figure 6–11. Sample representation of speech in noise testing using the QuickSIN, which presents sentences at signal-to-noise ratios (SNR) ranging from +25 dB to 0 dB. In this example, correct responses to "key" words" (five per sentence) are indicated in the right-hand column, with the total correct equal to 18 out of 30 key words. This score is subtracted from the normative score (25.5), resulting in an SNR Loss of 7.5 dB from the normal result, which may be used for counseling purposes and/or to demonstrate benefits of amplification.

satisfaction and benefit from amplification in real-world listening environments (Kochkin, 2002). Although a technical description of directional microphone performance is beyond the scope of the present chapter, it is important to remember they provide speech recognition benefits in noise only when speech and noise are spatially separated. Specifically, for most systems, optimal performance is achieved when the desired signal (speech) originates in front of the wearer (0 degrees), and noise is located on the sides (± 90 degrees) or from behind (180 degrees). Some hearing aid test systems provide a mechanism to verify directional microphone performance by measuring hearing aid output through the 2-cc coupler for sounds that are spatially separated in a small acoustically isolated test box. It is also possible to verify direc-tional microphone performance in situ by using probe microphone systems to compare hearing aid output for sounds originating from the front (0 degrees) with those occurring behind (180 degrees). Figure 6–12 demonstrates a system that is working properly; when the directional microphones are activated, hearing aid output for sounds from the front is much higher than for sounds occurring at 180 degrees. Although not intended to verify the actual magnitude of benefit that a patient is likely to encounter in real-world settings, it serves as an efficient technique for verification and counseling the patient regarding the benefits of directional microphones. Some audiologists use aided speech recognition in noise measures (see above) to compare omni-directional and directional microphone conditions.

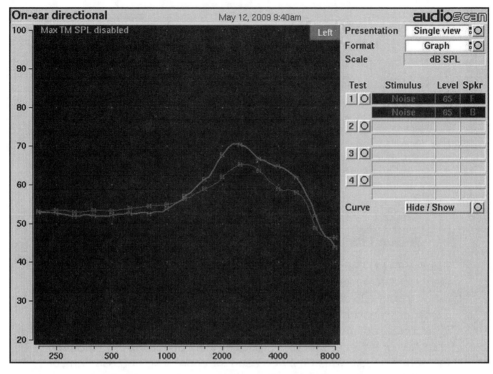

Figure 6–12. Real-ear measurement to assess benefits of directional microphones, depicting a reduction in energy for sounds occurring at from behind (180 degrees) versus in front (0 degrees), depicted as the thin line and thick line, respectively. In this example, the reduction in energy in the high-frequency region (above 1500 Hz) is approximately 5 dB, indicating improved amplification for sounds occurring from the front while reducing amplitude for sounds from behind the hearing aid user.

Self-Assessment Scales

The audiogram and speech recognition measures provide necessary, but not sufficient, information for selection of the appropriate hearing aid style and type for individual patients. Self-assessment scales, including the Abbreviated Profile of Hearing Aid Benefit (Cox & Alexander, 1995) or the Client Oriented Scale of Improvement (Dillon, James, & Gillis, 1997) have proven useful for profiting assessment, and also for determining hearing aid benefit by comparing aided to unaided performance. The Abbreviated Profile of Hearing Aid Benefit (APHAB) is a 24-item questionnaire that is divided into four subscales: Ease of Communication (EC), Background Noise (BN), Reverberation (RV), and Aversive Sounds (AV). Each subscale has six questions that pertain to that subscale; normative data exist for each subscale and also for a "global" benefit score comprising the average of the EC, BN, and RV subscales.

The Client Oriented Scale of Improvement (COSI) allows the patient to identify, prior to intervention, between one to five specific listening situations that they would like to improve with amplification. Subsequent to being fit, the patient rates the degree to which hearing aids resolved the difficulty according to how much better or worse he or she performs in those environments. Although it is more difficult to establish normative benefit data for the COSI than for the APHAB, it specifically targets only those listening situations that present difficulties for a given individual. As a result, both types of self-assessment measures have found some support clinically. Many clinicians administer these metrics at either the first (typically 1-2 weeks) or second (typically 30 days) postfitting visit.

Summary

Initial verification of hearing aid performance is an extremely important part of the hearing aid selection and fitting process. Digital hearing aids offer incredible technology to meet the needs of hearing-impaired persons, but at this point in time, they do not fit themselves. Appropriate fitting strategies, in combination with aural rehabilitation and (perhaps most importantly) realistic expectations for benefit, will optimize patient outcomes.

References

Berger, K. W., Hagberg, E. N., & Rane, R. L. (1977). *Prescription of hearing aids*. Kent, OH: Herald.

Byrne, D., & Dillon, H. (1986). The National Acoustics Laboratories' new procedure for selecting the gain and frequency response of a hearing aid. *Ear and Hearing, 7*, 257-265.

Cox, R. M., & Alexander, G. C. (1995). The abbreviated profile of hearing aid benefit. *Ear and Hearing, 16*(2), 176-186.

Dillon, H., James, A., & Ginis, J. (1997). Client Oriented Scale of Improvement (COSI) and its relationship to several other measures of benefit and satisfaction provided by hearing aids. *Journal of American Academy of Audiology, 8*(1), 27-43.

Dreschler, W. A., Vershuure, H., Lidvigsen, C., & Westermann, S. (2001). ICRA noises: Artificial noise signals with speech-like spectral and temporal properties for hearing instrument assessment. International Collegium for Rehabilitative Audiology. *Audiology, 40*(3), 148-157.

Hawkins, D. B., & Cook, J. A. (2003). Hearing aid software predictive gain values: How accurate are they? *Hearing Journal, 56*(7), 26-34.

Hearing Industries Association. (2008). Available at http://www.hearing.org

Hirsh, I. J., Davidson, E. G., Silverman, S. R., Reynolds, E. G., Eldert, E., & Benson, R. W. (1952). Development of materials for speech audiometry. *Journal of Speech and Hearing Disorders, 15*, 321-337.

Killion, M. C., Niquette, P. A., Gudmundsen, G. I., Revit, L. J., & Banerjee, S. (2004). Development of a quick speech-in-noise test for measuring signal-to-noise ratio loss in normal-hearing and hearing-impaired listeners. *Journal of the Acoustical Society of America, 116*, 2395-2405.

Kochkin, S. (2002). MarkeTrak VI: 10-year customer satisfaction trends in the US hearing instrument market. *Hearing Review, 9*(10), 14-25, 46.

Lybarger, S. F. (1944, July 3). *U.S. Patent application SN 543, 248*.

Lybarger, S. F., Preves, D. A., & Olsen, W. O. (1999). A bit of history on standards for acoustical measurements of hearing aids. *American Journal of Audiology, 8*, 3-5.

Mason, D., & Popelka, G. R. (1986). Comparison of hearing aid gain using functional, coupler, and probe-tube measurements. *Journal of Speech and Hearing Research, 29*, 218-226.

Nilsson, M., Soli, S. D., & Sullivan, J. A. (1994). Development of the Hearing in Noise Test for the measurement of speech reception thresholds in quiet and in noise. *Journal of the Acoustical Society of America*, *95*, 1085–1099.

McCandless, G. A., & Lyregaard, P. E. (1983). Prescription of gain/output (POGO) for hearing aids. *Hearing Instruments*, *34*(1), 16–21.

Pearsons, K. S., Bennett, R. L., & Fidell, S. (1977). *Speech levels in various noise environments*. EPA-600/1-77-025. U.S. Environmental Protection Agency.

Preves, D. A., Beck, L. B., Burnett, E. B., & Teder, H. (1989). Input stimuli for obtaining frequency responses of automatic gain control hearing aids. *Journal of Speech and Hearing Research*, *32*, 189–194.

Shaw, E. A. G. (1974). Ear canal pressure generated by a free sound field. *Journal of the Acoustical Society of America*, *56*, 1848–1861.

Tillman, T. W., & Carhart, R. (1966). An expanded test for speech discrimination using CNC monosyllabic words: Northwestern University auditory test No. 6 (USAF School of Aerospace Medicine Report SAM-TR-66-55). In J. B. Chaiklin, I. M. Ventry, & R. F. Dixon (Eds.), *Hearing measurement: A book of readings* (2nd ed., pp. 226–235). Reading MA: Addison-Wesley.

7

Hearing Aid Amplification in Pediatric Patients

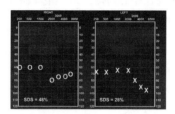

MARGARET E. WINTER, M.S., CCC-A

A fundamental principle of pediatric hearing care is that no child is too young for a hearing test. A fundamental corollary of this principle is that, when a potentially handicapping hearing loss is discovered, even if it is within the first few weeks of life, immediate steps toward auditory habilitation are essential. The ultimate linguistic success of a child with hearing loss rests less on early identification, per se, than on early intervention.

Approximately 95% of deaf infants are born to hearing families. It is likely, therefore, that a majority of parents of deaf children will wish to take all possible steps to help their children to hear as normally as possible and to learn to communicate using spoken language.

The development of fluent formal language through any modality is of paramount importance. Although sign language can, in many instances, provide an excellent foundation to facilitate the development of oral language once the child has auditory access to speech as well as appropriate education and therapy, the goal of most hearing parents is to be able to communicate with their children in their own language. The first step toward realizing this goal is the fitting of amplification.

Identification and Device Fitting

Before newborn hearing screening, it was relatively rare for otolaryngologists to see young infants with known hearing loss. As little as 25 years ago, the average

age of identification of handicapping hearing loss was approximately 2½ years, by which time a diagnosis of hearing loss was seldom a surprise to parents who may have suspected the problem for many months. Awareness among physicians that hearing loss can be documented even in newborns is still not universal. Professionals who work with young deaf children still all too frequently hear reports from parents that their suspicions were met with indifference or disdain by their primary doctors. Some physicians who are aware that hearing can be assessed at birth may still be unaware that amplification can and should be fit within the first few weeks of life to minimize the effects of auditory deprivation on the development of oral language.

In 1998, Christine Yoshinaga-Itano and colleagues published a study that became a catalyst for the development of many newborn hearing screening programs throughout the country (Yoshinaga-Itano et al., 1998). In it, they showed that children whose hearing losses were identified before the age of 6 months fared better in terms of language development than children identified after 6 months of age, given the provision of early intervention services within 2 months of identification for both groups. A majority of newborns in the United States now are screened shortly after birth and the follow-up process for children who do not pass incorporates multiple disciplines, including audiologists, primary care physicians, otolaryngologists, and educators. Physicians can now expect to see babies on their caseloads who have failed newborn hearing screenings and they will need to know how to assist the parents of these children in obtaining the services needed to confirm and document the degree of hearing loss and provide amplification,

if appropriate. They also will need to support parents in gaining access to educational and therapy services. The otolaryngologist will be expected to provide medical clearance for hearing aid fitting if there are no medical contraindications and the hearing loss is not treatable medically. She or he will see the child periodically for examination and possibly for treatment of otitis media and/or cerumen that interferes with the use of the hearing aids or with the audiologist's ability to take good ear impressions. She or he will work with parents to determine, insofar as possible, the cause of the hearing loss and to rule out other significant medical conditions associated with the hearing loss. Referrals to the primary care physician may come through the newborn screening program; referrals to the otolaryngologist may come through the program or through the audiologist who performs the diagnostic procedures. That same audiologist may continue to see the child for many years. In some cases, it will be the physician who refers the child to the audiologist. It is prudent, therefore, for physicians, audiologists, and the other professionals who may see these young infants to have open communication and mutual respect for one another's particular skills and opinions.

Qualifications for Pediatric Audiologists

Assessment of hearing of very young children requires a multiple-test-battery approach by experienced clinicians. These clinicians must be able to use a variety of tests to form as complete a picture of the child's auditory abilities as possible at any given stage of his or her growth. A particular weakness in many newborn screening programs is the paucity of audiologists who specialize in the evaluation and habilitation of infants. In urban areas, pediatric audiology may be readily available; in more rural areas, audiologic services may be difficult to come by at all and pediatric specialty services nearly impossible. It may be necessary, and perhaps preferred both by families and by audiologists with only adult patients, for these very young children to be referred to programs that are a distance away at least through the processes of fitting of hearing aids and establishment of a stable audiogram. Where this is not possible, there are certain minimum requirements for audiologists who wish to, or agree to, fit hearing aids on very young children.

1. They must be willing to proceed with amplification as soon as the diagnosis is made and medical clearance is received from the otolaryngologist. They must understand how auditory brainstem responses (ABR) and/or auditory steady state responses (ASSR), otoacoustic emission (OAE) results, tympanometry, acoustic reflexes, and behavioral observation should be coordinated and interpreted so that the appropriate amount of gain and output can be selected.

2. They must be comfortable enough with babies and their parents to take good ear impressions and be familiar with the styles and materials appropriate for very small ears. They will need to be available to take ear impressions very often as the baby outgrows his molds, which can be frequent. (Physicians must be aware that cerumen that only partially blocks the ear canal, which they would otherwise not find necessary to remove, may need to be removed in order for the audiologist to get a good impression.)

3. They must be aware that the acoustic characteristics of an infant's ear differ significantly from adults' and that the application of hearing aid fitting formulas geared toward young children, specific to their age, are essential. As the baby grows, the fittings will need to be regularly re-evaluated and adjusted.

4. They must be familiar with appropriate test techniques for young children through the preschool years, so that they can obtain accurate, ear-specific, frequency-specific physiologic and behavioral audiometric thresholds at the earliest possible age. This information will influence the fine tuning of the hearing aids as the child grows and more information about the baby's auditory abilities becomes available. They must display the ability to approach assessments with knowledge of young children and flexibility of procedure, as young children rarely conform to textbook expectations.

5. They should be familiar with appropriate referral sources, since a significant percentage of children with hearing loss also have other disabilities that must be followed by professionals from other disciplines.

6. They must be able and willing to communicate findings clearly to parents and to answer the many questions that families will have about their child's hearing and their child's future. It should go without saying that all professionals working with the families of young hearing impaired children must be aware of the enormous distress this diagnosis will cause parents. With very early diagnosis comes the benefit of early intervention, but identification of hearing impairment —an invisible handicap that may not be in any way evident to parents of a young infant—is usually a shock. Parents require time to process the information given

them and time to understand the ramifications of hearing loss in their child's life and their lives as a family. Parents of deaf children frequently remember that they were given no useful information by the professionals who identified their baby's hearing loss; this is probably not entirely true and is more likely indicative of stunned parents' inability to process the information immediately. It is helpful for families to hear and read explanations repeatedly and in various forms, and a cooperative working relationship among physicians, audiologists, educators and therapists will facilitate parents being able to take positive action to help their children.

What Constitutes Handicapping Hearing Loss for Children

Adults with postlingual hearing loss usually have established language fluency when their hearing was still within the normal range. Speech is extremely redundant, and even a degraded signal may be understandable to a post-lingually deafened adult (witness our general ability to be able to communicate on cell phones even when the signal is very poor). Some hearing loss may be manageable without amplification by adults, who may be savvy enough to manipulate their environment to compensate for mild or frequency specific hearing loss, and to recognize when they have missed or misunderstood critical information. By contrast, any degree of hearing loss—mild, frequency-specific, unilateral, as well as more severe degrees of bilateral loss—is handicapping to a young child, especially when the onset is prior to the establishment of fluent oral language skills. Children need

to hear well both in order to recognize spoken language as well as to develop oral language from the outset. A much higher fidelity signal is required for children in this learning process. A vast amount of language is learned by children incidentally, and normal hearing in both ears is required to maximize their ability to overhear a broad range of vocabulary and complex language constructs being used at home and at school. Furthermore, children are not only using their hearing to learn language but also to learn social skills and to achieve academically, often in disadvantageous acoustic environments. All hearing impaired persons have greater difficulty discriminating speech in noisy environments, and classrooms, lunchrooms, and playgrounds are certainly not quiet places. Children, not being aware of the impact of their hearing deficits, or else disinclined to call attention to themselves, frequently are unable to compensate even for mild hearing loss without technological help and human support.

Hearing aids can benefit children with all degrees, types, and configurations of hearing loss. In our society, hearing loss is often equated with aging and infirmity, and evidence of hearing loss may be viewed as fodder for ridicule among schoolchildren. Therefore, some parents view hearing aids as stigmatizing, especially when they do not see strong evidence that their child's hearing loss is handicapping. Physicians have been known to support this notion, usually at the expense of the child, often because they are accustomed to working primarily with adults who can function much better in daily life with mild to moderate hearing loss than children can. Although hearing aids initially may call unwanted attention to a child if parents and teachers do not provide a supportive atmosphere toward acceptance, there is nothing much more stigmatizing to a child than struggling in school and having difficulty on the social scene, leading to strong feelings of general inadequacy. Children with any degree of hearing loss are working harder to focus and maintain attention than children with normal hearing, and amplification can help to alleviate this struggle. At the very least, children with hearing loss, even minimal loss where parents refuse amplification, should be evaluated frequently to determine the stability of the loss, and close attention should be paid to their progress in school. Children in primary grades are usually nurtured and assisted by teachers and classroom aides; older children may begin almost imperceptibly to flounder as the auditory demands on them become greater.

Unilateral Hearing Loss

Many children and adults with varying degrees of unilateral hearing loss succeed in school and in the workplace with minimal handicap. There is, however, a plethora of literature documenting subtle negative effects of unilateral loss on academic achievement (e.g., Lieu, 2004). Children with unilateral loss have poor ability to localize sounds and have greater difficulty discriminating speech in noisy environments. In particular, children who may already be at risk academically because they have even mild learning disabilities, language delay, recurrent otitis media, and/or attention deficits may be more greatly impacted by unilateral loss.

Profound unilateral loss is unlikely to be directly aidable with conventional amplification, both because of the degree of impairment and also because in a sig-

nificant number of cases there is a low tolerance for loud sound. A hearing aid therefore not only provides no functional benefit but can be uncomfortable as well. Lesser degrees of sensorineural hearing loss where some ability to discriminate speech can be demonstrated may indeed benefit from a hearing aid, as may predominantly conductive hearing loss.

CROS (contralateral routing of signals) systems, which have been used for many years by some adults with unilateral loss to attempt improve localization ability, typically are not recommended for children. Use of a bone-anchored hearing aid (BAHA) may provide more promise than CROS aids for children with unilateral loss and is discussed in greater detail below. At this time, the device that provides the clearest benefit in the classroom to children with unilateral loss is the FM system, in any of its many configurations. FM technology is also discussed below.

Conductive Overlay

Children who wear hearing aids during most of their waking hours are often especially susceptible to cerumen impaction. Although this may not cause a large threshold shift, any decrease in hearing for children with permanent hearing loss is significant. Cerumen can plug up earmolds and can increase acoustic feedback—which is problematic enough in very small ears, even when cerumen is not a factor—and ear canals must be clear for good earmold impressions to be taken. A maintenance program of cerumen management may need to be recommended by the physician.

Otitis media may be brief and occasional or it may be frequent, long lasting, or chronic. Serous otitis media is often not treated medically, (American Academy of Pediatrics, 2004) in an effort to reduce the unnecessary use of antibiotics, and where episodes of otitis media cause minimal or no hearing loss and/or resolve quickly there is generally no expected handicap. Otitis media frequently does cause mild hearing loss, though, and where this loss is persistent or occurs repeatedly, it is logical to assume that speech/language and academic delays can result. Rather surprisingly, much of the literature on this subject does not show a clear correlation between otitis media and language delay, (Simpson et al., 2007) and yet most pediatric audiologists can point to numerous clinical cases of children whose language development begins to soar immediately following PE tube placement. Where resolution of otitis media is not speedy, it is wise to obtain audiometric information, consider the child's level of language development, and weigh the risks and benefits of medical treatment.

Even more vigilant medical attention is essential for children with sensorineural or nonfluid-related conductive hearing loss who develop otitis media. The mild loss resulting from middle ear fluid in children with normal hearing inevitably becomes a much more significant handicap in children who wear hearing aids. Under the best of circumstances the detection levels of children who use amplification are usually at least slightly outside the normal range; children with severe loss may be boosted only to the level of moderate loss with their hearing aids, often even less in the high frequencies. A conductive overlay of 20 to 40 dB due to otitis media may push these children outside the long-term average speech spectrum such that, until the fluid is

resolved, they are unable to detect speech sounds at conversational levels. Children with profound but aidable thresholds will be pushed beyond the aidable range completely (Figure 7–1). Treatment of otitis media that is more aggressive than watchful waiting may be required for these children. At the very least, as long as the fluid persists, audiologic testing should be conducted regularly to determine the degree of adjustment that should be made to the gain and output of the hearing aids.

Hearing Aids, Features and Styles

Infants and young children with aidable hearing impairment are most often fit with behind-the-ear (BTE) style hearing aids. In-the-ear (ITE) styles are almost always inappropriate for a variety of reasons: they are a swallowing hazard, they are ineffective for more than mild hearing loss in very small ears, they usually lack some of the features that are important for young children such as direct audio input that enables the coupling of FM devices to the hearing aid, and they require frequent recasing as the child's ears grow. (Exceptions to this rule might occasionally be a child with absent or severely malformed pinnas who otherwise has conventionally aidable hearing; in these cases, ITE aids can be considered with full awareness of the practical drawbacks.) ITE styles may be appropriate for some school-aged children. The decision of style must be made with consideration of the child's preferences, the size of the ear canal (a completely in-the-canal style may either not be possible to make for a very small canal or else it will not

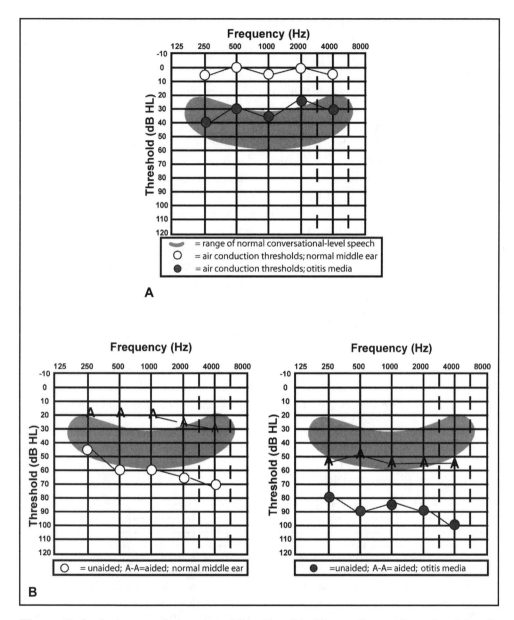

Figure 7–1. A. A normally hearing child with mild otitis media may be only minimally handicapped by the associated conductive hearing loss. **B.** A child who gets good benefit from a hearing aid with normal middle ear function may barely be able to detect conversational-level speech with even a mild conductive overlay. Children with greater degrees of hearing loss are even more adversely affected.

fit completely in-the-canal), the degree of hearing loss, and the recommended features of the hearing aid.

It is important to note that evidence of profound hearing loss in infants should not lead the physician to assume that the child will gain no benefit from hearing aids. No response on ABR does not necessarily indicate an absence of measurable hearing, (Luxford et al., 2004) because most ABR equipment is incapable of stimulating at the highest levels of an audiometer and ABR results do not match behavioral results precisely. Therefore, no response to click stimuli at 90 dB nHL might still be consistent with a flat hearing loss of 90 dB HL or so, which could be very usable residual hearing. It is reasonable to assume that a child with no true auditory responses on an audiogram will be unable to achieve benefit from hearing aids that would enable him or her to hear the components of speech. However, it is not possible to predict from a pure tone audiogram showing at least some residual hearing what functional benefit an individual child will gain from amplification. Figure 7–2 demonstrates one example of two children with very similar audiometric data, one of whom has always attended mainstream education and is now excelling in the second grade, and the other of whom—despite early auditory therapy and early oral education —has no functional oral language and communicates exclusively through sign.

Children with severe to profound hearing loss may have the potential to benefit from hearing aids even where adults with the same pure tone audiogram may not. Fitting formulas geared specifically to children consider high frequency information more critical than formulas geared toward adults, because children require this auditory information to learn to discriminate as many of the frequency components of speech as possible. Adults, by contrast, are able to make sense of limited information because of their already established knowledge of spoken language and may find high-frequency amplification useless or annoying.

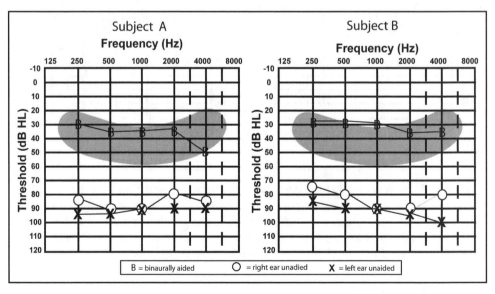

Figure 7–2. Subject A, an 8-year-old boy identified at age 1 yr, 4 months, is now at the top of his class in mainstream second grade; oral language is age-appropriate. Subject B, an 11-year-old boy identified at 2 years, began a sign program after 2 years of being unable to develop functional language in an oral program. *Oral language potential cannot be predicted by the audiogram alone.*

Young infants and children require flexible, adjustable amplification, and digital technology has been a boon to effective fittings of this population. Initial settings of any hearing aid based on ABR and/or ASSR thresholds will need to be modified as the child grows physically and as more precise frequency-specific information is obtained over time. Flexible amplification often can compensate for changes in ear canal volume and in hearing levels, either caused by progressive loss or intermittent decreases due to otitis media, so that parents are not required to invest thousands of dollars for new hearing aids before the expected life of the initially fit aids is reached. Multiple-band instruments are far more effective in addressing precipitous, reverse-slope, or otherwise unusual configurations of hearing loss than the minimally adjustable instruments of the past. Digital feedback control mechanisms can help children stay "on the air" between the time molds begin to be outgrown and the time they can be replaced. Features such as volume control, automatic directionality, and noise reduction/speech enhancement algorithms may or may not be appropriate for a child at the time of the initial fitting but may be appropriate within a year or two, depending on the child's age. Digital technology allows these features to be activated or deactivated in the programming software or restricted to certain programs in a multimemory device.

Bone Anchored Hearing Aids

The BAHA system uses an osseointegrated titanium implant coupled to an externally worn sound processor to transmit sound via bone conduction to the inner ear. It is applicable in the general population both to bilateral conductive or mixed hearing losses where air-conduction amplification is not appropriate and to unilateral hearing loss where direct amplification is not effective. Multiple studies demonstrate the effectiveness of the BAHA in addressing bilateral conductive hearing loss, especially where atresia and/or microtia prevent the use of conventional hearing aids, and research with pediatric recipients indicates excellent benefit and a high level of satisfaction (Seemann et al., 2004).

Currently the Food and Drug Administration approves this surgical procedure for appropriate candidates 5 years of age and over. However, babies identified with hearing loss secondary to middle ear anomalies such as atresia, and who have conductive or mixed hearing losses with bone conduction thresholds ranging from normal to as poor as ~40 dB HL, can be fit with a BAHA sound processor attached to a soft headband, which provides good-quality bone conduction amplification until the child attains the approved age for surgery. After surgery, the same processor (or perhaps an upgraded version) can be affixed to the abutment of the implanted device, obviating the need for a headband of any kind. Reported benefits of the BAHA speech processors over most bone conduction hearing aids are their digital signal processing and the availability of choice of omni-directional or directional microphone technology, and they can be used with FM systems to further heighten benefit.

There is less literature at this time regarding the use of the BAHA in children to address unilateral, or single-sided, deafness. Studies involving adult subjects have shown a preference for the BAHA compared with contralateral routing of signals (CROS) amplification, both subjectively by the users and as evidenced by speech perception scores in both quiet and noise conditions (Niparko et al., 2003). As more children with unilateral loss receive the BAHA device, a better picture of overall benefit will be obtained.

FM Systems

All hearing-impaired persons can expect to encounter listening situations where background or competing noise makes understanding extremely difficult and where neither hearing aids nor compensatory strategies can completely address the problem. The classroom is certain to be one of these situations. The auditory information children are expected to process in the classroom is critical to their communicative, academic, and social development, and often current material is dependent upon the understanding of previously presented materials. Children in class may not even be aware of what information they are missing; asking the child if he or she understands is likely to elicit an affirmative response whether they understand or not. Children may be embarrassed to call attention to themselves and may not communicate to the teacher that they are not following the material well. FM technology provides an excellent way to address the issues of poor classroom acoustics and competing speech and noise in the classroom.

In all FM configurations, the teacher or talker must use a microphone and a transmitter. Typically, the microphone is worn on the lapel or on a lavaliere and the transmitter is worn on a belt or in a pocket. Alternatively, a microphone/transmitter can be passed from speaker to speaker, as in a small group project setting. The students may have personal receivers attached directly to their hearing aids or cochlear implants, or they may have a small speaker on their desk or table. An arrangement that projects the FM signal through speakers situated throughout the classroom is called a sound field system, and it benefits all students, not just the child with hearing loss. FM systems enable the student to hear the teacher's voice via the receiver regardless of the teacher's physical position in the classroom (face not visible, back turned, or strolling the aisles of the room), reducing the impact of competing noise in the room.

The best configuration of the system will depend on the age and language facility of the student, the type of amplification the child uses, and the specific listening demands of a particular class or school. Children who are too young to report static or interference or a poor quality signal, or young children with cochlear implants whose systems cannot be monitored by the teacher or audiologist (because they cannot listen through the child's implant), may be best served by either a sound field or portable speaker system. Children who do not sit at a desk and who may change stations during the class session might benefit from either type of system and the specifics of their needs should be carefully considered before any purchase. Children who are linguistically competent and are mobile within the classroom, or who play field or other sports, may be fit with personal FM receivers attached to their hearing aids or implants.

FM systems not coupled to hearing aids or cochlear implants may also benefit children with minimal hearing loss, fluctuating hearing loss (including from otitis media), learning disabilities, attention deficit disorders, and unilateral hearing loss, and several companies manufacture systems specifically geared toward assisting children with normal hearing in one or both ears.

Cochlear Implants

An abundance of research and clinical evidence demonstrates that the best pediatric candidates for cochlear implantation are (a) very young children (below school age, and preferably before preschool age) if they are prelingually deaf and have no auditory-oral skills, (b) older children who have had normal hearing and lost it due to illness or injury, (c) children or youth who have had progressive loss, or (d) children or youth who have developed functional speech perception and oral language skills with hearing aids but can be expected to benefit from the better access to high frequencies that a cochlear implant allows.

Although many factors contribute to success with cochlear implants—and many often unknowable variables impede it—we do know time is of the essence. When a very young child is determined to be an implant candidate, and when the parents are philosophically in favor of cochlear implantation, it is almost always best to move ahead immediately rather than wait for newer technology. The benefits of early implantation have far outweighed the benefits of the technological progress of these devices, and young children have been shown to make excellent use of all different cochlear implant makes and models and have learned to develop speech and language skills with many different types of processing strategies. Older prelingually deaf children who do not already communicate through the auditory-oral modality are much less likely to develop functional oral skills after they receive the implant. Older children who do have a strong auditory oral foundation are best implanted at the point at which it can be determined that they are good candidates rather than postponing the decision until the child has lost further ground academically and linguistically.

The otolarygologist who is not also an implant surgeon is advised to be familiar with the general candidacy criteria for pediatric cochlear implants and to know the locations of the nearest and best cochlear implant programs with pediatric experience. Most pediatric cochlear implant programs use a multidisciplinary team approach to determining candidacy, so a diagnosis of severe to profound hearing loss is not sufficient information for a physician to be able to recommend a cochlear implant. Rather, the physician should make the earliest possible referral to a cochlear implant center if his or her patient appears to meet the basic candidacy criteria and should in all cases of doubt contact the implant center directly for advice on how best to steer the family for appropriate services.

Summary

Early diagnosis, advances in hearing aid and implant technologies, and availability of publicly funded early start services have enabled thousands of children with hearing loss to flourish linguistically and educationally. These services and devices are of limited value unless they are provided early and consistently. The physician is in a position to influence the promptness of intervention and to have a tremendous impact on the family's ability and willingness to follow through with appropriate recommendations and thus maximize their children's opportunities for success.

References

American Academy of Pediatrics. (2004). Clinical practice guideline: Diagnosis and management of acute otitis media. *Pediatrics*, *113*(5), 1412–1429.

Lieu, J. E. (2004). Speech-language and educational consequences of unilateral hearing loss in children. *Archives of Otolaryngology-Head and Neck Surgery*, *130*, 524–530.

Luxford, W. M., Eisenberg, L. S., Johnson, K. C., & Mahnke, E. M. (2004). Cochlear implantation in infants younger than 12 months. *Elsevier International Congress Series*, *1273*, 376–379.

Niparko, J., Cox, K., & Lustig, L. (2003). Comparison of the bone anchored hearing aid implantable hearing device with contralateral routing of offside signal amplification in the rehabilitation of unilateral deafness. *Otology and Neuorology*, *24*, 73–78.

Seemann, R., Liu, R., & Di Toppa, J. (2004). Results of pediatric bone-anchored hearing aid implantation. *Journal of Otolaryngology*, *33*(2), 71–74.

Simpson, S. A., Thomas, C. L., van der Linden, M. K., MacMillan, H., van der Wouden, J. C., & Butler, C. (2007). Identification of children in the first four years of life for early treatment for otitis media with effusion. *Cochrane Database of Systematic Reviews.* Issue 1 Art. No. CD004163. DOI: 10.1002/14651858.CD004163.pub2.

Yoshinaga-Itano, C., Sedey, A. L., Coulter, D. K., & Mehl, A. L. (1998). Language of early- and later-identified children with hearing loss. *Pediatrics*, *102*(5), 1161–1171.

Medical Reasons for Hearing Aid Failure

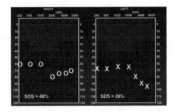

M. JENNIFER DEREBERY, M.D.

It is the rare patient who looks forward to wearing hearing aids. The most common barriers to successful amplification are patient denial, patient reluctance and cost. Cosmetic concerns, unrealistic expectations, patient dexterity, and level of hearing loss are also significant issues that the physician and audiologist/dispenser must confront in virtually every patient who receives a recommendation for amplification.

In contrast to these "usual suspects," this chapter deals with certain medical conditions that offer additional unique challenges to successful air conduction hearing aid use. These conditions all require physician recognition and intervention if amplification is to be helpful.

Dermatophytid (ID) Reaction

The dermatophytid (ID) reaction is dermatitis secondary to an allergic sensitivity to a distal fungal reaction. In order to develop an ID reaction, the individual must first have a primary focus of fungal infection in the body. The most common site would be in the finger or toenails as onchomycosis, or mucosal in the vagina or pharynx (thrush). Fungal antigens are hematologically spread, with the eventual development of immediate Type I Gel and Coombs IgE-mediated hypersensitivity.

The presenting symptom of this allergic reaction is a dermatitis, which often develops on the hands, auricle, or external auditory canal (Derebery & Berliner, 1996). It is important to note that the primary fungal infection is not in the ear canal. The fissured canal and postauricular area represents the "target organ" of the allergic reaction. Culture of the ear generally will reveal gram positive organisms and little, if any, fungi.

The patient will present with "chronic external otitis" which, in the case of the hearing impaired, may prevent successful air conduction amplification. The external canal, concha, and/or the postauricular area may be much fissured and weep a serous discharge. The external auditory canal frequently is swollen, and the skin eventually may become thickened and lichenified. Pruritis and pain are common symptoms, although the pain involved is not as severe as in an acute otitis externa. Patients may also have a conductive hearing loss secondary to swelling of the external auditory canal.

The differential diagnosis does include malignancy, and a biopsy or a high-resolution CT scan should be taken in severe cases. Although malignant external otitis is also in the differential diagnosis, the patient with an ID reaction is more likely going to complain of severe itching and more moderate discomfort than the severe pain usually associated with malignant external otitis.

Treatment is threefold. First, identify the primary focus of fungal infection. The author has found the most common location to be the toenails (Derebery & Berliner, 1996). Dermatologic referral usually is necessary to ensure eradication. However, treatment must extend beyond antifungal medications to include immunomodulation for successful resolution of otologic symptoms.

Second, the patient should be tested for an immediate hypersensitivity to the dermatophytic fungi trichophyton, candida, and epidermophyton. Testing may be either by skin testing or in vitro, and patients should be desensitized with allergy immunotherapy to those antigens to which they react. The author will "empirically" suggest to patients that they avoid eating fermented food in the diet for a period of several weeks to months as well.

Third, any significant secondary bacterial infections should be treated with topical or oral antibiotics.

Case Report of Typical Presentation

The patient was a 28-year-old Caucasian female presenting with a 2-year history of bilateral conductive hearing loss and "chronic external otitis." Her audiogram is shown in Figure 8–1. Biopsy of the external canal was negative, and a CT scan was normal. Prior treatments were unsuccessful and had included multiple antibiotics by mouth, intravenously and orally, topical antibiotic otic drops, and topical and oral steroids.

Physical examination revealed marked fissuring of postauricular areas, concha, and external auditory canals (Figure 8–2). The external auditory canal was swollen virtually shut, and there was a clear, serous discharge noted in the external canals and postauricular sulci. She also was noted to have onchomycosis (Figure 8–3).

Treatment included oral antifungal agents, desensitizing allergy immunotherapy to the reactive fungi, and dietary elimination of yeast-containing foods.

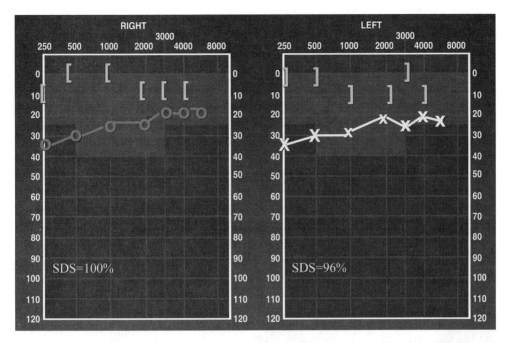

Figure 8–1. Audiogram of 28-year-old patient with persistent chronic otitis externa as a result of an ID reaction.

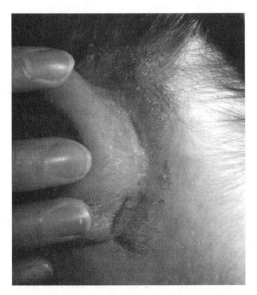

Figure 8–2. Physical examination of the ear showing persistent "chronic otitis externa" as a result of an ID reaction.

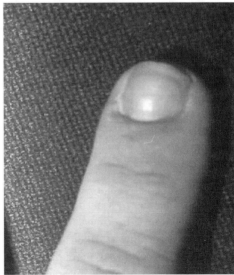

Figure 8–3. Onchomycosis of finger as site of fungal infection in patient with ID reaction.

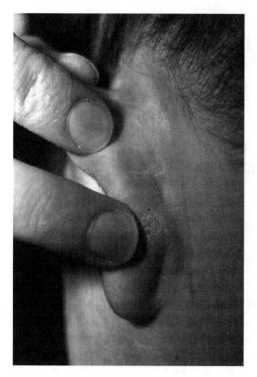

Figure 8–4. Appearance of ear of same patient following six weeks of treatment.

Figure 8-4 shows the appearance of her ear 6 weeks after starting treatment. Her dermatitis resolved with continued treatment, as did her conductive hearing loss.

Allergic Reaction to Hearing Aid Earmolds and Materials

Chronic external otitis in the hearing aid wearer may be caused by a number of conditions, including a "friction rub" from a poor fitting mold, malignancy, poor aural hygiene, seborrhea, psoriasis, and atopic dermatitis. Symptoms that suggest an immune reaction to the hearing aid include irritation and weeping eczema. Although one typically does not think of

an immune reaction to an inert material such as a hearing aid mold, allergic contact dermatitis has been reported in 23.5 to 42.5% of hearing aid users (Onder et al., 1994). The source of the reaction is not always the hearing aid per se, but may result from the use of topical medications to treat an infected ear or the preservatives in the medication, or nickel in earrings or jewelry in close proximity to the hearing aid.

The reader is reminded that, although we use the word "allergic" contact dermatitis, the immunology of these reactions is not the classic immediate Type I Gel and Coombs hypersensitivity response of which we usually think. These reactions represent a delayed hypersensitivity, and they may take some time to develop in a patient who was formerly able to wear the hearing aid without difficulty. Although removing the hearing aid will improve the symptoms, improvement may not be "immediate" and may take several days to a few weeks to resolve when the hearing aid is not worn.

The most common substances used as hearing aid materials are methacrylic plastics, but silicone or polyvinyl chloride may also be used (Meding & Ringdahl, 1992). The acrylic shell of a hearing aid mold is cured by ultraviolet light treatment, or by the addition of polymers. If polymerization is incomplete, uncured acrylics may leach through the shell, contact the skin, and result in eventual sensitization. After the electronic components have been integrated inside the shell, a plastic face plate is bonded in place using cyanoacrylate adhesives or it is solvent bonded with methylmethacrylate monomer. Other substances found in the adhesives used to bond components may contain potential reactants such as silicone, or p-tert butylphenol formaldehyde. Additional potentially sensitizing substances used in the manufacturing process include phthalates, benzoyl peroxide, hydoquinone, cellulose ester plastics, vinyl plastics, and aromatic amines (Sood & Taylor, 2004).

Patients wearing hearing aids who subsequently develop persistent "chronic external otitis" in the distribution of the hearing aid should receive dermatologic referral and patch testing to rule out sensitization to the hearing aid mold and other possible antigens (Figure 8–5). Patch testing typically will involve a "standard" tray of suspects, to which should be added various acrylics, glues, and additives. It is often necessary to contact the hearing aid manufacturer for specific identification of the components.

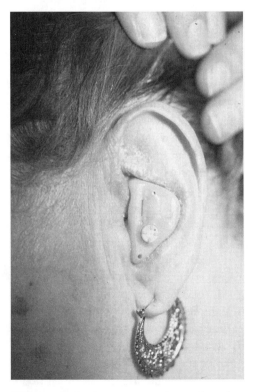

Figure 8–5. Allergic reaction to hearing aid.

Treatment will be substitution of a less or nonreacting material. In some cases, this may require using a different manufacturer's product, as it is not always technically possible to substitute shell materials. It may also be possible to have the canal portion of the hearing aid coated with inert 14 karat gold to lessen reactivity.

Ménière's Disease

Although uncontrolled vertigo is considered the most disabling symptom of Ménière's disease (MD), by definition, all of these affected patients also suffer from sensorineural hearing loss (SNHL) at some point in their disease course, with most having some degree of permanent hearing loss. The measured hearing levels can fluctuate greatly at different time points, making successful amplification particularly challenging. Although these patients, or those affected with cochlear hydrops without vertigo, would most definitely benefit from amplification, this is a group that will frequently tell the otolarygologist that "I tried hearing aids, and they didn't work for me." Among the unique challenges in successful amplification of patients with MD are reduced dynamic range, rising audiometric configuration, reduced speech discrimination, fluctuating pure-tone thresholds, significant pressure or fullness, tinnitus, and episodic vertigo, which is occasionally accompanied by Tullio's phenomena (Johnson & House, 1979). Additionally, as MD is most frequently unilateral or asymmetric if bilateral, this adds to the inherent amplification challenges posed.

The availability of digital signal processing (DSP) in place of earlier analog signal processing has proven exceptionally beneficial in fitting difficult audiometric configurations such as those in patients with MD. The larger number of bands/channels of compression allows much greater precision in shaping the frequency gain/output response necessary to comfortably fit the reduced dynamic range common in MD.

Fortunately, most patients with MD do not develop severe or profound losses in the affected ear and are candidates for traditional amplification. However, the fluctuating nature of MD creates a unique challenge to successful hearing aid use. Namely, which audiometric configuration should be used for programming? A "normal" non-MD patient fit with amplification does not have hearing fluctuations. There is a reasonable expectation that the hearing loss in question will progress only slowly with time, if at all. This measured level of hearing is used to determine the frequency-gain response of the "baseline" program, after modification to fit a prescriptive target, binaural summation, any conductive or mixed component of loss, and so forth. This baseline level is presumed to be the most beneficial for listening. Typically, when we think of "programmable capability," we mean different programming strategies available to improve sound perception in noisy, as opposed to ideal quiet background situations. This stable baseline level is adjusted for quiet situations by the use of omnidirectional microphones (Program 1) or more noisy situations by use of directional microphones (Program 2). Beyond this, other "custom" programs may be added for listening to music, telephone, or some other specific activity. However, the initial baseline audiogram is the starting point for any other listening activity that is anticipated.

In contrast, for the patient with MD, the actual baseline can fluctuate widely from day to day, or even from hour to hour. Additionally, the basic audiometric profile of a patient with MD can vary greatly, from the "classic" low frequency loss seen in 71% of MD, to a flat (20%), up sloping (6%) or the very uncommon "trough" seen in 3% (Johnson & House, 1979). With such a wide variety of "baseline hearing" to choose from, which level of hearing loss should be considered as the starting point for amplification? Patients with MD should be encouraged to come in for an audiometric evaluation on a "typical" as well as a "bad" day of hearing to obtain audiometric data to characterize both the configuration and degree of hearing loss. This allows separate programming of the differing frequency gain/output responses specific for the level of amplification in a given pattern of hearing loss. As intuitively obvious as this would sound, the author is amazed by the number of patients with MD seen that present with a history of unsuccessful amplification of their hearing loss, with only one reference audiogram—which may be more than a year old—and was used as the sole basis for a hearing aid evaluation.

Additionally, as Valente et al. note, with each fluctuating level of hearing loss, there is also great variability in dynamic range (Valente, Mispagelm, Valente, & Hullar, 2006). Because of the known variability of intersubject loudness discomfort level (LDL) (up to 30 dB for the same hearing level), they recommend individual measurement of LDL in estimation of dynamic range, rather than the usual reliance on the "predicted" LDL obtained from group data. The use of this individually measured, rather than the "normalized" LDL, which is computed from patients presenting with more common causes of hearing loss such as noise exposure or presbycusis, typically results in output from the hearing aid being 10 to 15 dB lower than would have been predicted. Although they do not report whether this has been confirmed as increasing satisfaction in patients such as those with MD, with a known reduced dynamic range, conceptually, this is a reasonable step to take in this patient population. The physician is encouraged to discuss this with the audiologist and dispenser with whom he or she works to aid this most challenging group of patients.

In the case of the patient with unilateral MD with a profound hearing loss, reduced dynamic range, or very poor speech discrimination, the best approach will be to take advantage of the better hearing ear. If there is another cause of hearing loss in the non-MD ear, this should be improved with appropriate amplification or, if conductive, surgery to maximize communicative ability. Additional improvement may be obtained by the use of a CROS (contralateral routing of sound), BiCROS, or BAHA (bone-anchored hearing aid).

CROS and BiCROS amplification are offered by a number of manufacturers, and are available in the original wired or in a wireless configuration. Fortunately, DSP is available in all of the new wireless models, with the newest models also having directional microphones. Interestingly, Valente et al. (2006) have noted that the best acceptance of CROS amplification in the unilaterally impaired patient is found in those who have some degree of high-frequency hearing loss in the better hearing ear, rather than normal hearing. This is apparently due to a reduction in the "tinny" quality of the amplified sound that is a common complaint when presented to a normal hearing ear.

It has been this author's experience that a far greater acceptance in this patient group has been seen in those with severe unilateral MD and normal or near normal hearing in the uninvolved ear treated with a BAHA rather than a CROS or BiCROS. The BAHA involves the surgical implantation of a titanium screw and attached abutment to the cortical bone of the mastoid of the impaired ear. After a sufficient healing period (3 months in the adult, 6 months in the pediatric age group), a sound processor is attached to the abutment for signal processing. Originally analog, the newer devices use DSP. Depending on the model, dual microphones are available either on the processor itself, or as an optional fitting to the analog instrument. At the time of this writing, it is not clear if the dual microphone capability actually enhances the perception of speech in noise in the unilaterally impaired patient. Key to successful use of the BAHA is the hearing threshold of the better hearing ear, which must be normal, or with no more than a 25 to 45 dB pure-tone average (PTA), depending on which model is used. Recently, bone conduction through a device worn on the upper molar has been presented (Popelka et al., 2009). Whether this will prove to be an effective future treatment option for single-sided deafness remains to be seen.

Autoimmune Inner Ear Disease (AIED)

Most types of hearing loss will progress slowly if at all. The exceptions to this generalization are sensorineural hearing loss (SNHL) secondary to ototoxicity, Ménière's disease with its fluctuations, sudden SNHL and autoimmune inner ear disease (AIED). The first publications on AIED were by Lehnhardt in the European literature in 1958 (Lehnhardt, 1958). McCabe (1989) renewed interest in this entity in 1979, with his case reports suggesting that this type of SNHL was potentially treatable by medical means.

AIED is defined as a very rapidly progressive SNHL, most typically bilateral, that is due to a presumed immune attack against the inner ear or structures. The actual pattern of hearing loss may vary. Initially, it may present unilaterally, with the eventual development of bilateral loss. It may present as a very rapidly progressive—as opposed to "usual" fluctuating case of MD. Another clinical picture may be of the patient with a prior "dead" ear or profound hearing loss from a presumed viral infection, sudden, traumatic or other cause, who later develops steroid-responsive SNHL in the only remaining hearing ear.

The diagnosis of AIED is suspected in patients with one or both ears showing a rapidly progressive SNHL that is otherwise unexplained, and responds to immunomodulation. McCabe's initial clinical description noted that these patients would progress to deafness if not recognized and treated with steroids or other immunosuppressive medication. This author has found that few patients do lose all serviceable hearing with or without effective pharmacotherapeutic intervention, but that the rapid changes in hearing can be extremely difficult for the patient to cope with, as well as present some unique challenges in amplification.

Although it is beyond the scope of this chapter to review the diagnosis of AIED, at the present time, the diagnosis usually is made by ruling out other forms of hearing loss such as an acoustic neuroma or ototoxicity, as well as documenting a history of rapidly progressive sensorineural hearing loss. The diagnosis may be made with or without an in vitro test such as a nonspecific autoimmune marker, or a Western blot assay for heat shock protein 70.

How much hearing loss is too much and warrants a possible diagnosis of AIED? The author has found the diagnostic criteria used by the American Academy of Otolaryngology-Head and Neck Surgery in the published double-blind, randomized, placebo-controlled trial of methotrexate for treatment of AIED to serve as a useful clinical template to diagnose this condition (Harris et al., 2003). This study used the following audiometric criteria to support the suspected clinical diagnosis of AIED when other causes had been ruled out: An otherwise unexplained SNHL that decreased over a 1 to 3 month period of time by 15 dB at one frequency, 10 dB at two consecutive frequencies, or a greater than 12% decrease in speech discrimination.

When they initially present for a hearing aid evaluation, some of these patients will be referred in for an otolaryngic evaluation and are noted to require frequent reprogramming for significant changes in hearing threshold. Others may present with a known diagnosis of MD and be noted to progress much more rapidly than is typical with this syndrome. Others may have been treated with a course of prednisone with a marked improvement in hearing that they subsequently lose when they have tapered or stopped the prednisone.

The author has seen patients with AIED progress from a mild to profound loss bilaterally in 3 months. Clearly a patient with this rapid a hearing loss would present a tremendous challenge with amplification. Although it is beyond the scope of this chapter to review the literature on pharmacologic interventions for AIED, the following suggestions may prove helpful in monitoring treatment results in this group of patients.

If a patient with rapid hearing loss chooses to be treated with prednisone or other immunomodulating medications, hearing must be monitored on a regular basis to assess efficacy. Audiometric evaluation at least every 1 to 3 months is recommended. The reader is encouraged to use his or her own objective standard of how much progression is unacceptable and apply it to the "baseline" audiogram obtained prior to pharmacotherapy to assess whether or not a particular medication or regimen is truly beneficial. The author uses the reverse of the audiometric criteria noted above to define AIED as the criteria for improved hearing after pharmacologic intervention, with the caveat that there should be no further reduction of hearing by the following amounts at any frequency between 250 and 6000 Hz: 15 dB worse at one frequency, 10 dB or worse hearing at two consecutive frequencies, or a greater than 12% decrease in speech discrimination.

Using these specific reference points is less important than choosing *some* objective measure for defining what is both improved as well as reduced hearing, and monitoring on a frequent enough basis to allow continued pharmacologic intervention, if this is desired by the patient, as well as any appropriate changes in level of amplification. Ideally, patients whose hearing is stable should be monitored with audiograms at least every 3 to 4 months to watch for early evidence of progressive loss. Those being treated with pharmacotherapy or immunomodulation should be followed at least monthly to assess response to treatment and tapering of steroid. The audiometric results must be shared with the audiologist or dispenser in order to assure the best possible amplification outcome. These are patients who will require long-term, regular monitoring of their hearing, much as the patient who presents to the primary care physician with diabetes mellitus or unstable hypertension requires for his or her medical condition.

The following case report will serve to illustrate the complexities of treating this problem.

Case Report of Typical Presentation

The patient was a 26-year-old African American female medical student who presented with episodic vertigo for 6 weeks, and sudden bilateral sensorineural hearing loss, which had occurred 4 weeks prior. Her audiogram is shown in Figure 8–6. She was treated with prednisone 60 mg per day for 14 days, with a subsequent tapering over an additional 14 days, and noted improved hearing (Figure 8–7). When the prednisone was discontinued, her hearing began to both decrease and fluctuate (Figure 8–8). She developed a fever of unknown origin and tachycardia. Her hearing loss continued to progress when she was referred to our office for treatment (Figure 8–9). She was again given prednisone 60 mg per day, and promptly developed diabetes. At this point, rheumatologic evaluation was recommended. She was started on azulfidine, with a rapid taper of the prednisone. Audiometric studies after start of azulfidine showed improved hearing (Figure 8–10).

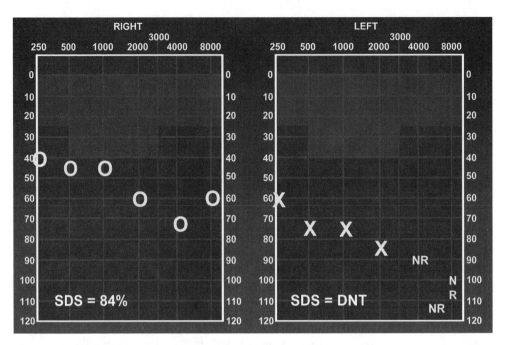

Figure 8–6. Initial audiogram of a 26-year-old female with AIED.

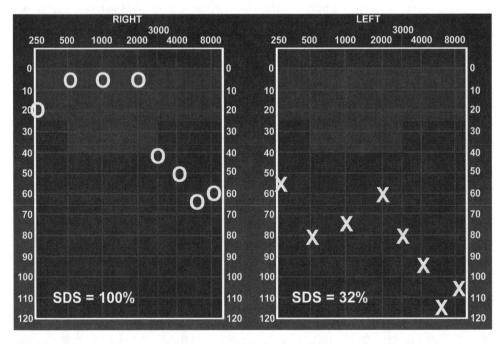

Figure 8–7. Audiogram of same patient following 28 days of prednisone treatment and tapering.

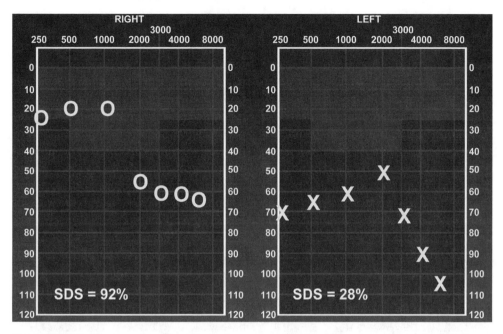

Figure 8–8. Audiogram of same patient two months after cessation of prednisone treatment.

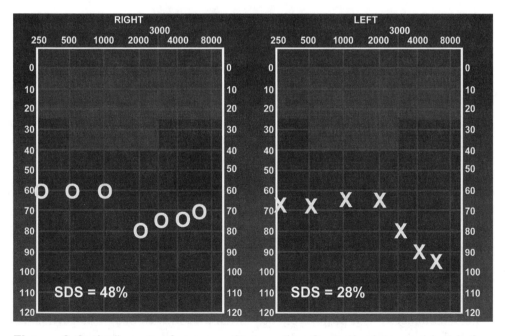

Figure 8–9. Audiogram of same patient another 2 months later and just before starting treatment with azulfidine.

105

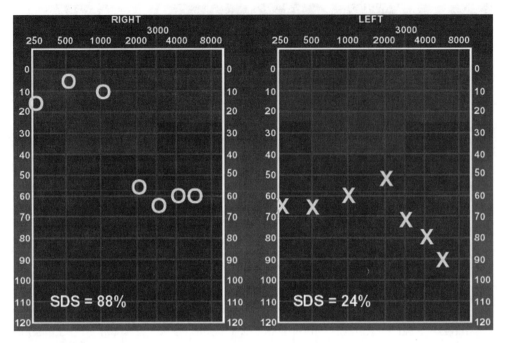

Figure 8–10. Audiogram of same patient after start of azulfidine (two months after prior audiogram).

She was able to taper her prednisone, as her dosage was increased on azulfidine; to a maximum of 500 mg qid. Her diabetes resolved. At the current time, she is maintained on prednisone 5 to 8 mg per day; with stable hearing. She is successfully wearing a hearing aid in her right ear, and has been able to finish medical school.

Analgesic Ototoxicity

Rapidly progressive SNHL secondary to ingestion of large doses of narcotic was first reported by Radziminski in 1963. Later reports of hearing loss observed with concomitant ingestion of propoxyphene (Lupin & Harley, 1976), heroin (Polpathapee & Tuchida, 1984), or hydrocodone (Freidman et al., 2000). Hydrocodone is a semisynthetic narcotic-containing anal-

gesic, antitussive similar to codeine, which is highly addictive. The usual prescribed dose is less than eight tablets per day. There is a wide variety in the doses associated with subsequent ototoxicity, but the reported range is from 8 to 60 tablets per day (Friedman et al., 2000).

There is a variable clinical presentation, but Friedman et al. (2000) report that 67% of patients will present with a new onset of bilateral sensorineural hearing loss that often is initially felt to be a sudden loss. The hearing loss will subsequently progress over several days to weeks, with 83% of patients eventually developing a profound loss. Dizziness is infrequent and is reported in 17%. Although often treated with oral or transtympanic steroid, the loss is not steroid responsive. Hearing will stabilize if the analgesic medication is stopped, but will progress to deafness if the analgesic is continued.

The pathophysiology has yet to be clearly defined, as there are no temporal bone specimens at present, but the susceptibility is most likely genetic or idiosyncratic. The sensorineural hearing loss is most likely cochlear in origin, as those patients who develop deafness and subsequently receive a cochlear implant usually are very successful recipients, with postoperative discrimination scores ranging from 64 to 100% correct.

The otolaryngologist usually is consulted in the case of analgesic ototoxicity, either by the referring primary care physician or the audiologist or hearing aid dispenser who is unable to attain a satisfactory hearing aid fit and becomes aware of the rapid progression of loss.

The differential diagnosis of analgesic ototoxicity is AIED, sudden SNHL, perilymphatic fistula, and acoustic neuroma. It is the author's observation that patients will rarely self-report taking hydrocodone or other analgesics on drug intake forms, and the treating physician should ask specifically if they are taking these medications as well as the amount in any patient with an unexplained rapidly progressive SNHL. The only hope to stabilize hearing and subsequently receive amplification is by identifying drug intake and having the patient stop it immediately.

Case Report of Typical Presentation

The following case history illustrates the challenges in treating this condition by amplification. A 50-year-old Caucasian male who suffered from chronic back pain developed a rapidly progressive bilateral hearing loss, worse in the right ear, and was referred for evaluation and audiometric testing in November 2005 (Figure 8–11). He admitted to taking Vicodin on a daily basis, eventually disclosing that he was taking approximately 60 tablets per day. He was treated with prednisone 60 mg/day for one month, and stopped his Vicodin with prompt referral to a drug rehabilitation program. He had no response to prednisone, and was noted to have mild progression of his hearing loss in his only hearing left ear until the hydrocodone was completely discontinued (Figure 8–12).

He is successfully using a hearing aid in the left ear and is no longer taking Vicodin. He has declined treatment with a BiCROS hearing aid.

Superior Semicircular Canal Fistula

Superior semicircular canal (SSCC) fistula is a dehiscence of the bony roof of the superior semicircular canal. The resulting "third window" increases transmission of sound energy through the vestibule with a resulting decrease in acoustic energy and an increase in bone conduction. Many if not most of these patients will present with a low frequency conductive hearing loss, which is often misdiagnosed as otosclerosis, with patients being referred for either surgery or amplification (Minor, 2005).

In addition to the hearing loss, other common symptoms can include vertigo, oscillopsia, and dizziness with sound stimulation (95%), especially when the sound has been amplified such as with a hearing aid. Dizziness or vertigo may also occur with Valsalva maneuver. Hennebert's sign (nystagmus from pressure in the external auditory canal) or Tullio's phenomena (nystagmus in the vertical

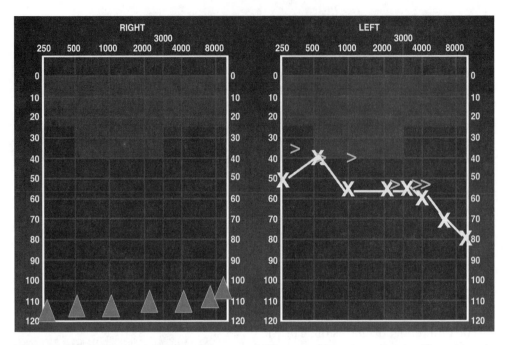

Figure 8–11. Presentation audiogram of 50-year-old male patient with analgesic ototoxicity (Vicodin).

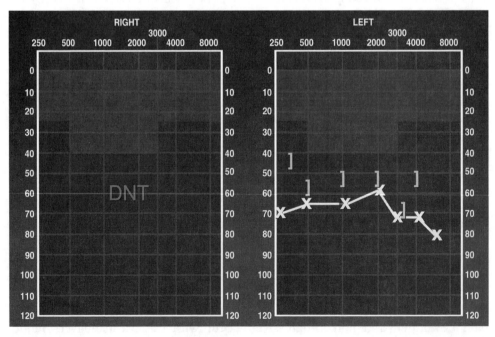

Figure 8–12. Audiogram of same patient 7 months later, after completely discontinuing Vicodin use.

plane) also have been described. Another frequent finding in 50% of individuals is "conductive hyperacusis," hearing the sound of one's own feet or eye movements on the affected side (Minor, 2005).

The etiology of SSCC fistula is likely a congenital developmental defect. Dehiscence and thinning has been found in 1% of temporal bones (Hirvonen et al., 2003). It is usually bilateral, and most affected individuals will develop symptoms during middle age. Prior head trauma is found in approximately 23% of affected individuals (Minor, 2005).

The differential diagnosis of SSCC fistula includes otosclerosis, congenital syphilis, perilymphatic fistula, hypermobile stapes syndrome, patulous eustachian tube, Ménière's disease, and benign positional vertigo. Audiometric testing will reveal a low to mid-frequency conduc-tive hearing loss, or hearing in the normal range with a mild air-bone gap. At times, bone conduction thresholds can be "super normal" or better than 0 dB (Figure 8–13). The acoustic reflex is normal, which can help distinguish a SSCC fistula from otosclerosis. An VNG will yield normal results, whereas VEMP testing may show reduced thresholds on the involved side. Confirmative diagnosis of suspected SSCC is with a high resolution CT scan of the temporal bones using 5-mm cuts (Figure 8–14).

The successful treatment of SSCC can take different forms. For some patients, explanation and avoidance of loud sound stimulation may suffice. Insertion of a PE tube may offer relief from pressure-induced symptoms such as dizziness with sound stimulation. Surgical repair can be performed through a middle cranial fossa

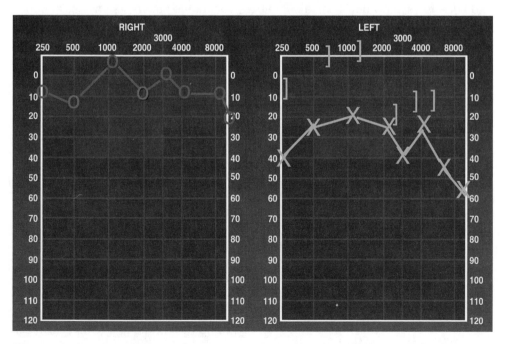

Figure 8–13. Audiogram of a patient with superior semicircular canal fistula, showing some "supernormal" thresholds.

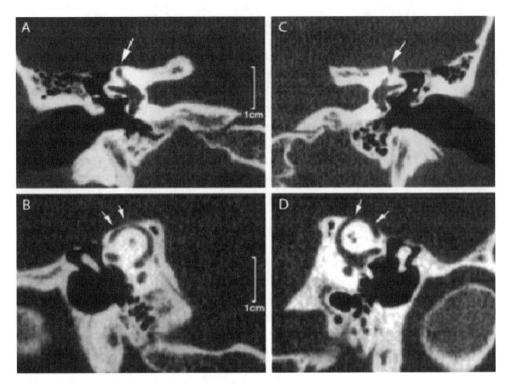

Figure 8–14. CT scan of a patient with superior semicircular canal fistula (**A**, **B**, **C**, and **D**). Arrows show dehiscence of the bony roof of the superior semicircular canal.

approach, and may entail resurfacing the dehiscent area, with a 63% success rate, or plugging of the SSCC with an 88% successful outcome (Minor, 2005).

Patients with SSCC dehiscence, whether operated on or not, will need long-term follow-up. In addition to the conductive loss, approximately 10% will develop a delayed onset SNHL, which may make amplification essential whether or not they have had surgery.

Patulous Eustachian Tube

The occlusion effect of hearing aids can cause variable amounts of annoyance in patients. However, in patients who have a patulous eustachian tube and hearing loss requiring amplification, the occlusion effect can be extreme, and the discomfort it causes should not be underestimated. In contrast to most patients, those with a patulous eustachian tube often will remark that they hear better and are most comfortable wearing a hearing aid when they have a cold or upper respiratory infection.

A patulous eustachian tube develops when there is a depletion of the fat pad of the cartilaginous eustachian tube. The classic predisposing factor is weight loss, which may sometimes be only a few pounds, or chronic illness with wasting. There is a female predominance of 75%, and the condition often is associated with pregnancy or oral contraceptive use. It may also develop in men who receive estrogen therapy for the treatment of prostate cancer (Doherty & Slattery, 2003).

The presenting symptom is aural fullness, usually but not always bilateral, that is improved in the supine position or during times of upper respiratory infection. The symptom can be severe, and may lead to depression. It is sometimes possible to visualize the movement of the tympanic membrane with otoscopy of the patient in a sitting position. Audiometric studies may or may not show a mild conductive component. Tympanometry may reveal mild excursions with breathing. Tinnitus is frequently seen in patulous eustachian tube, and can add to the distress experienced.

The differential diagnosis of a patulous eustachian tube includes eustachian tube dysfunction, Ménière's disease, cochlear hydrops, and otitis media with effusion. A careful history, querying specifically for changes in symptoms when lying down or illness, autophony, or autorespiration, will usually help distinguish this condition from others regardless of the audiometric findings.

The treatment of a patulous eustachian tube should be first directed toward any predisposing factors such as hormonal treatment or weight loss. It is the rare American patient that we actually encourage to eat more to improve health, but this is one of those exceptional conditions. Myringotomy and placement of a PE tube will improve symptoms in 50% (Chen & Luxford, 1990). Potassium iodide drops taken orally TID may cause some local changes in mucous viscosity and may be of benefit in some (Dyer & McElveen, 1991). Premarin 25 mg in 30 cc normal saline may also be used as a nasal drop, with three drops being applied in the affected side TID. Some patients may

need to have the dose titrated down if they develop uncomfortable symptoms such as breast tenderness secondary to systemic estrogen absorption. The hearing aid earmold itself will require significant venting to lessen the occlusion effect, which may be problematic in patients requiring significant low frequency gain. Poe has described successful surgical correction of the patulous eustachian tube in some patients (Poe, 2007).

Summary

Most patients with significant hearing loss are able to obtain good or adequate amplification. However, some particular problems involving the outer, middle, or inner ear that present unusual challenges for hearing aid use. Understanding these problems can lead to greater success and patient satisfaction with hearing amplification.

References

Chen, D. A., & Luxford, W. M. (1990). Myringotomy and tube for relief of patulous Eustachian tube symptoms. *American Journal of Otolaryngology, 11*(4), 272-273.

Derebery, M. J., & Berliner, K. I. (1996). Foot and ear disease—the dermatophytid reaction in otology. *Laryngoscope, 106*(2, Pt. 1), 181-186.

Doherty, J. K., & Slattery, W. H., 3rd. (2003). Autologous fat grafting for the refractory patulous eustachian tube *Otolaryngology-Head and Neck Surgery, 128*(1), 88-91.

Dyer, R. K., Jr., & McElveen, J. T., Jr. (1991). The patulous Eustachian tube: Management options. *Otolaryngology-Head and Neck Surgery, 105*(6), 832-835.

Freidman, R. A., House, J. W., Luxford, W. M, Gherini, S., & Mills, D. (2000). Profound hearing loss associated with hydrocodone/acetaminophen abuse. *American Journal of Otolaryngology, 21*(2), 188-191.

Harris, J. P., Weisman, M. H., Derebery, J. M., Espeland, M. A., Gantz, B. A., Gulya, A. J., et al. (2003). Treatment of corticosteroid-responsive autoimmune inner ear with methotrexate: a randomized controlled trial. *JAMA, 290*(14), 1875-1883.

Hirvonen, T. P., Weg, N., Zinerich, S. J., & Minor, L. B. (2003). High-resolution CT findings suggest a development abnormality underlying superior canal dehiscence syndrome. *Acta Otolaryngolologica, 123*(4), 477-481.

Johnson, E. W., & House, J. (1979). Meniere's disease: Clinical course, auditory findings, and hearing aid fitting. *Journal of American Audiological Society, 5*(2), 76-83.

Lehnhardt, E. (1958). Sudden hearing disorders occurring simultaneously or successively on both sides. *Laryngology, Rhinology, and Otology, 37*(1), 1-16.

Lupin, A. J., & Harley, C. H. (1976). Inner ear damage related to propoxyphene ingestion [Letter]. *Canadian Medical Association Journal, 114*(7), 596.

McCabe, B. F. (1979). Autoimmune sensorineural hearing loss. *Annals of Otology, Rhinology, and Laryngology, 88*(5, Pt. 1), 585-589.

Meding, B., & Ringdahl, A. (1992). Allergic contact dermatitis from the earmolds of hearing aids. *Ear and Hearing, 13*(2), 122-124.

Minor, L. B. (2005). Clinical manifestations of superior semicircular canal dehiscence. *Laryngoscope, 115*(10), 1717-1727.

Onder, M., Onder, T., Ozunlu, A., Makki, S. S., & Gurer, M. A. (1994). An investigation of contact dermatitis in patients with chronic otitis externa. *Contact Dermatitis, 31*(2), 116-117.

Poe, D. S. (2007). Diagnosis and management of the patulous Eustachian tube. *Otology and Neurotology, 28*(5), 668-677.

Polpathapee, S., Tuchida, P., & Chiwapong, S. (1984). Sensorineural hearing loss in a heroin addict. *Journal of the Medical Association of Thailand, 67*(1), 57-60.

Popelka, G. R., Derebery, J., Blevins, N. H., Murray, M., Moore, B. C., Sweetow, R. W., et al. (2009). *Preliminary evaluation of a novel bone conduction device for single sided deafness.* Accepted for publication.

Radziminski, A. (1963). The status of hearing after the administration of narcotic remedies. *Acta Otolaryngologica, 56,* 473-476.

Sood, A., & Taylor, J. S. (2004). Allergic contact dermatitis from hearing aid material. *Dermatitis, 15*(1), 48-50.

Valente, M., Mispagelm, K. M., Tchorz, J., & Fabry, D. (2006). Effect of type of noise and loudspeaker array on the performance of omnidirectional and directional microphones. *Journal of the American Academy of Audiology, 7*(6), 398-412.

Valente, M., Mispagelm K., Valente, L. M., & Hullar, T. (2006). Problems and solutions for fit amplification patients with Meniere's disease. *Journal of the American Academy of Audiology, 17*(1), 6-15.

The Management of Tinnitus in the Hearing-Impaired Patient

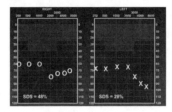

JOHN W. HOUSE, M.D.

Tinnitus is defined as a sensation of sound in the ears or head. The tinnitus may be unilateral, bilateral, or located in the head. The patient describes it as ringing, roaring, bells, crickets, seashell sound, like escaping steam, and so on. The patient's tinnitus maybe present constantly or intermittently.

In discussing tinnitus, it is important to understand that tinnitus is a symptom and not a disease. Therefore, it is important that the etiology of the tinnitus is determined and that serious pathology is ruled out. In addition, the hearing loss may be caused by a correctable condition such as cerumen impaction or infection. In cases of unilateral tinnitus, we feel that magnetic resonance imaging (MRI) may be indicated to rule out an acoustic neuroma or other cerebellar pontine angle lesions.

Types of Tinnitus

There are two types of tinnitus: subjective and objective. Only the patient hears the subjective type of tinnitus; with objective tinnitus, the sound may be heard by an observer. Subjective tinnitus is far more common and accounts for more than 98% of tinnitus patients.

The rare objective tinnitus may be either vascular or muscular. Vascular tinnitus is described as a rhythmic pulsation, which is synchronous with the heartbeat. The tinnitus maybe caused by arterial, venous, or from a vascular tumor, such as a glomus tumor. It also can be associated with a central brain lesion or hydrocephalous.

Muscular tinnitus has three causes: the middle ear muscles (stapedial or tensor tympani muscle spasm) or palatal myoclonus. The patient with either stapedial or tensor tympani muscle spasm describes the sensation of a clicking sound in the ear. This type of tinnitus may be associated with a subjective sensation of movement of the tympanic membrane, usually described as a fluttering feeling. Typically, it is unilateral and intermittent. Muscular tinnitus occurs rarely, and this author has found that it usually is not considered bothersome once the situation has been described and explained to the patient. On rare occasions, it may be necessary to section the tendons to these muscles to give the patient relief.

The patient with palatal myoclonus describes the sound as an intermittent staccato popping in the ear. The rhythmic contraction of the levator palatini muscle causes this form of tinnitus. The eustachian tube is normally closed except during swallowing. The levator palatini muscle elevates the palate and opens the eustachian tube with swallowing. The opening of the eustachian tube causes a popping sensation in the ear. If the patient is symptomatic during the visit, the examiner actually can visualize the rhythmic contraction of the soft palate. This movement of the palate is synchronous with the popping in the ear.

About 80 to 85% of patients with hearing loss, regardless of cause, will have associated subjective tinnitus. Most patients who report tinnitus have a sensorineural type of hearing loss. A few tinnitus patients have a conductive loss or normal hearing. Most patients are able to ignore their tinnitus, but a small percentage of patients find their tinnitus to be of great concern. In my experience, about 5% of patients are quite disturbed by their symptom. The tinnitus interferes with their sleep at night or their concentration during the day (Goodhill, 1953).

Treatment of Tinnitus

Because tinnitus is a symptom, there is not a universal treatment. In 1953, Victor Goodhill, M.D. put it well: "Any management which is based upon a single panacea for the treatment of a symptom and not a disease will result in failure."

Many treatments have been proposed and performed for subjective tinnitus. In our experience, most patients respond well to an evaluation followed by an explanation and reassurance. Some of the treatments for tinnitus include medications, biofeedback (and other relaxation techniques), surgery, counseling, cognitive behavioral therapy, tinnitus maskers, electrical stimulation, tinnitus-retraining therapy, customized acoustic neural stimulus, transcranial magnetic therapy, and hearing aids.

Medications

Some patients respond to low dose tranquilizers such as alprazolam, or antidepressants such as amitriptyline. The patients who find these helpful are either anxious or depressed. In these cases, counseling also may be helpful.

Surgery

Surgery may be helpful if the patient has a surgically correctable condition. In our experience patients with otosclerosis who undergo a stapedectomy may have relief or improvement of their tinnitus. We found that about 50% have complete relief, 25% partial relief, 20% no change and 5% are worse (House, 1981; House & Brackmann, 1981).

As in other conditions associated with hearing loss, about 80% of patients with acoustic neuromas have associated tinnitus. Tinnitus is the first symptom in about 11% of these patients. (House & Luetje, 1979). When the tumor is removed through the translabyrinthine approach, the cochlear nerve is resected with the tumor. Despite removing part of the inner ear and the cochlear nerve the patient's tinnitus is unchanged. (House & Luetje, 1979). Because of this and other studies of cochlear nerve sections, we know that subjective tinnitus is central in origin and therefore does not respond to cutting the cochlear nerve. This central origin of the tinnitus is the reason tinnitus may respond to therapies such as biofeedback, cognitive therapy, centrally acting medications, or tinnitus retraining therapy. It is also the reason patients find that increased stress, lack of sleep, or depression aggravate the tinnitus.

Tinnitus Retraining Therapy and Customized Acoustic Neural Stimulus (Neuromonics)

The relative loudness of a person's tinnitus is low and therefore various sounds, such as environment sounds often will cover up the tinnitus. In addition, many patients report that the tinnitus is not noticeable during their normal daily activity unless they stop to listen for it. Therefore, training the brain to ignore the tinnitus is one approach that has had some success in selected patients. Pawel Jastreboff, Ph.D., first proposed Tinnitus Retraining Therapy (TRT) (Jastreboff & Jastreboff, 2000, 2003). TRT uses a combination of low level, broadband noise and counseling to achieve habituation of tinnitus. Jastreboff reports success in that the patient no longer is aware of his or her tinnitus except if they focus on it.

More recently, Paul Davis, Ph.D., devised a treatment that he calls Neuromonics. (Davis, Wilde, Steed, & Hanley, 2008). A small, lightweight device with headphones delivers precisely designed music embedded with a pleasant acoustic neural stimulus. These sounds, customized for each user's audiologic profile, are theorized to stimulate the auditory pathway to promote neural plastic changes. Over time, these new connections help the brain to filter out tinnitus disturbance, providing relief from symptoms.

Both TRT and Neuromonics may be an adjunct to hearing aids as a way of helping patients to understand and better cope with their tinnitus. In our practice, we have used both modalities of treatment for tinnitus successfully in patients for whom hearing aid fitting alone was insufficient to help them cope with their tinnitus.

Tinnitus Maskers

In the 1970s Jack Vernon, Ph.D., proposed masking as a treatment for the symptom of tinnitus. Most patients with tinnitus are aware of the relief from their tinnitus when in the presence of background noise. Dr. Vernon noted that the shower sound or a fountain particularly tended to block out the tinnitus. This association led to the development of the tinnitus masker. The masker resembles a hearing aid that emits a soft sound tuned to the frequency of the patient's tinnitus. Patients with an associated hearing loss may also benefit from the tinnitus instrument. The tinnitus instrument amplifies sound (especially in the speech frequencies) and additionally provides masking sounds in the range of the patient's tinnitus. Trained personnel who have experience with fitting hearing aids and assessing tinnitus patients fit both the masker and the tinnitus instrument in a hearing aid dispensary.

Hearing Aids

During our early work with tinnitus maskers, we observed that many patients received relief of their tinnitus when wearing hearing aids. Because of this, we often recommend hearing aids for patients complaining of tinnitus and hearing loss, even in those whose hearing loss is mild. This is especially true when the hearing loss is primarily in the higher frequencies. With the development of open fit hearing aids, we are able to amplify only the higher frequencies while allowing the lower frequencies to enter the ear canal without amplification. We have had many patients with mild hearing loss whose only complaint was tinnitus benefit from properly fitted hearing aids.

Even though hearing aids only help to mask the tinnitus while being worn, some patients report that the tinnitus has become less bothersome at night after their hearing aids have been removed. We feel this is because they have a reduction in their stress level during the day. Prior to obtaining hearing aids they were struggling with the hearing loss and blaming their inability to hear on their tinnitus. We explain to the patient that the hearing loss causes the tinnitus, not the tinnitus causing the loss. Once patients understand this and use the hearing aids they are better able to cope with the tinnitus.

Profoundly hard of hearing or deaf patients cannot benefit from hearing aids. These patients' maybe candidates for cochlear implantation. In our experience, cochlear implant patients with tinnitus report that their tinnitus is reduced while using their implants. Of 64 of our cochlear implant patients, 53% reported improvement in their tinnitus, 36% reported no change, 8% felt it was worse, and 3% had no opinion (House, J., 1984).

Conclusion

Because tinnitus is a symptom, there is not a universal cure. Patients complaining of tinnitus require an evaluation to determine the etiology of the tinnitus. The underlying cause of the tinnitus symptom should be treated, although in the majority of cases the cause is not treatable as such. A thorough explanation of the problem will, in most cases, satisfy the patient. If the tinnitus remains a problem for the patient, many courses of treatment may be offered. We have found that if a hearing loss exists (most cases) hearing aids can be very effective in reducing the severity of the tinnitus. With increased hearing ability many patients find their tinnitus is no longer a problem.

References

Davis, P. B., Wilde, R. A., Steed, L. G., & Hanley, P. J. (2008). Treatment of tinnitus with customized acoustic neural stimulus: A controlled clinical study. *ENT Journal, 86*(6), 330–339.

Goodhill, V., Rehman, I., & Brockman, S. (1953). Objective skin resistance audiometry; the electro-audiogram (EAG). *Transactions of the Pacific Coast Oto-ophthalmological Society Annual Meeting, 34*, 215-240.

House, J. W. (1981). Management of the tinnitus patient. *Annals of Otology, Rhinology, and Laryngology, 90*(6, Pt. 1), 597-601.

House, J. (1984). Effects of electrical stimulation on tinnitus. *Journal of Laryngology and Otology, 98*(Suppl. 9), 139-140.

House, J. W., & Brackmann, D. E. (1981). Tinnitus: Surgical management. *CIBA Symposium Foundation, 85*, 204-212.

House, W. F., & Luetje, C. M. (1979). *A history of acoustic tumor surgery: 1800-1900, early history* (Vol. 1). Baltimore: University Park Press.

Jastreboff, P. J., & Jastreboff, M. M. (2000). Tinnitus retraining therapy (TRT). *Journal of the American Academy of Audiology, 11*(3), 162-177.

Jastreboff, P. J., & Jastreboff, M. M. (2003). Tinnitus retraining therapy for patients with tinnitus and decreased sound tolerance. *Otolaryngology Clinics of North America, 36*(2), 321-336.

10

The Role of Hearing Aids in the Management of Tinnitus

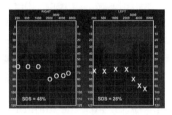

PAWEL J. JASTREBOFF, PH.D., SC.D., M.B.A.
MARGARET M. JASTREBOFF, PH.D.

A perception of sound without the presence of a physical sound that can be linked to this perception is known as tinnitus. Therefore, tinnitus is a phantom auditory perception, analogous to phantom pain or limb phenomena. Typically, it is described as ringing, buzzing, hissing, humming, whistling, roaring sound, perceived in the ears or the head. The majority of people who experience tinnitus are not negatively affected by it. Despite that, the number of people who have bothersome tinnitus requiring professional attention, that is, clinically-significant tinnitus, is still substantial. The latest epidemiologic studies estimate that approximately 8% of general population in the United States (i.e., 24 million Americans) has bothersome tinnitus (Hoffman & Reed, 2004). The etiology of tinnitus frequently is idiopathic and there are no proven mechanisms of tinnitus. Thus, most therapeutic approaches are based on clinical observations and focus on treating patients' complaints.

About 80% of people with clinically significant tinnitus have hearing loss (Davis & El Rafaie, 2000), and it has been reported that 50 to 70% of individuals with hearing loss report tinnitus as well (Del & Ambrosetti, 2007; Jastreboff & Jastreboff, 2003a; Sheldrake & Jastreboff,

2004). Because of observations such as these, for many decades, hearing aids have been commonly prescribed for the relief of tinnitus with the first such report published in 1947 (Saltzman & Ersner, 1947). The reports of effectiveness of hearing aids alone for tinnitus have been quite varied, from stating that they lack effectiveness to reports of up to 50% of patients experiencing some relief while using them (Del & Ambrosetti, 2007; Searchfield, 2005; Sheldrake & Jastreboff, 2004; Trotter & Donaldson, 2008). Creating an additional challenge for utilizing hearing aids for tinnitus management, decreased sound tolerance affects a significant proportion of tinnitus patients as well (Jastreboff & Jastreboff, 2004). Careful analysis of potential mechanisms involved in tinnitus treatment by the use of sound could help to optimize the use of hearing aids as a part of treatment for tinnitus.

Tinnitus and Sound

There are several observations related to tinnitus and ambient sound. Patients with tinnitus often report that their tinnitus seems louder and more intrusive in quiet, or when their ears are blocked. In the opposite sound environment situation, it is a common observation that ambient sounds help patients with tinnitus. These practical observations can be explained by results obtained from research of the auditory system.

Effects of Decreased Sound Input on the Auditory System and Tinnitus

It has been shown that majority of subjects develop temporary tinnitus when put in an extremely quiet environment (Heller & Bergman, 1953; Tucker et al., 2005). When tinnitus patients remain for some time in a quiet environment, it has been observed that the gain in their auditory system increases, resulting in the enhancement of the tinnitus signal (Gerken, 1979; Gerken et al., 1984, 1985; Gerken, Simhadri-Sumithra, & Bhat, 1986). At the same time, it is well established that all of our senses react not to the absolute value of a stimulus, but rather to the difference between the stimulus and background. Consequently, the strength of any signal in the nervous system is related to its difference with background neuronal activity (Jastreboff & Hazell, 2004). Considering the tonotopic organization of the auditory pathways and the fact that about 80% of tinnitus patients have some form of hearing loss (Hoffman & Reed, 2004), most often affecting high-frequency range, parts of the auditory pathways that correspond to the frequency range with hearing loss, are understimulated. More detailed explanation of the relation of tinnitus and hearing loss is provided by the discordant dysfunction theory, which postipulates that, not simplistically, the hearing loss itself, but rather the difference in the functional properties of the outer and inner hair cell systems is responsible for tinnitus emergence (Jastreboff, 1990, 2004; Jastreboff & Hazell, 2000).

On the other hand, by increasing the background neuronal activity, it is possible to decrease effectively the strength of the tinnitus-related neuronal activity within the auditory pathways and, subsequently, in all systems involved in processing the tinnitus signal (Jastreboff & Hazell, 2004). The increase of the background neuronal activity in the auditory pathways may be achieved by enhancing input to the cochlea, which could be accomplished by enhancing the auditory environment, and/or amplifying it by the use of hearing aids.

Effects of High Level of Sound Input on Tinnitus

It has been recognized since Itard's publication in 1825 that sounds can suppress ("mask") the perception of tinnitus (Stephens, 2000). Use of the term "masking" to describe the suppression of tinnitus perception has been widespread in the literature. Notably, the term "neural suppression" seems to be more appropriate than "masking," as disappearance of tinnitus perception does not follow rules of acoustic masking, which reflects the interaction of two traveling waves in the cochlea. Specifically, there is no phenomenon of a critical band; typically tinnitus perception can be suppressed equally easily by tones from a wide frequency range (there is no "V" type of suppression curve); and typically, it is possible to achieve suppression of tinnitus by stimulating the contralateral ear. In fact, it is sometimes easier to suppress tinnitus by stimulation of the contralateral ear than by stimulation of the ipsilateral ear (Jastreboff & Hazell, 2004).

Masking therapy was popularized in the 1970s by Vernon (Vernon & Schleuning, 1978). The goal of this approach was a total suppression of tinnitus perception. High-intensity noise generators were used, or a combination of such a generator with a hearing aid, which was then termed a "tinnitus instrument." Typically, however, the sound level required to consistently suppress tinnitus perception for longer than a few minutes is high, which severely limited the use of "tinnitus masking therapy" (Penner, 1983). Its effectiveness was reported from none (e.g., the same as placebo) (Erlandsson, Rongdahl, Hutchins, & Carlsson, 1987) to 50–60% (Vernon & Meikle, 2000).

This discrepancy might be perhaps due to the fact that early reports showing a high success rate of masking therapy used as a criterion of success the use of a masking devices by a patient for a minimum time of at least 6 months, rather than any direct evaluation of the lessened impact of tinnitus on patients lives or reduction in tinnitus severity as an outcome measure (Vernon, Griest & Press, 1990; Vernon & Schleuning, 1978). In a limited number of cases, residual inhibition (i.e., decrease/disappearance of tinnitus after short, high-intensity sound) was observed. Typically, residual inhibition lasts only seconds to a few minutes, which preclude its clinical usefulness. It is commonly reported that loud sounds cause a worsening of tinnitus for minutes, hours, or even days. Therefore, for patients experiencing tinnitus who also need to use hearing aids, it is necessary to consider some limitation of amplification to avoid this phenomenon. This restriction on amplification is made even more pronounced by the presence of decreased sound tolerance. Both hyperacusis (abnormal amplification of signals within the auditory pathways) and misophonia (abnormal activation of the limbic and autonomic nervous systems as a consequence of conditioned reflexes developed to certain categories of sounds) frequently accompany tinnitus (Jastreboff & Jastreboff, 2002, 2007). Worsening of tinnitus by sound evokes misophonia (Jastreboff & Jastreboff, 2002), which in turn triggers sound avoidance, overprotection of the ear, and subsequently further worsen tinnitus, thus creating a vicious cycle. To avoid this when decreased sound tolerance is present, lower maximal gain and higher compression in the setting of hearing aids is recommended.

The Effect of a Sound on the Strength of the Tinnitus Signal

As mentioned earlier in this chapter, the general principle of both the perception as well as the processing of all signals within the brain is that the strength of a perceived signal depends on the difference between this signal and background, rather than on the absolute value of the signal. As examples, the light of a candle will be perceived as stronger when it is in a dark room as compared to being viewed in a room illuminated by sunlight; the sound of music will be perceived as louder in a quiet environment as compared with the same physical level of music listened to in a car. Therefore, by increasing the average level of ongoing neuronal activity by increasing the average level of background sound, it is possible to achieve a decrease in the strength of the tinnitus signal. Although only rarely it is possible to suppress tinnitus perception in a consistent manner, some decrease of the tinnitus signal is always possible by enriching the auditory background and/or providing amplification of the auditory background by the use of hearing aids. This effect is used in a variety of therapies utilizing sound, such as in relief therapy (a recent version of "masking therapy") in which any level of a sound which provides immediate easing of tinnitus is recommended (Henry et al., 2006).

Plastic Changes of the Auditory System Induced by Sound

The auditory system undergoes plastic modifications depending on the presence, level, and spectrum of a sound (Popelar, Erre, Aran, & Cazals, 1994; Willott, 1996).

Indeed, modifications of the cortical representation of various frequencies have been shown after exposure to sound (Keeling, Calhoun, Kruger, Polley, & Schreiner, 2008; Yu, Sanes, Aristzabal, Wadghiri, & Turnbull, 2007) and as a result of the presence of tinnitus (Muhlnickel, Elbert, Taub, & Flor, 1998). Moreover, the extent of tinnitus-caused shifts of cortical representation has been shown to have a strong positive correlation with the subjective strength of tinnitus, (Muhlnickel et al., 1998) offering the first objective, physiologic documentation of the presence of tinnitus.

The most common plastic modification of the auditory pathways is the change in the gain of the auditory system induced by the modification of the average level of sound to which subjects are exposed over some period of time. Specifically, when the level of signal stimulating the auditory nerve is low (as a results of, e.g., otosclerosis, cerumen accumulation, overuse of ear plugs, etc.), the gain increases (Gerken et al., 1985; Gerken, Simhadri-Sumithra, & Bhat, 1986). As a result, the tinnitus signal is amplified as well, and tinnitus is perceived as louder. When, however, the auditory system is stimulated over some period of time, the opposite effect occurs, and the internal gain decreases, thus yielding a subjective reduction of tinnitus. These effects are frequency dependent.

As an example, a given patient may have normal hearing in the low- and middle-frequency range, but significant hearing loss for higher frequencies. In that case, areas of the auditory pathways that process high frequency sounds will be understimulated, and result in enhancement of the tinnitus signal (whose pitch typically is the same frequency[ies] as those areas with hearing loss) will occur.

Potential Mechanisms of the Action of Hearing Aids on Tinnitus

The majority of patients with tinnitus have some hearing loss requiring the use of hearing aids. It was noted that some patients reported improvement of their tinnitus while using their hearing aids, which is one reason why hearing aids commonly are used as a first approach to help patients with tinnitus. Unfortunately, hearing aids typically are dispensed without particular consideration of the potential mechanism(s) of their effects on tinnitus, and counseling related to tinnitus is limited to advising that the use of hearing aids should help by masking tinnitus.

For the optimal implementation of hearing aids for tinnitus treatment, it is important to recognize the potential mechanisms through which hearing aids may affect tinnitus in a positive manner. Moreover, understanding these mechanisms may help in avoiding situations, known from clinical practice, whereby the use of hearing aids actually induces or worsens tinnitus. It is important to recognize that hearing aids are merely sound amplifiers, and that, in the absence of external sounds, they cannot provide relief of tinnitus, except through a placebo effect. They work by enhancing the level and spectrum of sound reaching the inner ear, and subsequently increasing stimulation of the auditory pathways. Thus, in the case of use by those patients suffering from tinnitus, they act as a tool to implement a sound therapy, in addition to their role of improving speech understanding and decreasing the "strain to hear."

The "strain to hear" phenomenon, that is, attempts to understand speech, increases tinnitus through two mecha-nisms: the increase of general stress level, and by increasing the gain within the auditory system. It well recognized that stress commonly increases tinnitus (Jas-treboff & Hazel, 2004). As the majority of tinnitus patients have hearing loss that interferes with their ability to understand speech, particularly in noisy situations, their general stress level is increased, affecting their perception of tinnitus as well. Straining to understand results in an increase of the gain within the audi-tory pathways. Properly selected and fit-ted hearing aids decrease strain to hear, leading to a subsequent decrease in the strength of tinnitus. For these reasons, proper counseling is essential, as fre-quently patients blame their tinnitus, rather than their underlying hearing loss, for their problems with communication.

During the recent past, the impact of the placebo effect in medical treatments is much more recognized (Ioannidis, 2008; Khan, Redding, & Brown, 2008; Kirsch et al., 2008). Some positive effect of hear-ing aids on tinnitus may reflect the pla-cebo effect as well. Patients have a feeling that something is being done for them that is presumably worthwhile as it costs a substantial amount of money.

Generally, sounds of nature and music have been recognized as effective in the reduction of stress, lessening of sleep problems, promotion of learning, im-provement of well-being, and induction of positive changes in cognitive function. Sounds (music) that are associated with positive memories are particularly helpful. Hearing aids may enhance these positive effects by increasing the pleasurableness and/or acceptability of these sounds. There are a number of specific, currently utilized tinnitus treatments involving sound, for example, masking/relief ther-apy, Tinnitus Retraining Therapy (TRT), music therapies, Neuromonics, Phase Shift Tinnitus Reduction, desensitization, pink noise therapy, Dynamic Tinnitus Mitigation system, and Auditory Integration Training. For all of these treatments, the adjunctive use of properly fitted hearing aids should be beneficial. The optimal implementation of hearing aid setting and use, however, depends on the specific therapy utilized. For example, in the case of masking therapy, the emphasis would be toward achieving the maximally acceptable amplification of the sound, whereas for TRT therapy, stress would be given toward the avoidance of the negative simulation of the limbic and autonomic nervous systems by additional sounds, which would be done by initially starting treatment with underamplification and higher compression, and then by gradually increasing to the point of maximal amplification. (More detailed comments are presented in a subsequent section.) These treatments differ in specific recommendations regarding the type of sound and its use as well, but the main difference is in the form of accompanying counseling provided to the patient.

Practical Considerations for the Use of Hearing Aids in Patients Suffering From Tinnitus

For all tinnitus therapies involving sound, the use of hearing aids for patients who also have hearing loss is potentially beneficial. Generally, the use of hearing aids will provide enhanced stimulation for the frequency ranges corresponding to the hearing loss, which were under-stimulated before amplification, and subsequently will decrease the strength of the tinnitus signal, providing that the sounds of the

frequencies in question are present in the environment. Hearing aids amplify environmental sounds and provide increased stimulation of the auditory pathways. As discussed above, the increased stimulation of the auditory pathways decreases the strength of the tinnitus signal, thus providing some relief from tinnitus. Additionally, hearing aids decrease the "strain to hear" and decrease the stress related to understanding. As stress typically increases tinnitus, by decreasing the stress level, some improvement in tinnitus may be achieved.

For nearly all the various sound therapies, the fitting and use of hearing aids are the same as in patients who do not suffer from tinnitus; therefore these therapies are not discussed further in this chapter. The comments and recommendations presented in the following section are based on the neurophysiologic model of tinnitus, as implemented in Tinnitus Retraining Therapy (TRT).

Outline of the Principles of Sound Therapy Utilized in TRT

Briefly, TRT involves counseling and sound therapy, both based on the neurophysiological model of tinnitus, with sound therapy aimed at consistent decrease of the strength of the tinnitus signal (Jastreboff & Hazell, 2004). The rules of comfort and avoidance of suppression of tinnitus are used to restrict the upper level of the sound signal used. All patients are advised to avoid silence and to be exposed to some form of sound 24 hours a day, 7 days a week. Improving the hearing abilities and restoring the symmetry of auditory stimulation via a wide range in the frequency sounds is always recommended and attempted. The frequent presence of decreased sound tolerance (our data from Emory University indicates that 30% of patients with tinnitus suffer from hyperacusis, and about 60% with misophonia (Jastreboff, & Jastreboff, 2002) must be taken into account during evaluation and fitting. Current TRT protocol is geared toward using at least two types of sound: sounds of nature (particularly gently flowing water, such as a brook, stream, or creek), and a broadband noise (provided by sound generators or combination devices). Furthermore, music is used in the majority of patients, primarily to treat misophonia (Jastreboff & Hazell, 2002, 2004).

Specific Modifications in the Selection, Fitting, and Use of Hearing Aids

In contrast to the more common use of hearing aids to improve communication, patients suffering from significant tinnitus are advised to use their hearing aids all the time, except when sleeping. The use of hearing aids should not evoke negative reactions. Thus, avoidance of the occlusion effect, as well as the overall comfort of hearing aids is of paramount importance in treating the patient who also suffers from significant tinnitus. Consequently, the preference is to the use of digital hearing aids with the receiver in the ear.

Asymmetric auditory stimulation results in decreased functionality of the unaided side, (Silverman, Silman, Emmer, Schoepflin & Lutolf, 2006) as well as plastic modification of the auditory system (Hwang, Wu, Chen, & Liu, 2006). Therefore, the use of hearing aids is recommended to preserve or restore symmetrical stimulation of the auditory system (Jastreboff & Hazell, 2004; Sheldrake & Jastreboff,

2004). When the hearing loss is asymmetrical, then the setting of the hearing aids should be aimed at restoring symmetry, if at all possible. In the case of unilateral deafness, utilization of multisensory integration and the consequent fitting of CROS, BiCROS, or transcranial stimulation are recommended (Jastreboff & Hazell, 2004). The creation or enhancement of any asymmetric stimulation of the auditory pathways would push the tinnitus signal toward the understimulated side, thus making treatment more difficult. Likewise, in order to preserve the symmetry of the auditory stimulation, it is necessary to use bilateral hearing aid fitting in cases of bilateral hearing loss.

It is recommended that the setting of hearing aids be gradually modified in a stepwise fashion, with the initial setting biased toward underamplification and a higher level of compression used, to prevent an overstimulation by sound. The same principle applies to adjusting the frequency range of amplification. According to the neurophysiologic model of tinnitus, it is beneficial to provide amplification of high-frequency sounds, preferably at least up to 10 kHz (understanding the limitation imposed by both technology and the specifics of hearing loss in a given patient). In patients who have a long-term, high-frequency hearing loss; the prompt amplification of such high frequencies could, unfortunately, evoke feelings of overload and discomfort. Therefore, expansion toward higher frequencies should be done gradually, with constant dialogue with the patient as to his or her acceptance of hear aids setting and the comfort of their use in everyday situations.

The level of even enriched auditory background sound is relatively low, and natural environmental sounds, which are typically soft, are utilized as well, as part of sound therapy for tinnitus. Therefore, if hearing aids have programs aimed at "noise elimination," these programs must be disabled as a part of tinnitus treatment. Expansions (i.e., the more rapid reduction of hearing aid gain for sound levels below the knee point) should be turned off as well, and low-compression knee point (at or below 40 dB SPL) are recommended (Searchfield, 2005). These steps enable amplification of low level environmental sounds, and those provided by table-top sound machines, to the level that can be perceived by patients. Directional microphones can be beneficial by improving understanding in noisy situations; however, they tend to attenuate sound stimulation in quiet environments. Thus, multiprogrammable hearing aids are preferred with omni-directional characteristics being used while the wearer is in a quiet environment. Automatic volume control is preferable; otherwise patients will have a tendency to manipulate the volume, thereby attracting attention to both their hearing loss as well as tinnitus. If various levels of amplifications are desirable, the use of multiple programs would solve the need for variable amplification.

Notably, there is a small group of patients whose tinnitus is suppressed as soon as they switch the hearing aids on (Sheldrake & Jastreboff, 2004). Presumably, the environmental background sound amplified by hearing aids is sufficient to suppress tinnitus perception in these individuals. Unfortunately, in many of these patients, bothersome tinnitus eventually returns as soon as they take their hearing aids off. These patients need additional, specific help to solve this problem (Sheldrake & Jastreboff, 2004).

Real-ear measurements (REM) (e.g., speech mapping, which is used to deter-mine the level and spectrum of sound provided by sound generators in cases where combination instruments are used) are recommended as a part of fitting and follow-up procedures to improve optimization of the proper fitting of hearing aids. At the same time, attention should be paid to the comments provided by patients regarding their own perception of the sounds amplified by hearing aids, and we should treat this feedback as superior to technical measurements alone. As a routine, during the initial fitting appointment and subsequent follow-up visits, after programs of hearing aids have been set, we advise that patients should go outside of the clinic to evaluate the function of their hearing aids in the "normal environment," and then return for any further corrections of the settings, if they are necessary. The need for this procedure is enhanced by attempts to expand amplification above the 6- to 8-kHz range, and the resulting increased tendency to induce feedback.

For the majority of patients suffering from tinnitus who also have hearing loss, combination instruments (i.e., devices with an independently controlled hearing aid, as well as a sound generator combined in one shell) are considered to be optimal, as they provide amplification in addition to supplying a well-controlled source of sound. At the present time, available devices provide a broad band noise; however, in principle, other sounds, (e.g., sounds of nature), could be even more beneficial. Combination instruments currently available in the United States are still being developed, and are not perfected yet. The authors have had excellent results with combination instruments. Although setting these combination instruments requires specific knowledge and even more extensive education of patients, they are extremely helpful when used properly. Briefly, the hearing aid portion is set by the professional as for when hearing aids are used alone, while the level of the sound generator is controlled by the patient him- or herself, who is advised to follow the specific set of instructions which will assure that the sound would not induce annoyance, will not cause suppression of the perception of their tinnitus while being sufficiently above the threshold of perception (to avoid effects of stochastic resonance) (Jaramillo & Wiesenfeld, 1998; Jastreboff & Jastreboff, 2000; Morse & Evans, 1996).

It is not necessary to be at "mixing point" (i.e., the beginning of partial suppression of tinnitus, when patients can still separate their perception of tinnitus from an external sound, but when the perception of tinnitus and external sound start to mix, blend together) to be successful with TRT. The majority patients set their sound generators below "the mixing point" level due to the limitations imposed by the need to remain below the annoyance level. The use of REM to determine the level of sound provided by the sound generator alone or sound generators being part of combination instruments is highly recommended. The authors report that the results of almost 1000 REM measurements reveal that, on average, patients are using sound at the level of 8.5 dB SL (personal communication).

Worsening of Tinnitus Induced by Hearing Aids

Although infrequent, there are clear cases whereby tinnitus worsens as a result of the use of hearing aids. This worsening may result from the inappropriate selection, programming, or fitting of the hearing aids. Most frequently, it occurs with an occlusive fitting for patients with good low-frequency hearing thresholds. While environmental sound in quiet backgrounds has a majority of its energy below 200 Hz, the physical limitations (size of moving parts producing sound waves) of hearing aids cannot amplify sound below 200 Hz. Therefore, for low-frequency sound, an occlusive hearing aid will act as an earplug, enhancing (worsening) tinnitus due to the mechanisms described above.

Worsening of tinnitus can also occur when hearing aids evoke discomfort for any reasons (e.g., physical discomfort of the fitting within the ear canal, overamplification, distortion, etc.). These factors enhance the negative activation of the limbic and autonomic nervous systems caused by tinnitus, and, additionally, attract attention to the ears and anything else even remotely related to hearing, including tinnitus. As a consequence, patients will experience a worsening or their tinnitus.

Older Versus Modern Hearing Aids

Substantial progress has occurred in the technology, as well as the use of hearing aids over last decade. Older, analog hearing aids were large and difficult to ignore, with poor esthetic appeal. Fitting these models tended to be more occlusive in nature, as they lacked an effective anti-feedback feature. The maximal amplification of high frequencies was low, often not exceeding 4 kHz. Older style analog hearing aids, however, tended to have a high level of internal noise, and thus acted unintentionally acted as basic combination instruments, albeit with a fixed level of noise generators.

The combination of hearing aid and sound generator, devices that were termed "tinnitus instruments," was physically large, with powerful noise generators and low-quality hearing aids. They were not suitable for use in modern sound therapies.

Last, but not least in importance, unilateral fitting was more prevalent in the past, enhancing rather than deceasing, the asymmetrical stimulation of the auditory system.

Modern, digital hearing aids, particularly those with a receiver in the ear, offer substantial advantages over the older hearing aids, including: (1) expansion of the frequency range up to 10 kHz; (2) utilization of compression allowing for the enhancement of low level sounds; (3) increased popularity of open fit with receiver in-the-ear technology, which is partly allowed by the incorporation of effective antifeedback programs; (4) increasing awareness of the importance of auditory rehabilitation and more extensive counseling; (5) much better combination instruments; (6) more focus on comfort and acceptability of instrumentation; (7) increasing popularity of bilateral fitting and therefore restoration of symmetric stimulation; and (8) improved procedures assisting in hearing aids fitting (e.g., REM and better algorithms for selecting the parameters of the initial fitting). All these advantages and improved aesthetics of hearing aids have enhanced the acceptability as well as the use of hearing aids for cases of milder hearing loss compared to the past.

Paradoxically, not all new developments are beneficial for the use of hearing aids as part of the treatment of tinnitus. Technologic progress in miniaturization created the popularity of completely-in-canal (CIC) hearing aids, which in some cases where venting was inadequate actually enhanced tinnitus. The modern tendencies to improve speech understanding in noise, and remove the perception of low level noise, promotes the incorporation and expansion of a variety of noise reduction programs, which may be counterproductive from the standpoint of sound therapies useful for tinnitus. Similarly, the increased popularity of multiple microphones has decreased the use of omni-directional characteristics, which are actually preferable for sound therapies. Finally, a tendency to provide patients with effort-free hearing aids has resulted in the creation of a variety of self-adaptable programs, which change the parameters of hearing aids, according to the external sound environment. One can argue that, from the point of view of the neurophysiology of hearing, these programs make the use of hearing aids more difficult and may additionally have a detrimental effect on the use of devices for the treatment of tinnitus. An analogous example would be an attempt to use glasses that would automatically change the optical power of its lens depending on the angle of a head position, with a resulting change from "reading" to "distance" glasses. The recent promotion of binaural "asymmetrical fitting," whereby one hearing aid is set in an omni-directional mode, while the other uses a directional microphone, indicates the recognition of some of the problems encountered with adaptive devices. These adaptive programs may cause an unwanted increase in attention to hearing and to tinnitus, further decreasing stimulation by the low level background sounds desirable for tinnitus treatment.

Otolaryngologic Concerns Regarding Tinnitus and the Use of Hearing Aids

In practice, only a few otolaryngiologic conditions linked to tinnitus could be helpful in improving tinnitus by medical or surgical means, (Jastreboff & Jastreboff, 2003a) with those most common being caused by conductive hearing losses (e.g., otitis media, cerumen impaction, ossicular stiffness/discontinuity, otosclerosis). Nonsurgical approaches to the patient with tinnitus as a chief complaint are suggested to consider as a first line of treatment, as even an otherwise successful operation may still enhance tinnitus (Ayache, Earally, & Elbaz, 2003) whereas a failed operation would pose an even greater chance of worsening the symptom (Jastreboff & Hazell, 2004). Therefore, for patients with conductive hearing loss such as otosclerosis who also have bothersome tinnitus, it is suggested to consider of the use of hearing aids, as these could be as effective as surgery, without the risk of worsening tinnitus.

All types of sensorineural hearing losses (e.g., associated with Ménière's disease vestibular schwannoma, sudden hearing loss, etc.) need to be treated according to whatever is the current state of the art of treatment. However, it is important to recognize that these procedures or treatment for hearing loss, and/or vertigo might not be beneficial in improving tinnitus as seen in a majority of the cases of Ménière's disease or vestibular schwannoma. Hearing aids however, when appropriate, can be used as part of sound therapy treatment and provide benefits. When TRT is used, it is recommended that medical/surgical and TRT treatments be conducted simultaneously.

Conclusions

Hearing aids can be an effective tool when incorporated as a part of sound therapy used in tinnitus treatment. Their role is to increase background sound, decrease the contrast between tinnitus and background sound, restore the symmetry of stimulation of the auditory system, decrease the "strain to hear," as well as increase understanding and thus decrease the frustration, and decrease the focus and attention paid to tinnitus and the ears in general. Patients' education related to hearing and tinnitus is crucial, and proper, intensive counseling is essential to achieve positive results and maximize the usefulness of hearing aids in tinnitus treatment. The selection, programming, and fitting of hearing aids for patients with tinnitus are different from "standard procedures" and require specific knowledge and extra time.

References

Ayache, D., Earally, F., & Elbaz, P. (2003). Characteristics and postoperative course of tinnitus in otosclerosis. *Otology and Neurotology, 24*(1), 48–51.

Davis, A., & El Reface, A. (2000). Epidemiology of tinnitus. In R. S. Tyler, (Ed.), *Tinnitus handbook* (pp. 1–23). San Diego, CA: Singular, Thomson Learning.

Del, B. L., & Ambrosetti, U. (2007). Hearing aids for the treatment of tinnitus. *Progress in Brain Research, 166,* 341–345.

Erlandsson, S., Ringdahl, A., Hutchins, T., & Carlsson, S. G. (1987). Treatment of tinnitus: A controlled comparison of masking and placebo. *British Journal of Audiology, 21,* 37–44.

Gerken, G. M. (1979). Central denervation hypersensitivity in the auditory system of the cat. *Journal of the Acoustic Society of America*, *66*, 721-727.

Gerken, G. M., Saunders, S. S., & Paul, R. E. (1984). Hypersensitivity to electrical stimulation of auditory nuclei follows hearing loss in cats. *Hearing Research*, *13*, 249-259.

Gerken, G. M., Saunders, S. S., Simhadri-Sumithra, R., & Bhat, K. H. V. (1985). Behavioral thresholds for electrical stimulation applied to auditory brainstem nuclei in cat are altered by injurious and noninjurious sound. *Hearing Research*, *20*, 221-231.

Gerken, G. M., Simhadri-Sumithra, R., & Bhat, K. H. V. (1986). Increase in central auditory responsiveness during continuous tone stimulation or following hearing loss. In R. J. Salvi, D. Henderson, R. P. Hamernik, & V. Colletti, (Eds.), *Basic and applied aspects of noise-induced hearing loss* (pp. 195-211). New York: Plenum..

Heller, M. F., & Bergman, M. (1953). Tinnitus in normally hearing persons. *Annals of Otology*, *62*, 73-93.

Henry, J. A., Schechter, M. A., & Zaugg, T. L., Griest, S., Jastreboff, P. J., Vernon, J. A., et al. (2006). Outcomes of clinical trial: Tinnitus masking vs. tinnitus retraining therapy. *Journal of the American Auditory Association*, *17*(2), 104-132.

Hoffman, H. J., & Reed, G. W. (2004). Epidemiology of tinnitus. In J. B. Snow (Ed.), *Tinnitus: Theory and management* (pp. 16-41). Hamilton, London: B. C. Decker.

Hwang, J. H., Wu, C. W., Chen, J. H., & Liu, T. C. (2006). Changes in activation of the auditory cortex following long-term amplification: an fMRI study. *Acta Otolaryngologica*, *126*(12), 1275-1280.

Ioannidis, J. P. (2008). Effectiveness of antidepressants: An evidence myth constructed from a thousand randomized trials? *Philosophy, Ethics, and Humanities in Medicine*, *3*, 14.

Jaramillo, F., & Wiesenfeld, K. (1998). Mechanoeletrical transduction assisted by Brownian motion: a role for noise in the auditory system. *Nature and Neuroscience*, *1*(5), 384-388.

Jastreboff, M. M., & Jastreboff, P. J. (2002). Decreased sound tolerance and Tinnitus Retraining Therapy (TRT). *Australian and New Zealand Journal of Audiology*, *21*(2), 74-81.

Jastreboff, P. J. (1990). Phantom auditory perception (tinnitus), mechanisms of generation and perception. *Neuroscience Research*, *8*, 221-254.

Jastreboff, P. J. (1995). Tinnitus as a phantom perception: Theories and clinical implications. In J. Vernon, A. R. Moller (Eds.), *Mechanisms of tinnitus* (pp. 73-94). Boston, London: Allyn & Bacon.

Jastreboff, P. J. (2004). Tinnitus retraining therapy. In J. B. Snow (Ed.), *Tinnitus: Theory and management* (pp. 295-309). Hamilton, London: B. C. Decker.

Jastreboff, P. J., & Hazell, J. W. P. (2004). *Tinnitus retraining therapy: Implementing the neurophysiological model*. Cambridge, UK: Cambridge University Press.

Jastreboff, P. J., & Jastreboff, M. M. (2000). Potential impact of stochastic resonance on tinnitus and its treatment. *Association for Research in Otolaryngology*, *5542*, 216.

Jastreboff, P. J., & Jastreboff, M. M. (2003a). Tinnitus and hyperacusis. In J. B. Snow, Jr., J. J. Ballenger (Eds.), *Ballenger's otorhinolaryngology head and neck surgery* (16th ed, pp. 456-775). Hamilton, Ontario, Canada: B. C. Decker.

Jastreboff, P. J., & Jastreboff, M. M. (2003b). Tinnitus Retraining Therapy for patients with tinnitus and decreased sound tolerance. *Otolaryngologic Clinics of North America*, *36*(2), 321-336.

Jastreboff, P. J., & Jastreboff, M. M. (2007). Tinnitus and decreased sound tolerance: Theory and treatment. In G. Huges & M. Pensak (Eds.), *Clinical otology* (3rd ed., pp. 487-497). New York: Thieme Medical.

Keeling, M. D., Calhoun, B. M., Kruger, K., Polley, D. B., & Schreiner, C. E. (2008). Spectral integration plasticity in cat auditory cortex induced by perceptual training. *Experimental Brain Research*, *184*(4), 493-509.

Khan, A., Redding, N., & Brown, W. A. (2008). The persistence of the placebo response in antidepressant clinical trials. *Journal of Psychiatric Research*, *42*(10), 791-796.

Kirsch, I., Deacon, B. J., Huedo-Medina, T. B., Scoboria, A., Moore, T. J., & Johnson, B. T. (2008). Initial severity and antidepressant benefits: A meta-analysis of data submitted to the Food and Drug Administration. *PLoS Medicine*, *5*(2), e45.

Morse, R. P., & Evans, E. F. (1996). Enhancement of vowel coding for cochlear implants by addition of noise. *Nature Medicine*, *2*(8), 928-932.

Muhlnickel, W., Elbert, T., Taub, E., & Flor, H. (1998). Reorganization of auditory cortex in tinnitus. *Proceedings of the National Academy of Sciences USA*, *95*(17), 10340-10343.

Penner, M. J. (1983). The annoyance of tinnitus and the noise required to mask it. *Journal of Speech and Hearing Research*, *26*, 73-76.

Popelar, J., Erre, J-P., Aran, J-M., & Cazals, Y. (1994). Plastic changes in ipsi-contralateral differences of auditory cortex and inferior colliculus evoked potentials after injury to one ear in the adult guinea pig. *Hearing Research*, *72*, 125-134.

Saltzman, M., & Ersner, M. S. (1947). A hearing aid for the relief of tinnitus aurium. *Laryngoscope*, *57*, 358-366.

Searchfield, G. D. Hearing aids and tinnitus. (2005). In R. S. Tyler (Ed.), *Tinnitus treatment clinical protocols* (pp. 161-75). New York: Thieme Medical.

Sheldrake, J. B., & Jastreboff, M. M. (2004). Role of hearing aids in management of tinnitus. In: J. B. Snow (Ed.), *Tinnitus: Theory and management* (pp. 312-315). Hamilton, London: BC Decker.

Silverman, C. A., Silman, S., Emmer, M. B.,

Schoepflin, J. R., & Lutolf, J. J. (2006). Auditory deprivation in adults with asymmetric, sensorineural hearing impairment. *Journal of the American Academy of Audiology*, *17*(10), 747-762.

Stephens, D. (2000). A history of tinnitus. In R. S. Tyler (Ed.), *Tinnitus handbook* (pp. 437-448). San Diego, CA: Singular, Thomson Learning.

Trotter, M. I., & Donaldson, I. (2008). Hearing aids and tinnitus therapy: A 25-year experience. *Journal of Laryngology and Otology*, *122*, 1052-1056.

Tucker, D. A., Phillips, S. L., Ruth, R. A., Clayton, W. A., Royster, E., & Todd, A. D. (2005). The effect of silence on tinnitus perception. *Otolaryngology-Head and Neck Surgery*, *132*(1), 20-24.

Vernon, J., Griest, S., & Press, L. (1990). Attributes of tinnitus and the acceptance of masking. *American Journal of Otolaryngology*, *11*, 44-50.

Vernon, J., & Schleuning, A. (1978). Tinnitus: A new management. *Laryngoscope*, *88*, 413-419.

Vernon, J. A., & Meikle, M. B. (2000). Tinnitus masking. In R. Tyler (Ed.), *Tinnitus handbook*. San Diego, CA: Singular, Thomson Learning.

Willott, J. F. (1996). Auditory system plasticity in the adult C57BL/6J mouse. In R. J. Salvi, D. Henderson, F. Fiorino, & V. Colletti (Eds.), *Auditory system plasticity and regeneration* (pp. 297-316). New York: Thieme Medical.

Yu, X., Sanes, D. H., Aristizabal, O., & Wadghiri, Y. Z., & Turnbull, D. H. (2007). Large-scale reorganization of the tonotopic map in mouse auditory midbrain revealed by MRI. *Proceedings of the National Academy of Sciences USA*, *104*(29), 12193-12198.

11

Nutritional Supplements for the Hearing-Impaired Patient

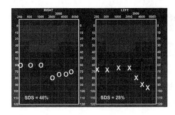

MICHAEL J. A. ROBB, M.D
MICHAEL D. SEIDMAN, M.D.

Introduction

Nutraceutical is defined as "food, or parts of food, that provide medical or health benefits, including the prevention and treatment of disease" (DeFelice, 2002; Kalra, 2003). The purpose of this chapter is to review the scientific evidence of select nutraceuticals that suggest these natural compounds either help prevent mitochondrial dysfunction and/or possess anti-inflammatory activity that may offer potential benefits to both hearing as well as general health. Current otologic nutraceutical research is summarized in the areas of ototoxicity, presbycusis, and noise-induced sensorineural hearing loss.

Optimum health and wellness are dependent on many factors, including a healthy diet, exercise, avoidance of tobacco products, maintaining appropriate weight, and, where appropriate, supplementation with multivitamins, minerals, and essential fatty acids. The diet should be nutrient rich, not solely energy rich. Exercise need not be vigorous; moderate, regular exercise confers health benefits. Multivitamin and mineral supplements are a simple way of ensuring adequate

RDA (recommended daily allowance) intake of important micronutrients, especially in those at risk for deficiencies such as the poor, adolescents, the obese, and the elderly (Ames, 2006). Additionally, antioxidants may play an exciting and synergistic role in helping to prevent, minimize, alleviate, or even reverse certain disease entities.

Today, many patients welcome suggestions regarding natural interventions that may improve their auditory symptoms or at least slow the rate of ongoing reductions in hearing sensitivity. Studies over the past 25 years have shown that several antioxidants have the potential to favorably impact hearing. The research on otoprotection stems primarily from animal studies but some human data exist. Although controversial, the overwhelming body of evidence suggests that there are numerous health benefits to be gained from antioxidants. These antioxidants are readily available over the counter in FDA-registered Drug Establishment, USP (United States Pharmacopeia), and GMP (Good Manufacturing Practice) grades.

This chapter does not intend to minimize the importance of a well-balanced multivitamin and mineral formula, essential fatty acids, regular moderate exercise, normal sleep, and a healthy lifestyle. The aim of this chapter is to introduce the hearing specialist to several nutraceuticals receiving much attention at present in the laboratory and the clinic for their ability to improve mitochondrial health, scavenge reactive oxygen species, and reduce markers of bio-inflammation. Diverse mechanisms of action and clinical applications are discussed, including examples of how these natural compounds may favorably impact general as well as hearing health. Safety, tolerability, interactions with prescription medica-

tions, and supplemental dosage ranges are also reviewed.

Mitochondrial Function

To understand many pathophysiologic processes that affect the human body, the reader must first have an understanding of the processes of oxidation and reactive oxygen species, respiration, and mitochondrial function. This basic biochemistry, pivotal in the process of aging, hearing loss, cardiovascular disease, neurodegenerative disorders, oncogenesis, and other human disorders, is reviewed in the following paragraphs.

The process of aging is associated with many molecular, biochemical and physiologic changes. Such changes include increased DNA damage, reduced mitochondrial function, and an increase in inflammatory markers, decreased cellular water concentrations, ionic changes, vascular insufficiency, and a reduction in cellular membrane integrity. All of these pathophysiologic changes further predispose the body to increases in free radical production, cellular demise, organ failure, and ultimately, systemwide failure.

There are many proposed factors that contribute to the aging process. These include: reduced red blood cell velocity, altered vascular plasticity, and increased vascular permeability (Prazma et al., 1990; Seidman, Khan, Dolan, & Quirk, 1996); reduced oxygen and nutrient delivery, and waste elimination (Gacek & Schuknecht, 1969; Harkins, 1981; Hoeffding & Feldman, 1988; Rosenhall, Pederson, & Dotevall, 1986); and genetic mutations and a significant increase in the production of reactive oxygen species (ROS), also known as free radicals. Concomitant with the increase in ROS is a reduced production or function of the endogenous enzymes that protect the cell from ROS damage including superoxide dismutase, catalase, and glutathione peroxidase. These ROS have been shown to be responsible, in part, for producing mitochondrial DNA (mtDNA) damage by causing deletions in the mitochondrial genome. These deletions (mtDNA del) are an important component of the age-associated diminution in auditory sensitivity. Specific deletions are directly proportional to aging, such as an increased frequency of the "common" aging deletion—4977 base pairs—in presbycusic human temporal bones (Markaryan, Nelson, & Hinojosa, 2008; Seidman, 2000; Seidman, Khan, Bai, Shirwany, & Quirk, 2000). When mtDNA deletions reach a certain level, the mitochondria become bioenergetically inefficient. This reduced efficiency can be measured in different ways. One such method is by measuring reductions in the specific enzymes (cytochrome oxidase [COX], succinate dehydrogenase [SDH], and nicotinamide adenine dinucleotide [NADH]]). Another method is by using flow cytometry to measure reductions in mitochondrial membrane potentials (MMP), which serves as a measure of mitochondrial function and finally, by the measurement of specific deletions or point mutations in the mitochondrial DNA genome. Such reductions in mitochondrial function and increases in mtDNA deletions have been identified within heart, brain, liver, and skeletal muscle samples in aged rats, mice, monkeys and humans (Corral-Debrinksi et al., 1991; Cortopassi & Arnheim, 1990; Hattori et al., 1991; Seidman, Quirk, Nuttall, & Schweitzer, 1991; Wallace, 1992). Aging involves the progressive accumulation of metabolic and physiologic changes associated with an increasing susceptibility to disease.

There are many hypotheses in the current literature providing explanations for senescence. In the authors' opinion, three of the most convincing theories are the telomerase theory of aging, the dysdifferentiation hypothesis of aging, and the membrane hypothesis of aging (MHA), which is also referred to as the "mitochondrial clock theory" of aging.

The telomerase theory of aging suggests that there is a reduction in telomere length over time. The end of a chromosome is made up of a structure called the telosome. The tip of the telosome is a region of DNA repeat sequences and associated proteins collectively known as the telomere. It is hypothesized that DNA transcription and replication are affected by position effects mediated by the telomere. Reduction in the length of the telomere and alterations in its chromatin assembly may explain the instability that occurs during senescence as well as the immortalization process in vitro (Pommier, Lebeau, Ducray, & Sabatier, 1995). In tumor-derived cell lines, telomeres are maintained by the ribonucleoprotein enzyme, telomerase. However, telomerase activity is repressed in practically all normal human somatic cells. Thus, there is an inherent problem of end-replication creating a tendency toward progressive telomere shortening. Cumulatively, this predilection leads to limited replicative capacity, chromatin instability, and eventually, cellular senescence. Viral oncogenes or certain somatic mutations can block cellular aging, probably by activating telomerase. Therefore, telomere shortening is effectively prevented, which appears to be an important mechanism for sustaining the cellular growth of tumors (Shay & Wright, 1996). Low level telomerase activity also has been demonstrated in normal human T and B cells; this also has been shown to decrease with aging (Hiyama et al., 1996). Although many aspects of telomerase activity remain undefined, it has been hypothesized that the balance between telomere shortening and telomerase activity may underlie cellular aging processes. Using this line of reasoning, although unproven, changes in telomeres may also predispose to the development of presbycusis.

The dysdifferentiation theory suggests that aging is a continuum of programmed differentiations leading to either a cessation of normal gene activity or a systematic activation of genes whose effects are deleterious to cellular function. Support for this theory is provided by apoptosis (programmed cell death) studies in *C. elegans* (earthworm). These experiments elegantly elaborated the genetic mechanisms responsible for controlling cell death. The maintenance of homeostasis for cellular metabolism and function consumes a large fraction of total body energy expenditure. This is engineered by the delicate balance between cellular proliferation and death. The *Bcl-2* gene exists in progenitor and long-lived cells and appears to have a key function in the cells of the developing embryo. The gene appears to prevent oxidative damage to cellular organelles and lipid membranes. Studies have demonstrated that *Bcl-2* protects cells from the toxicity of H_2O_2 or t-butyl hydroperoxide in a dose-dependent manner (Hockenberry, Otlvai, Yin, Milliman, & Korsmeyer, 1993; Kane et al., 1993). *Bcl-2* deficient mice demonstrate changes expected of more rapid cell death, including fulminant lymphoid apoptosis of systemic organs (Korsmeyer, Yin, Oltvai, Veis-Novack, & Linette, 1995). *Bcl-2* also inhibits other types of apoptotic cell death, implying a common mechanism of lethality. Moreover, studies have demonstrated that *Bcl-2* protects

cells from H_2O_2 and menadione-induced oxidative deaths (Hockenberry, Oltvai, Yin, Milliman, & Korsmeyer, 1993; Oltvai, Milliman, & Korsmeyer, 1993). Another protein that appears to operate as an accessory to *Bcl-2*, is a 21 kd protein referred to as *Bax*. In experiments by Hockenberry and colleagues, the suggested model of the ratio between *Bcl-2* and *Bax* appears to determine survival or death following an apoptotic stimulus. Specifically, elevated expression of *Bcl-2* appears to be preventative, whereas that of *Bax* favors the apoptotic process. It is intriguing to realize that a trigger for the *Bax* gene is the ROS (Moon et al., 2002).

Lastly, the membrane hypothesis of aging, also known as the mitochondrial clock theory of aging, states that senescence is related to decreasing effectiveness of cellular protective and reparative mechanisms. This yields biochemical and metabolic errors, which progressively accumulate resulting in cell death (Sohal & Allen, 1985). The membrane hypothesis of aging (MHA) further postulates that cellular senescence is attributable to cross linking action of free oxygen radicals within the cellular membrane. Additionally, ROS lead to lipid peroxidation, polysaccharide depolymerization, nucleic acid disruption, and oxidation of sulfhydryl groups with subsequent enzyme inactivation (Southorn & Powis, 1988). Therefore, the MHA suggests that ROS induced cell membrane structural damage is the primary mediator in cellular aging (Zs-Nagy & Semsei, 1984; Zs-Nagy, Cutter, & Semsei, 1988).

Careful analysis of the above mechanisms suggests that certain aspects of the three leading theories of aging may be interrelated. In all three, free radical species lead to genetic and cellular alterations resulting in cellular dysfunction, and consequently senescence, or perhaps, in the ear, presbycusis. Specifically, the generation of ROS damages cellular integrity, which in turn may lead to alterations in gene expression including telomere shortening and activation of *Bax* genes resulting in apoptosis and aging. Potentially, treatments aimed at reducing the production of ROS could be used to decelerate the effects of aging, including presbycusis.

Diet

Essential Omega Fatty Acids (Fish Oil)

The typical American diet contains suboptimal amounts of vitamin D, E, fruits, vegetables, nuts, seeds, and omega-3 fatty acids, such as fish oil. Fast foods and other unhealthy meal habits are not that uncommon and significantly increase the amount of omega-6 fatty acids that are consumed. A proper diet (the Mediterranean diet best emulates our needs) should provide a ratio of omega six (n-6) to omega three (n-3) fatty acids of 2.3:1. This recommended ratio translates to 6.7 g n-6 and 2.9 g n-3 fatty acids per day in a 2000 kcal (8360 kJ) diet. Moreover, additional health benefits can be conferred upon patients if the ratio approaches 0.3:1. The typical American diet is out of balance with upper ratios reaching 25:1 and an average of 9.8:1 (Gao, Wilde, Lichtenstein, Bermudez, & Tucker, 2006; Holick & Chen, 2008; Kris-Etherton et al., 2000; Raper, Cronin, & Exler, 1992).

A proinflammatory state can result if there is an imbalance in the omega six versus three ratio. Prostaglandin E2 (PGE2) and leukotriene A4 (LTA4) are the common pro-inflammatory eicosanoids. Prostaglandin E3 (PGE3), thromboxanes and leukotriene A5 (LTA5) are the common anti-inflammatory eicosanoids. If omega-6 (i.e., linoleic acid and gamma linolenic acid) fatty acids predominate in the phospholipid structure of the cell, then inflammation may result. A balance between omega six and three is important to avoid shunting the eicosanoid pathway to a pro-inflammatory state (Maroon & Bost, 2006).

Caloric Restriction

Dietary restraint and antioxidants have been shown to possess health benefits and extend lifespan in numerous species. Mechanisms likely involved include maintaining a healthier microvascular supply, reduced formation of ROS, and ultimate slowing of the mitochondrial clock. From an otologic standpoint, long-term caloric restriction of 30% in rats maintains acute auditory sensitivities and minimizes the quantity of mtDNA deletions and outer hair cell loss. Mean auditory thresholds are at least 25 dB more acute than the placebo group over a 2½ octave high-frequency bandwidth. Antioxidant treated rats (vitamin E, C, melatonin) have improved auditory thresholds and fewer mtDNA deletions. The beneficial effect is partial and not as marked as with caloric restriction. In comparison, placebo subjects have worse auditory sensitivities, similar to human presbycusis patterns, and significantly more deletions and outer hair cell loss (Seidman, 2000).

Recent studies in our laboratory have focused on the effects of grape seed extracts, namely resveratrol, which demonstrate promise in reducing bioinflammation, reducing the generation of reactive oxygen species, and maintaining optimum mitochondrial function.

Physiologic improvements have been observed in cognitive ability, activity levels and auditory sensitivity in the animal model. It is believed that resveratrol and grape seed extracts may exert these effects via multiple biochemical pathways and they may also have caloric restriction mimetic activity (Seidman, Babu, Tang, Emad & Quirk, 2003; Seidman et al., in preparation).

Micronutrients (Vitamins and Minerals)

Busy young women, men working in manual labor, the widowed elderly, and the poor are just a few examples of people who may not realize that their diet is most likely inadequate. The World Health Organization estimates that micronutrient deficiencies affect 2.2 billion people. The quality of soil plays a significant role in the concentration of micronutrients in food. It has been suggested that a significant number of older adults fail to get amounts and types of food to meet essential energy and nutrient needs (Cid-Ruzafa, Caulfield, Barron, & West, 1999). Furthermore, deficiencies of vitamins and minerals are predicted to affect ~1/3 of all adults over the age of 65 (Chandra, 1997) and inadequate vitamin intake has been linked to chronic heart disease, cancer, and osteoporosis (Fairfield & Fletcher, 2002; Fletcher & Fairfield, 2002). Mitochondria are abundant in the cochlea; hence, balanced nutrition is extremely important when attempting to maximize mitochondrial health as the nervous system and its sensory organs undergo the physiologic changes associated with aging.

Allopathic physicians rarely review the diet and antioxidant supplementation of patients in any relevant depth (Seaman, 2002), a practice that probably reflects the lack of emphasis given nutrition in medical school and residency training. This is a lost opportunity for educating a patient about health and wellness. In the authors' clinical experience, patients who are specifically asked about their diets rarely report eating three to five servings of fruits and vegetables per day but rather average one or less servings. It has been estimated that the 95% of Americans have less than one helping of fruit or vegetables each day. Su and Arab (2006) examined the relationship between daily salad and raw vegetable consumption, select serum micronutrient levels, and adequate dietary intake in 9,406 women and 8,282 men aged 18 to 45 years and older than 55 years. Those who enjoyed salads, raw vegetables, and salad dressing had above-median levels of folic acid, vitamins C and E, lycopene, and alpha and beta carotene. Salad consumers also had a higher likelihood of meeting the vitamin C recommended daily allowance. These outcomes suggest that the nutrients in salad are well absorbed. The intake of the d-alpha-tocopherol form of vitamin E falls below standard recommendations in 90% of men and women in the United States (Ahuja, Goldman, & Moshfegh, 2004; Maras et al., 2004). Recall that there are several components of vitamin E and all have some importance including the mixed tocotrienols. Patients should be encouraged to increase their intake of green leafy vegetables, fresh fruits, whole grains, and nuts for the purposes of increasing not only multivitamin and mineral intake but also total antioxidant reserve. Overloading on a particular vitamin, mineral, antioxidant or oil is not recommended as toxicity may result. Moreover, synergism is known to exist amongst several antioxidants (i.e., alpha-lipoic acid and acetyl-L-carnitine) and dietary intake of balanced food groups likely possesses additional health benefits that no single oral supplement can provide. A balanced diet and oral supplement regimen offer patients the best chance of obtaining all of the required macro and micronutrients while keeping antioxidant status high.

Doctors are in a prime position to inquire and briefly review the dietary habits and supplement use of patients. The goal of such an intervention should be to educate patients on the potential benefits of multivitamins and chelated minerals (minerals bonded to an amino acid for marketedly enhanced absorption, i.e., calcium bis-glycinate citrate, or citrate malate instead of calcium carbonate), essential fatty acids, mitochondrial enhancers/antioxidants, exercise, sleep, and hormones when indicated for general health and wellness. Patients will also appreciate learning about more specific health benefits of nutraceuticals such as: anti-inflammatory and analgesic properties; synergistic anti-cancer and otoneuroprotective effects; anti-fatigue and mood enhancing effects; known safety and mild side effect profiles; and any pertinent research in progress. After initial counseling is delivered by the physician, nutritionists, pharmacists and nurses can render additional care regarding dietary modifications, balancing and optimizing nutritional supplementation and monitoring outcomes. Although patients may choose complementary and integrative physicians to join the treatment team, otolaryngologists can make more specific recommendations according to the current body of research on otoneuroprotection.

Multivitamins and Minerals

Vitamins and minerals are essential for numerous body functions including the immune system, neurotransmitter production, and neural integrity. The B complex vitamins, especially folate (vitamin B9), and cobalamin (vitamin B12), are particularly important for hearing health as levels have been shown to be significantly lower in elderly women with hearing impairment (Houston et al., 1999). The following nutrients are necessary to support health and wellness: vitamin B complex including: B1 thiamine, B2 riboflavin, B3 niacin, B5 pantothenic acid, B6 pyridoxine, B12 cyanocobalamin and/or methycobalamin, biotin, choline, folic acid, beta-carotene (vitamin A precursor), vitamin C, vitamin D, and vitamin E. Important minerals include calcium, iodine, magnesium, zinc, selenium, copper, manganese, chromium, molybdenum, boron, and potassium. Serology is available for these vitamin levels.

According to the National Health and Nutrition Examination Surveys (NHANES), the diet of many Americans is insufficient to provide adequate intake of all the recommended vitamins and minerals. Some common vitamin deficiencies in the United States include iron, vitamin D, C, and E, calcium, magnesium, zinc, pyridoxine (vitamin B6), folate, and biotin. Vitamin C levels are reduced in smokers (Ames, 2006). Supplementing with a multivitamin is easier than dietary modification for many people. Patients typically are supplementing with over the counter multivitamins. Some of these preparations may have suboptimal bioavailability and absorption characteristics, which may reduce health benefits. One such example is a lack of mineral chelation in most general formulae. Investing in a multivitamin formula that features chelated minerals is a wise alternative (i.e., calcium citrate vs. calcium carbonate or zinc monomethionate amino acid chelate instead of zinc sulfate). Side effects may also be lessened with chelated preparations. For example, the use of iron bisglycinate reduces constipation compared to the more common ferrous sulfate.

Vitamins A, C, and E plus magnesium have been proven to act synergistically to protect hearing in guinea pigs exposed to 4 kHz, 120 dB SPL, and 5 h octave-band noise. Otoprotective effects were observed with antioxidant pretreatment initiated just 1 hour prior to the onset of the noise trauma (Le Prell, Hughes & Miller, 2007).

Polypharmacy

There is an interesting direct effect of chronic prescription medication use that is often overlooked, namely, micronutrient depletion. Many commonly prescribed prescription medications (thiazide loop diuretics, statins, corticosteroids, proton-pump inhibitors, oral contraceptives, aspirin, and other medications) deplete the body of certain micronutrients such as zinc, magnesium, vitamin C, B vitamins, potassium, calcium, phosphorus, sodium, iron, co-enzyme Q10, and others, thus potentially compromising health.

Micronutrient deficiencies are more common in the elderly, pregnant and lactating women, infants, adolescents, dieters, anorexics, bulimics, and those abusing tobacco or alcohol. Chronic medication use and/or polypharmacy increase the risk for micronutrient deficiency. Blood levels of suspected micronutrient deficiencies may be followed and dietary modifications and supplementation implemented accordingly.

One key question doctors might start asking themselves while obtaining a patient history is "What are the micro-nutrients at risk for depletion in my particular patient based on the medication list?" The following texts can help: *Drug-Induced Nutrient Depletion Handbook* from Lexi-Comp's Clinical Reference Library (written by a panel of pharmacists and updated annually); *The Nutritional Cost of Prescription Drugs: How To Maintain Good Nutrition While Using Prescription Drugs* by Ross Pelton, R.Ph. and James B. LaValle, R.Ph. (Morton Publishing; 2000); and *Natural Medicines Comprehensive Database* (http://www.naturaldatabase.com), edited and updated annually in print and online by Jeff Jellin, Pharm.D, and Phil Gregory.

Smoking and Antioxidant Status

Cigarette smoking remains a significant health hazard despite worldwide efforts to educate people about the carcinogenic effects of nicotine, benzene, carbon monoxide, and other toxic aromatic amines in tobacco. Smokers have lower circulating antioxidant levels in their blood and may be deficient in vitamin C and provitamin A carotenoids. The most commonly studied antioxidants in this patient subset include vitamin A, C, E, selenium, and zinc (Alberg, 2002; Alberg et al., 2000). If a smoker is found to have presbycusis, consideration for increasing antioxidant defenses should be discussed. There are many vitamins and nutraceuticals that potentially promote health in smokers but one exception is beta carotene (precursor to vitamin A). Although an excellent antioxidant, clinical trials have demonstrated an increased risk of lung cancer in male smokers or asbestos-exposed persons who supplement with beta carotene at pharmacologic levels (Albanes et al., 1996; Greenwald, Anderson, Nelson, & Taylor, 2007; Heinonen, Huttunen, & Albanes, 1994).

Pycnogenol®

Cigarette filters inefficiently retain significant quantities of harmful toxins such as polycyclic aromatic hydrocarbons, heterocyclic amines and reactive oxygen species. Zhang et al. (2002) investigated whether the addition of pine bark to filters could neutralize free radicals and reduce adverse health risks. In a dose-dependent manner, Pycnogenol® (French maritime pine bark extract), a complex of approximately 40 water-soluble natural plant flavonoids, reduced acute toxicity by 70% and mutagenicity by 48% in rodents exposed to smoke for over 2 months. See Rohdewald (2002) for a comprehensive review of Pycnogenol® studies including mechanisms and potential therapeutic applications.

Quercetin

Quercetin is a flavonoid compound which is being studied as possibly giving some protective effect against the deleterious effects of smoking. This strong antioxidant prevents the oxidation of low-density lipoprotein (LDL cholesterol). It is found in a wide variety of fruits and vegetables, including onions, apples, kale, green tea, red cabbage, tomatoes, green beans, lettuce, grapes, potatoes, and green tea (Seidman & Moneysmith, 2006). Quercetin is not carcinogenic in humans (Okamoto, 2005).

Quercetin protects against the ill effects of the pro-oxidant nicotine in rats by modulating the extent of lipid peroxidation, augmenting antioxidant defenses

and reducing the extent of DNA damage. The protective effect of intragastric administered quercetin against nicotine-induced lung toxicity (2.5 mg/kg body weight subcutaneous nicotine injection, 5 days a week × 22 weeks) was compared with N-acetylcysteine (NAC), a potent antioxidant (Muthukumaran, Sudheer, Menon, & Nalini, 2008). Nicotine-induced antioxidant imbalance in circulation, lung, liver, and kidney of experimental male albino rats was assessed. Rats in the experimental nicotine group lost weight, whereas quercetin-treated rats gained weight despite nicotine exposure. Indicators of lipid peroxidation (i.e., thiobarbituric acid reactive substances, hydroperoxides, nitric oxide) were increased significantly in the nicotine-treated group and quercetin treatment reduced these pro-oxidant levels to near normal levels. Endogenous antioxidant status, as determined by levels of superoxide dismutase, catalase, glutathione peroxidase and reduced glutathione, was found to be significantly decreased in the nicotine-treated group and significantly increased in the quercetin treated groups. Quercetin also reduced the degree of DNA damage, as evaluated by comet assay, in the blood of the treated rats. Quercetin protected the blood, lung, liver, and kidneys of the rats against nicotine toxicity. The protective effects were comparable to those of N-acetylcysteine. Additional research on quercetin is in progress in the areas of allergies, cancer, inflammation, and cardiovascular disease.

Although no specific studies on quercetin and hearing protection have been conducted, this flavonoid has the ability to scavenge toxic reactive oxygen metabolites induced by nicotine. Many patients seen in the clinics, and especially the Veteran's Administration, continue to smoke against medical advice. These patients might welcome an oral supplement like quercetin, and possibly other synergistic antioxidants, to help the body fight against the toxins in tobacco such as benzene and carbon monoxide which are known to induce cochlear ischemia via vasoconstriction and release of free radicals.

Several other antioxidants have been studied and found to be protective against nicotine toxicity. Green tea polyphenol (epigallocatechin gallate, EGCG) suppresses inflammation, proliferation and angiogenesis in human bronchial epithelial cells exposed to cigarette smoke by inhibiting nuclear factor-kappa B (NFkB). NFkB controls the transcription of immune and inflammatory response genes (Syed et al., 2007).

Resveratrol (grape seed extract) protects against tobacco induced endothelial junction disruption and increased endothelial permeability in human pulmonary artery endothelial cells subjected to second-hand smoke (Low, Liang, & Fu, 2007).

Findings such as these are very encouraging as the prevalence of smoking remains high around the world and the carcinogenic effects of tobacco have been well described. Theoretically, the vasoconstriction that results from nicotine could diminish blood supply through the auditory/labyrinthine artery, trigger the release of ROS, and eventually hasten mitochondrial damage to the outer and inner hair cells, spiral ganglion and stria vascularis. Supporting this theory, it has been noted that the risk for accelerated hearing decline at 4000 Hz is increased in those who smoke and endure chronic daily occupational noise (Pouryaghoub, Mehrdad, & Mohammadi, 2007). Smoking dramatically increased the percentage of high-frequency sensorineural hearing loss (SNHL) in occupational noise-exposed workers by 45%. Patients who present with hearing concerns who decide to persist with their tobacco abuse should be fully educated regarding the potential otoprotective effects of select nutraceuticals under current study. The addition of tobacco to chronic noise exposure may render the otoprotective effects of certain compounds, in particular, NMDA glutamate antagonists, less effective or ineffective, thus reinforcing the need for patients to refrain from compounding the toxic effects of noise with tobacco (Chen, Kong, Reinhard, & Fechter, 2001). In the future, it is probable that several natural compounds will show pronounced activity in boosting the human body's defenses against tobacco-induced ROS formation and DNA damage.

These substances may be otoprotective in the absence of tobacco exposure as well. Animal studies using mitochondrial enhancers such as Co-Q10 (ubiquinone), resveratrol (grape seed extract), alpha lipoic acid, acetyl-L-carnitine, N-acetyl cysteine, and others have elucidated that the aging deletion and/or markers of free radical damage at the cochlear hair cell level can be significantly reduced when such enhancers are used (Coleman et al., 2007; Le & Keithley, 2007; Seidman et al., 2004; Seidman, in preparation).

Ototoxicity

Aminoglycosides are necessary to save lives of patients with multidrug resistant infections such as sepsis, pneumonia, and meningitis. Because the use of ototoxic medications is unavoidable in certain life-threatening situations, there is an urgent need to improve our understanding and willingness to use otoprotective and synergistic antioxidants to help counteract the toxic effects of life-saving antibiotics or chemotherapy. It is not common practice at this time for infectious disease specialists to augment the use of aminoglycosides with potent synergistic antioxidants, some of which also have antimicrobial action, for the purposes of reducing the risk of ototoxicity and nephro-toxicity. More studies in this arena are needed with particular emphasis on the ability of certain high-ORAC value (oxygen radical scavenging activity) nutraceuticals to prevent decline in otoacoustic emissions and audiometric thresholds during the course of ototoxic medication use (Baloh & Honrubia, 2001; Khan, Seidman, Quirk, & Shivapuja, 2000; Segal, Harris, Kustova, Basile, & Skolnick, 1999; Seidman, 1998).

The aminoglycosides and cisplatin chemotherapy are nephrotoxic and ototoxic. Certain aminoglycosides are more ototoxic than vestibulotoxic. Kanamycin and amikacin are primarily auditory toxic and gentamicin and streptomycin are the most vestibulotoxic. Despite using therapeutic doses guided by peak and trough monitoring, gentamicin can result in permanent bilateral vestibular loss presenting as disequilibrium, oscillopsia, increased risk of falls, hearing impairment and tinnitus. Hence, there is no predictable "safe dose" of gentamicin (Black, Pesznecker, & Stallings, 2004). Tobramycin is equally toxic to hearing and balance organs (Baloh & Honrubia, 2001). With the use of these agents, outer hair cells in the basal turn of the cochlea are injured resulting in high-frequency sensorineural hearing loss. Reactive oxygen species are generated and cascades of cell death and lipid oxidation reactions are activated (Rybak, 2007; Rybak & Ramkumar, 2007). Antioxidant enzyme activity is lower in guinea pigs exposed to amikacin, result-

ing in hearing loss (Klemens et al., 2003). The common mechanism of both ototoxic as well as noise-induced hair cell degeneration is the activation of caspase enzymes (Cheng et al., 2005).

N-methyl-D-aspartate (NMDA) antagonism of the excitatory glutamate receptor is otoprotective against aminoglycosides in animals (Baloh & Honrubia, 2001; Segal, Harris, Kustova, Basile, & Skolnick, 1999). Prescription medications that selectively inhibit NMDA receptors in an uncompetitive, voltage-dependent manner are now commercially available and FDA approved for dementia of the Alzheimer's type and alcohol abuse. Examples of these new NMDA antagonists include Namenda (memantine HCL) and Campral (acamprosate). Older examples include dextromethorphan and amantadine.

Essential oils are important components of a well-balanced nutritional supplement regimen and contain mechanisms that may translate into otoprotection. Linalool, a monoterpene component of essential fatty acids, possesses anticonvulsant properties. Research suggests that this anticonvulsant action of linalool is due to a direct, dose-dependent, noncompetitive inhibition at the NMDA receptor complex (Brum, Elisabetsky, & Souza, 2001). Other than studies on lecithin and presbyacusis, no studies have yet looked into possible protection from ototoxicity by the use of essential fatty acids (Seidman, Khan, Tang, & Quirk, 2002). If the other fatty acids also possess NMDA receptor antagonism, it is possible that these nutrients could provide some otoprotection by preventing glutamate excitotoxicity in the cochlea. Those undergoing treatment for life-threatening infections with ototoxic antibiotics may benefit from special attention paid to the essential oils composition in their total parenteral nutrition.

Patients undergoing chemotherapy will also benefit from careful consideration of nutraceuticals (botanical antioxidants) known to possess sensitizing and synergistic chemotherapeutic properties. Two such examples include the recent findings that resveratrol adds to the growth inhibitory/anticancer activity of cisplatin and doxorubicin in vitro and that resveratrol enhances the beneficial effects of ionizing radiation against cancer cells (Reagan-Shaw, Mukhtar, & Ahmad, 2008; Rezk, Balulad, Keller, & Bennett, 2006).

Antioxidants studied to date do not interfere with the serum levels of aminoglycosides. Antioxidants work synergistically with each other and with certain antibiotics. In the clinics or on the wards, synergism may allow for a reduction in the daily therapeutic dose of a given ototoxic medication. Treatment strategies that have been proven effective in animals will need to be reproduced in humans. Aqueous otoprotective solutions will be necessary for parenteral use in the hospital, outpatient infusion center or surgical center. The potential for hearing and balance preservation, in addition to antimicrobial synergism and anti-cancer properties, should be sufficient motivation to inspire private and public funding for more translational research into otoprotection and nutraceuticals.

Aspirin

Aspirin is a common salicylate anti-inflammatory that can induce tinnitus and hearing loss at high doses (Boettcher & Salvi, 1991), but, paradoxically, it recently has been shown to offer protection against aminoglycoside ototoxicity. A randomized, double-blind placebo controlled trial in humans receiving gentamicin for acute infections showed that aspirin protected against hearing loss without affecting serum levels of gentamicin or treatment course. Total gentamicin doses were approximately 1000 mg in each group (80–160 mg IV bid). Only 3% of the patients treated with 1 gram of aspirin three times a day for 2 weeks suffered significant hearing loss defined as greater than 15 dB threshold shift at 6 and 8 kHz versus 13% of those taking gentamicin without aspirin. Additionally, in the placebo group, the majority of the threshold shifts were 15 to 25 dB. The hearing loss was subclinical, indicating that the patients did not perceive any obvious subjective sensation or handicap from the high-frequency hearing loss. Tinnitus was not observed as a side effect in any of the patients in either group. Vestibular side effects were noted in only two patients; calorics and quantitative rotational chair studies were not undertaken (Chen et al., 2007).

Aspirin may also demonstrate some otoprotective effects against cisplatin. In albino guinea pigs, the antioxidant properties of subcutaneous aspirin administered 90 minutes before cisplatin exposure delivered partial protection to the outer hair cells (Hyppolito, de Oliveira, & Rossato, 2006).

Aspirin is not considered a nutraceutical as it is not derived from food. The nutraceuticals featured below likely have anti-inflammatory action without the long-term risk of gastritis or gastric ulcers that may be associated with aspirin use.

Magnolia Bark

Magnolia officinalis bark comes from the Magnolia tree in the mountains of China and Japan and has been used medicinally since 100 AD. Studies in animals have shown that the bark extract possess anxiolytic, muscle relaxant, anti-allergic, anti-asthmatic properties, anti-angiogenic, anti-invasive, and anti-proliferogenic activity against certain cancers (Tse, Wan, Shen, Yang, & Fong, 2005). It also increases hippocampal acetylcholine release in rats (Hou, Chao, & Chen, 2000). In cells deprived of glucose, two components of this bark, honokiol and magnolol, proved to be neuroprotective against glutamate excitotoxicity and hydrogen peroxide-induced mitochondrial injury, suggesting that both compounds may favorably impact neurodegenerative diseases. Honokiol was more specific and potent than magnolol at protecting mitochondria from glutamate excitotoxicity at the NMDA receptor (Lin, Chen, Ko, & Chan, 2005; 2006).

Honokiol and magnolol (a honokiol isomer) were studied in rat heart mitochondria after treatment with agents that induced lipid peroxidation. Adenosine diphosphate (ADP) and ferrous sulfate (FeSO4) were used to induce injury, whereas oxygen consumption and malondialdehyde (MDA) production served as markers to quantitate lipid peroxidation. The two bark extracts were found to have antioxidant activity 1000 times higher than alpha-tocopherol (Lo, Teng, Chen, Chen, & Hong, 1994).

Recent investigations into the anti-inflammatory, anti-angiogenesis, and anti-metastatic action of honokiol and magnolol reveal that it suppresses the nuclear transcription factor nuclear factor-kappa B (NF-kB) activation and gene regulation via IKappaB kinase. Honokiol also down regulates the expression of COX-2, metalloproteinase 9 (MMP-9), intercellular adhesion molecule (ICAM-1), and other inflammatory and carcinogenic gene products (Tse et al., 2005; Tse et al., 2007).

Magnolia bark extracts are commercially available and appear safe in humans for short-term use. Safety when using the bark longer than 6 weeks is unknown.

The supplement should be avoided during pregnancy and lactation. Sleepiness and drowsiness are potential side effects, especially when use is combined with alcohol, barbiturates, benzodiazepines, and other central nervous system depressants, or when magnolia is taken in large doses. Supplemental dosage range is 250 to 750 mg/day of 1 to 2% standardized honokiol and magnolol extract (NMCD, http://www.naturaldatabase.com, retrieved December 30, 2007).

The NMDA glutamate antagonistic and antioxidant properties of magnolia are very interesting as glutamate excitotoxicity is one mechanism of cell death in stroke, Alzheimer's, spinal cord ischemia, retinal ischemia, glaucoma, epilepsy, ototoxicity, noise-induced hearing loss, and possibly presbycusis. Otoprotection against noise may be possible using glutamate antagonists in the future, as preliminary evidence shows that selective NMDA blockers favorably impact hearing under noise conditions (Khan, Seidman, Quirk, & Shivapuja, 2000; Puel, Pujol, Tribillac, Ladrech, & Eybalinj, 1994). It is plausible that nutraceuticals possessing the ability to inhibit excessive calcium influx via selective and voltage-dependent NMDA receptor blockade may play a therapeutic role in ototoxicity, presbycusis, and noise-induced hearing loss.

D-Methionine

D-methionine is an essential amino acid containing sulfur and is found in animal protein. Protein synthesis and methylation of DNA and RNA depend on methionine metabolism. Over the past 10 years, oral methionine has been shown to be an excellent otoprotectant to the stria vascularis and the outer hair cells of the rat cochlea exposed to amikacin, gentamicin, carboplatin, and cisplatin. Outer hair cell and stria vascularis protection is achieved even at low doses and cochlear antioxidant enzyme levels are maintained with D-methionine. There is an added benefit of increased life span, weight preservation in rats, and, most importantly, no diminution of chemotherapeutic action or alteration of serum aminoglycoside levels (Campbell et al., 2007; Campbell, Meech, Rybak & Hughes, 2003; Campbell, Rybak, Meech & Hughes, 1996). Oral, round window, and intraperitoneal administration of D-methionine in chinchilla and rats 30 to 120 minutes before receiving an infusion of 16 mg/kg cisplatin confers virtually complete otoprotection—less than 10-dB threshold shifts and less than 10% loss of outer hair cells. The controls suffer marked, diffuse outer hair cell damage and threshold changes greater than 60 dB. Of particular note for future clinical applications, the oral intake of D-met is equally as effective as the intraperitoneal administration (Campbell et al., 2007; Korver, Rybak, Whitworth, & Campbell, 2002).

Methionine is safe for treating acetaminophen poisoning under medical direction. Intake of methionine above levels found in food may be unsafe as it causes increased levels of homocysteine, a cardiac and stroke risk factor. The supplement is contraindicated in pregnancy, lactation, atherosclerosis, cancer, and the genetic disorder methylenetetrahydrofolate reductase deficiency. There are no known interactions with medications. The dosage used for acetaminophen poisoning to prevent hepatoxicity and death is 2.5 grams every 4 hours for four doses. Oral supplement methionine dose is 120 to 1600 mg per day (NMCD, www.natural database.com, retrieved January 3, 2008). Caution is advised with L-methionine, which is readily available over the counter, as this isomer may be hazardous for those with ovarian cancer (Kathleen Campbell, personal communication, 2008).

Glutathione

Glutathione plays a key role in antioxidant and detoxification reactions in the cell and is found in fruits, vegetables, and meats. It is involved in DNA synthesis and repair, prevention of oxidative cell damage, metabolism of toxins and carcinogens, immune system function, protein and prostaglandin synthesis, amino acid transport, and enzyme activation. N-acetylcysteine is converted to glutathione in the liver. Glutathione ethyl ester (GSH) is more bio-available than glutathione. GSH ester offers protection to outer hair cells in rats against cisplatin but protection is not as robust as D-methionine and the effect wanes as dose is increased (Campbell, Larsen, Meech, Rybak, & Hughes, 2003).

The effect of glutathione cotherapy in guinea pigs exposed to gentamicin toxicity has been studied. In the test group, glutathione was administered via gastric lavage immediately prior to gentamicin injection. In the control group, progressive hearing loss was detected via auditory brainstem responses. Glutathione treatment slowed the progression of hearing loss and attenuated the hearing loss by up to 40 dB. Morphologically, the hair cells were preserved to a greater degree with glutathione treatment, and the antioxidant did not reduce the antimicrobial action of the gentamicin against *Staphylococcus aureus* and *Pseudomonas aeruginosa*.

Glutathione is safe for most adults. Potential side effects and medication interactions remain unknown. The antioxidant is contraindicated in pregnancy and lactation, and asthmatics should not inhale glutathione. The oral supplemental dose of L-glutathione ranges between 30 to 600 mg/day with typical doses of 50 to 250 mg per day. Inhalational, intramuscular, and intravenous forms are also in use. The glutathione precursor, N-acetylcysteine, may be more bio-available, as it appears that glutathione may be inactivated by peptidases in the gastrointestinal tract (NMCD, http://www.naturaldatabase.com, retrieved January 30, 2008).

N-Acetylcysteine

Feldman et al. (2007) researched the otoprotective potential of N-acetylcysteine (NAC), a potent antioxidant and amino acid L-cysteine derivative that crosses cell membranes, against gentamicin-induced ototoxicity. This randomized human study involved 40 patients receiving gentamicin for bacteremia associated with dialysis catheterization. Patients received the antibiotic with or without NAC. Both 1 and 6 weeks after completing gentamicin therapy, bilateral ototoxicity was significantly more prevalent in the control group. In those exposed to gentamicin with NAC, the most significant degree of otoprotection was observed in the higher frequencies. (See additional discussion of NAC under the noise-induced hearing loss section.)

Presbycusis

Presbycusis is defined as the progressive bilateral hearing loss of biological aging involving inherited processes resulting in the gradual accumulation of DNA errors and abnormal mechanisms of repair. In his classic paper, which expanded on the previous work of Crowe, Guild and Polvogt published in 1934, Schuknecht described his observations on the otopathology of four types of presbycusis:

sensory, neural, strial (metabolic), and cochlear conductive (mechanical) cited a human temporal bone study of 21 patients with downward sloping audiograms to determine patterns of cochlear structure degeneration. Using strict audiometric criteria and quantitative histopathologic (Gacek & Schuknecht, 1969; Schuknecht, 1964). Later, Schuknecht and Gacek (1993) described two additional categories of presbycusis, namely mixed and indeterminate presbycusis. Mixed included a fusion of morphologic findings and indeterminate was devoid of consistent morphology with a flat or abrupt high-frequency loss possibly secondary to cellular dysfunction rather than cell death. Nelson and Hinojosa (2006) conducted a human temporal bone study of 21 patients with downward sloping audiograms to determine patterns of cochlear degeneration. Using strict audiometric criteria and quantitative histopathologic methods, they found hair cell and ganglion cell loss in all patients. Inner hair cell loss was seen in 18 and stria vascularis loss in 10 patients. Degree of degeneration was correlated with severity of hearing loss and ganglion cell loss was correlated with audiometric slope.

Compelling evidence supports the idea that several metabolic processes underlie presbycusis in addition to structural changes at the cochlear hair cell, supporting cell, ganglion, and eighth nerve level. Such otoneurodegenerative mechanisms include: ROS generation secondary to prolonged relative microhypoperfusion to the cochlea, lipid peroxidation, generation of mtDNA deletions secondary to the chronic ROS insult, cellular and tissue dysfunction (mitochondrial overdrive), senescence, and cascading apoptotic and necrotic events leading to cell death. The same mechanisms likely apply to the cochlea stressed by acute or chronic noise with subsequent mito-chondrial overdrive, glutamate excito-toxicity, and ischemia/reperfusion injury, all three of which lead to generation of ROS, DNA and protein damage, lipid peroxidation, and, ultimately, loss of co-chlear structure and function (Henderson, Bielefeld, Harris, & Hu, 2006; Jiang, Talaska, Schacht, & Sha, 2007; Seidman, 2000; Seid-man, Khan, Bai, Shirwany, & Quirk, 2000). The authors believe that the membrane hypothesis of aging (MHA), or "mito-chondrial clock theory of aging," is no longer a theory, as there has been signif-icant basic science research to validate this effect. Thus, optimizing mitochondrial health, in addition to using appropriate ear protection and living a healthy lifestyle, may confer more resilient structure and function at the level of the cochlea, eighth nerve, brainstem, and cerebral cortex.

Supplementation with a balanced regi-men of vitamins, minerals, essential oils, antioxidants, and mitochondrial enhancers may prove to be an exciting strategy for people interested in preserving their hearing. If these nutritional supplements continue to prove successful in more ani-mal and human studies, the need for hear-ing amplification might be delayed or even forestalled in certain subsets of patients. Moreover, additional health ben-efits will likely be conferred outside of hearing health. The following nutraceuti-cals featured offer encouraging prelimi-nary evidence as to how cochlear vitality might be sustained throughout life.

Coenzyme Q10 (ubiquinone or ubiquinol)

Coenzyme Q10 is a vital, potent, and fat-soluble antioxidant with mitochondrial protection capabilities. The enzyme plays a key role in oxidative phosphorylation

and is the electron acceptor in complex I and II of the electron transport chain. Adenosine triphosphate (ATP) formation is dependent on coenzyme Q10. The human production of CoQ10 diminishes with age with levels starting to decrease as early as the third decade. For example, retinal lev-els of CoQ10 decline by 40% in humans between the ages of 30 and 80. Dimin-ished antioxidant reserves and a reduced rate of ATP synthesis are likely outcomes that may accelerate macular degeneration (Qu, Kaufman, & Washington, 2008).

Blood levels of coenzyme Q10 can be evaluated commercially, although ideal levels for hearing health are yet to be determined. One controlled study of early, untreated Parkinson's patients reveals that the serum levels of CoQ10 are signif-icantly lower and correlate with reduced platelet mitochondrial activity of com-plex I and complex II/III of the electron transport chain (Shults, Haas, Passov, & Beal, 1997). CoQ10 has documented potential for clinical usefulness in man-agement of the cardiac patient with car-diomyopathy, congestive heart failure, hypertension, and possibly other condi-tions including mitochondrial diseases and the adverse effects of polypharmacy. Cardiac ejection fraction can increase with CoQ10 oral supplementation from a mean of 22% up to 39% with clinical improvement corresponding to a change in New York Heart Association (NYHA) Class IV (severe) to II (mild) heart failure (Langsjoen & Langsjoen, 1999; Langsjoen, Langsjoen, Langsjoen, Willis, & Folkers, 1994). Levels thought to be ideal in those with cardiomyopathy and congestive heart failure are 2.5 micrograms/mL or greater. Current normal total serum coen-zyme Q10 reference intervals from the Laboratory Corporation of America are 0.37 to 2.20 mcg/mL.

Of particular importance is the fact that "statins" (HMG CoA reductase inhibitors responsible for the hepatic blockade of cholesterol synthesis and numerous cardiovascular health benefits) directly inhibit mevalonic acid formation and the production of CoQ10. This drug-nutrient interaction may result in lower CoQ10 levels in plasma, platelets, lymphocytes, skeletal, and cardiac muscle (Littarru & Langsjoen, 2007). Numerous studies have shown that CoQ10 levels can decrease markedly by 20 to 50% within 2 weeks in patients taking statins. Although generally well tolerated, a small percentage of patients experience statin-induced myopathy, myalgia, myoglobinuria and even rhabdomyolysis. Many more report unexplained fatigue and exercise intolerance within days to weeks of initiating statin therapy (Rundek, Naini, Sacco, Coates, & DiMauro, 2004). Fifty cardiac patients on statins for an average of 2 years experienced myalgia, fatigue, dyspnea, memory loss and peripheral neuropathy. Statin discontinuation and oral CoQ10 supplementation helped these patients overcome the adverse effects dramatically without impairing heart function or causing an increase in stroke or myocardial infarction (Langsjoen, Langsjoen, Langsjoen, & Lucas, 2005). The public and many physicians have not been widely informed of this adverse direct effect of statins on CoQ10. Due to the numerous cardiovascular benefits of statins, suggestions are being made to release lovastatin over the counter, making it more available and affordable for millions of patients at risk for stroke and cardiovascular disease (Fuster, 2007). If this outcome is realized, it will be crucial for patients to receive proper education on the direct adverse effects of statins on mitochondrial health.

Cadoni and colleagues (2007) prospectively investigated the association of idiopathic sudden sensorineural hearing loss (ISSNHL), coenzyme Q10 and cardiovascular risk factors in 30 hospitalized Italian patients and 60 controls. Main outcome measures included the evaluation of serum CoQ10 levels and cardiovascular risk factors (total cholesterol, low-density lipoprotein [LDL]), and homocysteine. The association between ISSNHL and CoQ10, total cholesterol, LDL, and HCY levels was evaluated. A significant association between ISSNHL and high total cholesterol ($p < 0.05$), high LDL ($p = 0.021$), and low CoQ10 ($p < 0.05$) levels was found. There was no significant association between ISSNHL and HCY levels. Low levels of CoQ10, high levels of total cholesterol, and LDL were found to be significantly associated with ISSNHL in the univariate analysis. In the multivariate analysis, low levels of CoQ10 and high levels of total cholesterol remained significantly associated with a high risk of sudden sensorineural hearing loss.

Angeli and colleagues (2005) assessed the otoprotective effect of CoQ10 on the hearing deficits of three patients with bilateral, nonsyndromic sensorineural hearing loss carrying the mitochondrial DNA 7445A→G mutation. Two patients (one with a familial history of hearing loss and the other sporadic) agreed to supplement with 75 mg of CoQ10 (ubiquinone) twice daily for 1 year. The third patient with familial history of hearing loss declined to participate in the study. Bone conduction pure tone thresholds from 500 to 4000 cycles/sec were obtained before and after diagnosis and CoQ10 treatment. The two cases with familial histories of hearing loss revealed marked differences in their rates of hearing progression. In the patient who did not supplement with CoQ10, hearing declined 11 dB after being diagnosed. The patient on CoQ10 did not experience any further hearing deterioration after 1 year of initiating supplementation. Prior to CoQ10 supplementation, the rate of hearing loss was 6 dB per year in the familial case who eventually decided to take the antioxidant. CoQ10-treated patients did not show any additional deterioration of their SNHL after 12 (familial case) and 13 months (sporadic case). The progression rate of SNHL was 6 dB/year in the 2 years prior to initiation of treatment in the familial case who received CoQ10 treatment. One year after being diagnosed with mitochondrial hearing loss, the patient who refused CoQ10 treatment exhibited an 11 dB deterioration of his hearing thresholds. No CoQ10 side effects were experienced. This exciting study suggests that the otoprotective potential of coenzyme Q10 may halt or significantly slow down the progression of sensorineural hearing loss associated with the mitochondrial $7445A{\rightarrow}G$ mutation and possibly other mitochondrial deletions in the future.

Shults and colleagues (2002) found that CoQ10 1200 mg/day was well tolerated and slowed the progression of Parkinson's disease in a controlled trial of 80 patients. The Unified Parkinson's Disease Rating Scale was used as the outcome measure. A larger trial in Germany using nanoparticular CoQ10 at a dosage of 300 mg did not find such neuroprotection (Storch et al., 2007). Despite the well-documented mechanisms of mitochondrial damage in neurodegenerative conditions such as Parkinson's, Huntington's, and amyotrophic lateral sclerosis (ALS, Lou Gehrig's disease), mitochondrial encephalomyopathies and cerebellar ataxias, more research is necessary to see if CoQ10 supplementation will prove effective in slowing or reversing the course of neurodegenerative diseases.

Smith and colleagues (2007) studied high dose CoQ10 in a transgenic mouse model of Huntington's disease and found that CoQ10 levels were reduced in the brains of diseased mice. Supplementation resulted in higher CoQ10 levels, improved grip strength and mobility, and a reduction in ROS markers. Moreover, less brain atrophy and Huntington inclusions and increased weight were observed in the CoQ10 treated group. Motor performance was also improved but survival was not prolonged in a study using CoQ10 and remacemide in the mouse model of Huntington's disease (Schilling, Coonfield, Ross, & Borchelt, 2001).

CoQ10 dosages in humans studied to date range between 150–3000 mcg/day. One hundred milligrams of ubiquinol is comparable to 200 mcg of ubiquinone or even more. Ubiquinol, the two-electron reduced product of ubiquinone, is more potent and is absorbed 2–8 times more than ubiquinone. The supplement is best ingested with a meal that contains some fat for increased absorption. Human Parkinson's studies used CoQ10, 2400 mg per day, combined with 1200 IU of vitamin E (d-alpha tocopherol) without any adverse effects attributed to CoQ10 (Shults, Flint Beal, Song, & Fontaine, 2004). Safety has been demonstrated for oral dosages of 300, 600, and even 1200 mg/kg for 13 weeks in rats. Neither death nor any toxicologic signs were observed in any group during the administration period. No changes in body weight, food consumption, ophthalmoscopy, hematology, blood biochemistry, necropsy, organ weights, or histopathology were detected in the toxicologic study. No deaths or signs of toxicity were observed (Honda et al., 2007). Ubiquinol studies in rats and dogs have found a no observed adverse effect level of 200 mg/kg/day in female rats, 600 mg/kg/day in male rats and more than 600 mg/kg/day in male and female dogs with no deaths reported (Kitano et al., 2008). Converting doses of study compounds from mg/kg animal body weight to mg/kg normalized for human body surface area (BSA) is the most appropriate method of extrapolating animal dosing to human dosing as suggested by the FDA (Reagan-Shaw, Nihal, & Ahmad, 2008).

Food sources of coenzyme Q10 include beef, salmon, herring, mackerel, sardines, peanuts, wheat germ, rice bran, soy oil, and organ meats. Cooking destroys concentrations of CoQ10 so food levels are typically low. Ubiquinone and ubiquinol Q10 formulations are commercially available. Dr. Frederick Crane first isolated CoQ10 from beef heart mitochondria in 1957 at the University of Washington-Madison. The chemical formula for CoQ10 was derived in 1958 by Professor Karl Folkers and colleagues at Merck. Presently, all CoQ10 is produced synthetically in Japan to exact human standards and distributed worldwide. Typical dosages range from 30 mg to 300 mg per day, whereas neurodegenerative studies report that doses up to 2400 mg per day are well tolerated by patients. Serum levels may not increase significantly at doses higher than 2400 mg/day and serum increases may be temporary despite prolonged supplementation (Hanisch & Zierz, 2003; Shults et al., 2004).

CoQ10 is well tolerated in adults and most children. Mild side effects include stomach upset, loss of appetite, nausea, vomiting, diarrhea, and allergic skin reactions. Blood pressure may be reduced so caution should be exercised in those with borderline hypotension. In those hypertensive patients on blood pressure med-

ication, it is possible that pressures may decline necessitating a reduction or discontinuation of the prescription medication. CoQ10 may decrease the effectiveness of warfarin (Coumadin) and increase clotting risk. Coumadin dosing and serology for optimum coagulation should be followed closely. Pregnant and breast feeding mothers should refrain from taking CoQ10 due to unknown effects on the fetus (NMCD, http://www.natural database.com, retrieved January 3, 2008).

Lecithin

Lecithin, a phospholipid, is a polyunsaturated phosphatidylcholine (PPC) molecule found in eggs, organ meats, legumes, wheat germ, and milk (Sanders & Zeisel, 2007). These molecules are high energy structural and functional components integral to the phospholipid bilayer of biologic membranes. They play a crucial role in cell signaling and membrane transport. The cellular content of PPC declines during the process of aging. There is mounting evidence that replacement can affect many physiologic processes. In 2002, the second author (M.D.S.) demonstrated the ability of oral PPC to improve mitochondrial membrane integrity and function and reduce age-related hearing loss significantly in rats. Threshold shifts ranged from 35 to 40 dB in the control subjects and only 13 to 17 dB in the lecithin-treated group. Lecithin preserved mitochondrial membrane potential and protected mitochondrial DNA in the stria vascularis and auditory nerve from oxidative damage. A lower ratio of the common aging deletion (mtDNA4834) to total mitochondrial DNA was detected in the experimental group (Seidman, et al., 2002).

Oral lecithin replacement increases serum choline, a precursor to the neurotransmitter acetylcholine. Choline is the precursor for PPC synthesis and is an essential nutrient. Acetylcholine and very low density lipoprotein are formed from dietary choline. Human intake of choline averages 600 mg/day for men and 450 mg/day for women. Dietary questionnaires yield lower estimates of choline intake around 250 to 500 mg/day. Choline deficiency has been associated with liver and muscle pathology, diminished learning and memory, increased risk for neural tube defects and hepatic carcinoma (Sanders & Zeisel, 2007).

Lecithin is safe for most people. Side effects include diarrhea, nausea, abdominal fullness, or pain. The phospholipid is contraindicated in pregnancy and lactation. There are no known medication interactions. Supplemental dosage range is 600-1200 mg per day, typically, with a tolerable range of 30 to 7,200 mg per day (NMCD, http://www.naturaldatabase.com, retrieved January 3, 2008).

Green Tea

Green tea is the beverage of choice in Asia and is known to confer numerous health benefits. Epigallocatechin gallate (EGCG) is the main polyphenolic, antioxidant component in green tea. In addition to free radical scavenging activity and reduction of lipid peroxidation—10 times greater than trolox, a vitamin E analogue (Zhang & Osborne, 2006), known mechanisms of EGCG action include reduction of inflammatory cytokines and mediators, reduction of NF-kappa B and AP-1 (Ahmad, Gupta, & Mukhtar, 2000; Tipoe, Leung, Hung, & Fung, 2007); protection against glutamate excitotoxicity (Fu & Koo, 2006); facilitation of presynaptic glutamate release via positive modulation of N and P/Q-type calcium channels (Chou, Huang, Tien, & Wang, 2007); signal modulation of cytochrome c, caspases, voltage-dependent anion channels and Bcl-2 (Jung et al., 2007); decreased production of matrix metalloproteinases, MMP-2 and MMP-9 (Ho, Yang, Peng, Chou, & Chang, 2007); reduction of Huntington protein aggregation (Ehrnhoefer et al., 2006); iron metal chelation at sites of neuronal degeneration, and reduction of amyloid precursor protein (Avramovich-Tirosh et al., 2007). L-theanine is thought to be the key amino acid in green tea with anxiolytic properties due to its ability to modulate GABA (A) receptor activity similar to the benzodiazepine chlordiazepoxide (Vignes et al., 2006).

Xie and colleagues (2004) conducted a controlled experiment on the otoprotective effects of EGCG on cultured in vitro spiral ganglion cells of mice concentrations. Spiral ganglion viability was decreased and apoptosis increased in the presence of H_2O_2. Manganese superoxide dismutase gene expression was up regulated with increasing H_2O_2 (2007). Interestingly, EGCG suppressed this upregulation by scavenging oxygen-free radicals and ultimately protected the cultured spiral ganglion cells.

Scientific research continues into the many remarkable anti-inflammatory and anti-cancer effects of EGCG. Green tea has the ability to inhibit the growth of oral cavity, head and neck, breast, lung, esophageal, gastric, pancreatic, hepatic, colon, prostrate, ovarian, and bladder cancer without affecting normal cells. Antiproliferation of tumor occurs via proteasome inhibition (Butt & Sultan, 2009; Dou et al., 2008; Masuda, Suzui, Lim, & Weinstein, 2003; Thangapazham, et al., 2007). Over the past 20 years, 70% of the chemotherapeutic drugs approved by the FDA have originated from nutraceuticals (Newman, Cragg, & Snader, 2003).

In vitro animal and some human clinical studies reveal many other health promoting effects of EGCG such as improved cognition, reduced LDL oxidation (Basu & Lucas, 2007); protection against ischemic retinopathy, oxidative stress-induced retinal degeneration, and ultraviolet retinal damage (Chiou, Li, & Wang, 1994; Yang, Lee, & Koh, 2007; Zhang & Osbourne, 2006; Zhang, Safa, Rusciano, & Osborne, 2007); myocardial tissue preservation after infarction (Devika & Stanely Mainzen Prince, 2008); and neuroprotection against Huntington's disease and possibly other neurodegenerative diseases like Parkinson's, Alzheimer's and amyotrophic lateral sclerosis (Avramovich-Tirosh et al., 2007). Although data are lacking in the area of cochlear hair cell and auditory nerve protection—with the exception of the spiral ganglion study—preliminary promising results from the ophthalmological and neurologic literature may serve as inspiration for more investigations into the potential otoprotective effects of green tea.

Safety data in animals reveal no genotoxic effects of EGCG and no adverse effects at dosages of 500 mg/kg/day in dogs (Isbrucker, Bausch, Edwards, & Wolz, 2006; Isbrucker, Ewards, Wolz, Davidovich, & Bausch, 2006). In human studies, reports of safety are varied. Over 10 case reports of liver injury associated with supplements containing *Camellia sinensis* (green tea) have been reported since 2003. The age of these predominantly female patients ranged from 25 to 53. Duration of exposure before symptom was 5 to 120 days. Accumulated dosage intake varied from 6 to 240 grams. Liver enzymes were abnormal. All patients recovered after ceasing intake of the green tea extract (Bronkovsky, 2006). In other studies, single oral doses up to 1600 mg are safe and well tolerated. The antioxidant is rapidly absorbed from the gut and the half-life is 1.9 to 4.6 hours (Ullmann et al., 2003, 2004). Side effects are mild and similar to placebo. Serology profiles do not reveal significant changes after drinking 8 to 16 cups of green tea daily for 4 weeks (Chow et al., 2003). A recommended daily allowance (RDA) for green tea has not been determined. If supplement capsules are preferred, a typical dose is 500 mg of standardized extract. As a beverage, four or five cups per day are recommended. White, red, and green teas contain the active EGCG antioxidant. Decaffeinated green tea is available.

Noise-Induced Hearing Loss

Noise trauma is a significant health hazard for approximately 50 million people in the United States working in machinery, manufacturing, construction, mining, commercial aviation, music, and other loud pursuits. Occupational noise is endured by an estimated 600 million people worldwide and accounts for 16% of disabling cases of hearing loss in the elderly. Military noise trauma accounts for 47% of current wartime evacuations and is the fourth leading reason for medical consultation upon the soldier's return (Kopke et al., 2007; Nelson, Nelson, Concha-Barrientos, & Fingerhut, 2005).

Moreover, tinnitus and abnormal sound sensitivity (hyperacusis) are likely associated with military noise trauma due to abnormal outer hair cell compression and amplification. The American Tinnitus Association reveals estimates that almost 50% of soldiers returning from the conflicts in Iraq and Afghanistan are reporting tinnitus. Tinnitus and hearing loss top the list of war-related health costs. According to *The Independent Budget* for the Department of Veteran Affairs—Fiscal Year 2009, a comprehensive budget and policy document created by veterans for veterans, since 2000, the number of veterans receiving service-connected disability for tinnitus has increased by at least 18% each year. The total number of veterans awarded disability compensation for tinnitus as of fiscal year 2006 surpassed 390,933. At this alarming rate, it is estimated that by 2011, there will be 818,811 veterans receiving military compensation for tinnitus, at a cost to American taxpayers of over $1.1 billion. One possible way of reducing the risk of hearing loss and tinnitus is by initiating otoprotection earlier in combination with hearing protection and rescue treatment with steroids and antioxidants within a 3-day to 6-week time window (Haynes, O'Malley, Cohen, Watford, & Labadie, 2007; LePrell, Yamashita, Minami, Yamasoba, & Miller, 2007). The aim of such intervention is to reduce discordant outer and inner hair cell damage, minimize hearing loss, and possibly prevent tinnitus from surfacing. It has been observed that tinnitus does not accompany all patients with hearing loss. The slope of the high-frequency noise notch is associated with the perception of tinnitus but tinnitus can also result from flat losses from blast trauma. The perception of tinnitus with or without hyperacusis is a growing problem for America's military personnel. It threatens their futures with potential long-term mood and sleep disruption, changes in cognitive ability, stress in relationships, and employability challenges. The Department of Veterans Affairs acknowledges that disability payments for tinnitus and hearing are increasing (Kopke et al., 2006).

Acoustic trauma causes a series of events leading to cochlear and nerve damage such as ischemic reperfusion injury, glutamate excitotoxicity with excessive calcium influx, ROS overproduction, DNA and protein damage, mitochondrial injury, lipid peroxidation, glutathione depletion, and inflammatory cascades (Henderson, Bielefeld, Harris, & Hu, 2006; Kopke et al., 2007). Numerous studies have investigated the potential mechanisms of outer, inner hair cell and cochlear nerve protection from free radical scavenger administration in animals. Human studies are underway looking into the ability of NAC either alone or in combination with acetyl-L-carnitine and other antioxidants to protect against noise-induced permanent threshold shifts (Duan et al., 2004; Kopke et al., 2006; Kopke et al., 2005).

Noise can cause increased ROS, cochlear damage, and loss of hearing through the induction of metabolic and mechanical stress, leading to apoptosis and necrosis. These stressors result in diminished cochlear blood flow, mitochondrial overdrive, glutamate and aspartate release at inner hair cell-afferent auditory nerve fiber junctions, damage to supporting structures, afferent dendrite swelling, outer hair cell and stereocilia dysfunction, and spiral ganglion neuronal death (Jager, Goiny, Herrera-Marschitz, Brundin, Fransoon, et al., 2000; Henderson et al., 2006; Miller, Brown, & Schacht, 2003; Pujol & Puel, 1999).

Four possible targets of therapeutic intervention exist, which could theoretically be of benefit: (1) ROS/antioxidant balance; (2) lipid peroxidation and sustained hair cell loss; (3) cochlear blood flow; and (4) apoptotic cell death. Although prevention remains of utmost importance, the goal is to find a practical intervention that preserves hearing after traumatic noise exposure (Henderson et al., 2006). Interestingly, cochlear "toughening" or "conditioning" effects do exist after moderate levels of noise exposure in chinchillas (i.e., 6h, 0.5 kHz octave band noise, 95 dB, 10 days) strongly suggesting an increase in antioxidant cochlear defenses that ultimately translate into 10 to 20 dB less permanent threshold shifts and hair cell damage when compared to controls receiving only high-level noise exposure without prior "conditioning" exposures (Henderson, McFadden, Liu, Hight, & Zheng, 1999). Henderson hypothesizes that the antioxidant cochlear defenses are up-regulated over time with moderate levels of "toughening" noise. He submits the possibility that "conditioning" upregulates the cochlea's antioxidant enzyme systems, thereby protecting the organ of hearing from free radical damage and metabolic stress byproducts. Threshold shifts and cochlear hair cell damage can be reduced after noise exposure when rats and/or chinchillas are treated with certain mitochondrial enhancers that increase antioxidant reserve such as D-methionine, alpha-lipoic acid, acetyl-L-carnitine, N-acetylcysteine, and resveratrol (Campbell et al., 2007; Coleman et al., 2007; Kopke, Coleman, Liu, Campbell, & Riffenburgh, 2002; Le Prell, Hughes, et al., 2007; Seidman et al., 2003).

Resveratrol
(trans-3, 4',5-trihydroxystilbene)

Resveratrol (grape seed extract) is a natural polyphenol antioxidant found in red wine, red grapes, grape juice, mulberries, peanuts, and numerous plant species. Fifty milligrams of grape seed extract is approximately equal to the resveratrol content of 75 glasses of red wine (the average glass of red wine has 640 mcg of resveratrol). This potent antioxidant possesses cardioprotective, chemopreventive, and anti-inflammatory properties (Cucciolla et al., 2007; Das & Das, 2007; Saiko, Szakmary, Jaeger, & Szekeres, 2008). Moreover, positive effects on age longevity, lipid levels, cancer prevention, and antiviral effects have been noted (Shankar, Singh, & Srivastava, 2007). Although alcohol can reduce LDL, it is the polyphenols in the grape seed that appear to have even more desirable properties. Resveratrol has the ability to promote nitric oxide production in vascular endothelium; inhibit platelet thromboxane; reduce leukotriene in neutrophils; modulate lipoprotein synthesis and secretion; promote longevity; and arrest tumor growth (i.e., neuroblastoma) and inhibit tumor initiation, promotion, and progression (Soleas, Diamandis, & Goldberg, 1997; van Ginkel et al., 2007). Various mechanisms account for these health benefits including inhibition of the synthesis and release of the following proinflammatory mediators: phospholipase, cyclo-oxygenase 1 and 2 (COX-1, COX-2), phosphodiesterase (eicosanoid synthesis), prostaglandins, activator protein-1 (AP-1), and transcription factors like nuclear factor kappaB (NFkappaB). Metabolism is via hydroxylation, glucuronidation, sulfation, and hydrogenation. Toxicity is limited at chemotherapeutic levels. Dosage range in humans is 25–200 mg per day (Das & Das, 2007; Shankar, Singh, & Srivastava, 2007; Soleas, Diamandis, & Goldberg, 1997; Draczynska-Lusiak, Chen & Sun, 1998; van Ginkel et al., 2007).

Seidman and colleagues (2003) studied the effects of resveratrol on hearing. Resveratrol proved otoprotective in 10 Fischer rats exposed to 24 hours of 105-dB noise with a bandwidth of 4500–9000 cycles/sec. Resveratrol was given via gavage for 3 weeks prior to the noise trauma and for an additional 4 weeks after the noise exposure. Normal saline (0.9% NaCl) was used for the controls. Auditory brainstem evoked responses were obtained up to 4 weeks after the noise trauma. Histologic analysis was performed. Cytocochleograms were obtained in 0.24-mm intervals along the basilar membrane. Mean outer hair cell loss was 1.3% in the control group and 0.48% in the resveratrol treatment group. Peak outer hair cell loss was 5.2% in controls from 7 to 9 kHz and 2.7% in the treated group from 7 to 8 kHz. Although both groups suffered outer hair cell damage, the loss was significantly less in the active group, especially the outer hair cells in the region between 6000 and 9000 cycles/sec, which corresponded to the region most susceptible to noise trauma. Additionally, threshold shifts in the resveratrol group were significantly less than the saline control group suggesting that resveratrol is otoprotective to cochlear outer hair cells exposed to noise trauma.

Possible risks and benefits of resveratrol supplementation at levels greater than that found in food and wine are still under analysis. The antioxidant is contraindicated in pregnancy, lactation, and possibly in those with breast cancer, uterine cancer, ovarian cancer, endometriosis, and uterine fibroids (NMCD, http://www.naturaldatabase.com, retrieved January 30, 2008). Recently, resveratrol has been shown to possess synergistic effects with chemotherapy and radiation in fighting human gynecologic cancer cell lines (Rezk, Balulad, Keller, & Bennett, 2006). Additionally, studies in the author's laboratory have shown that resveratrol can significantly increase the kill rate of glioma brain tumor cells in vitro (Jiang et al., 2005). Supplemental dosage range for resveratrol is 40–1000 mg per day (Seidman & Moneysmith, 2006).

Alpha-Lipoic Acid (ALA)

Alpha-lipoic acid is a mitochondrial co-enzyme that functions in the pyruvate dehydrogenase complex and is essential for proper energy cellular production. It is found in organ meats and green leafy vegetables. The reduced form, dihydrolipoic acid, is the antioxidant that prevents microsomal lipid peroxidation by reducing glutathione, recycling vitamin E, scavenging free radicals and inhibiting singlet oxygen. Enhanced mitochondrial potentials and increased energy production are facilitated by this process.

The benefits of ALA include healthy brain mitochondria, improved memory, cardioprotection, glucose uptake and insulin regulation, protection against cirrhosis, hepatitis C and mushroom poisoning, viral interruption and cell death in HIV, and recycling of vitamins C and E in the body (Liu, 2008; Packer, Tritschler, & Wessel, 1997; Packer, Witt, & Tritschler, 1995). In the mouse model of Huntington's disease, a neurodegenerative autosomal dominant disorder with chromosome 4 locus presenting with deficits in cognition, movement, mood, and caudate nucleus atrophy pathologically, alpha-lipoic acid prolongs survival significantly (Andreassen, Ferrante, Dedeoglu, & Beal, 2001).

ALA inhibits arterial leukocyte recruitment, an initiating step in atherogenesis, via action on TNF—alpha-induced NF-kappaB activation in human aortic endothelial cells. NF-kB is a transcription nuclear factor. Genes regulated by NF-kB are key mediators in inflammation. ROS are involved in the signaling events of NF-kB activation. Compounds that inhibit

NF-kB signaling also exert in vivo anti-inflammatory responses. ALA increases cellular glutathione levels and also acts as an iron and copper chelator. The iron and copper chelating mechanism of ALA is believed to be responsible for the anti-atherogenic activity (Zhang & Frei, 2001).

Seidman et al. (2000) investigated the effects of mitochondrial enhancers on rat hearing and mitochondrial function by orally supplementing their diet for 6 weeks with alpha-lipoic acid in group one (300 mg/kg/day) and acetyl-L-carnitine in group two (300mg/kg/day). The control group (group three) received a regular diet devoid of up-regulators of mitochondrial function. Hearing thresholds, and skeletal muscle, brain, liver, and stria vascularis and other cochlear tissue, and auditory nerve were analyzed for mtDNA deletions using polymerase chain reaction. Results revealed reductions in mtDNA aging and prebycusic in the rats nourished with ALA and ALCAR. ALCAR conferred significant hearing protection over all frequencies and ALA slowed down the progression of hearing loss.

Evidence to date reveals that ALA is safe for most adults. Rash and mild gastrointestinal upset may occur as side effects. Contraindications include pregnancy, breast-feeding, excessive alcohol use, thiamine deficiency, and thyroid disease. ALA may lower blood sugar, thus requiring frequent glucose monitoring and possible dosage adjustments of prescription medication. Supplemental ALA doses range from 100 to 1200 mg/day (NMCD, http://www.naturaldatabase.com, retrieved January 30, 2008).

Acetyl-L-Carnitine (ALCAR)

Acetyl-L-carnitine is an amino acid produced by the body and plays a key role in maintaining bio-energy and integrity by facilitating transport of fatty acids from the cytosol into the mitochondrial matrix. Cellular energy in the form of increased ATP production results from regulation of acetyl-CoA and the metabolism of sugars, lipids, and amino acids. Studies on heart mitochondria reveal that this energy process declines with age (Seidman et al., 2000).

Rat models of chronic untreated diabetic polyneuropathy show that ALCAR exerts neuroprotective effects (Sima, 2007). Randomized placebo-controlled trials in patients with chronic diabetic neuropathy demonstrate that ALCAR (500–1000 mg three times daily) reduces neuropathic pain, improves vibration perception and nerve fiber regeneration (Sima, Calvani, Mehra, Amato, & Acetyl-L-Carnitine Study Group, 2005).

In the chinchilla ear, if ALCAR is used in conjunction with NAC via intraperitoneal injection, permanent threshold shifts and hair cell loss are reduced 1 and 4 h postnoise exposure. Prolonged use of ALCAR up to 2 weeks postnoise exposure may prove to be of additional value to counteract the secondary oxidative effects of acute noise exposure (Coleman et al., 2007). Otoprotective synergism exists between ALA and ALCAR (Seidman et al., 2000) and possibly between ALCAR plus NAC in animals exposed to noise (Coleman et al., 2006; Kopke et al., 2005).

Acetyl-L-carnitine seems safe in adults. Side effects include stomach upset, nausea, vomiting, restlessness, and a fishy odor of the urine, breath, and sweat. Medication interactions may occur with blood thinners such as acenocoumarol and warfarin resulting in an enhanced anticoagulant effect. Treatment with concurrent anticoagulant dosing may require adjustments.

Supplemental ALCAR dosages range from 500 to 4000 mg/day, given in divided doses (NMCD, www.naturaldatabase.com, retrieved December 30, 2007).

D-Methionine

This glutathione-preserving antioxidant protects outer hair cells and the stria vascularis from gentamicin (Sha & Schacht, 2000) and cisplatin chemotherapy, a platinum-based ototoxin (Campbell et al., 1996; Campbell, Meech, Rybak, & Holmes, 1998). Moreover, D-met demonstrates virtually complete otoprotection against noise-induced hearing loss in the chinchilla (6 hours, 105 dB SPL, 4 kHz narrow band noise) up to day 21 postacoustic trauma when rescue treatment is implemented within 1 hour after noise trauma (Campbell et al., 2007). With treatment, mitochondrial glutathione levels are increased and the egress of glutathione from injured cells halted during periods of noise overexposure. Additional studies are in progress to delineate the window of opportunity for rescue with other types of noise exposure, including blast trauma. The D-met isomer is present in cheese and yogurt (fermented proteins) due to fermentation. In other parts of the world, acetaminophen toxicity is being treated with methionine up to 10 grams in a 12-hour time period. Although 1600 mg or less is a typical daily dosage, L-methionine 3 grams twice a day for 12 weeks was well tolerated in 12 HIV adults with vacuolar myelopathy (Di Rocco et al., 2004). No side effects of treatment with D-methionine, which is preferred and produces higher plasma levels, have been reported to date; however, racemic or L-methionine may cause toxicity (Campbell et al., 2007).

Glutathione

NAC is converted to L-glutathione in the liver, and is found in fruits, vegetables, and meats. Noise exposure induces a number of ROS, which induce vasoconstriction and potential cochlear ischemia. One such ROS marker and potent vasoconstrictor is 8-isoprostaglandin F (2-alpha). In guinea pigs, the cochlea was protected from vasoconstriction when glutathione monoethyl ester was infused prior to noise exposure (Miller, Brown, & Schacht, 2003). To test the ability of glutathione to limit cell damage induced by ROS, guinea pigs were fed a 7% low protein diet for 10 days, a diet sufficient to induce reduced tissue levels of glutathione. They were then treated with intraperitoneal glutathione (5 mg/kg body weight) 1 hour prior, immediately after, and 5 hours after noise exposure. The antioxidant was able to attenuate threshold shifts and limit hair cell loss (Ohinata, Yamasoba, Schacht, & Miller, 2000).

Glutathione is safe for most adults. Side effects are not known at this time. The supplement should be avoided in pregnancy and lactation. Patients with mild, stable asthma are cautioned not to inhale glutathione because it may induce cough, breathlessness, and marked functional bronchoconstriction due to sulfite inhalation (Marrades et al., 1997). No known drug interactions have been reported. Supplemental doses range from 30 to 600 mg per day, with a typical dose of 50 to 250 mg daily (NMCD, http://www.naturaldatabase.com

N-Acetylcysteine (NAC)

NAC is a precursor to glutathione and facilitates the recycling of other antioxidants including vitamins C and E. It offers additional cardioprotective effects by reducing homocysteine and lipoprotein (a) (Seidman & Moneysmith, 2006). This antioxidant is the standard antidote used to treat acetaminophen (Tylenol) poisoning.

In the presence of acrylonitrile, a known chemical contaminant that depletes glutathione and generates cyanide, hearing loss is potentiated in noise. NAC preserves glutathione levels in the rat liver and cochlea and protected nerve and hair cells. (Pouyatos, Gearhart, Nelson-Miller, Fulton, & Fechter, 2007). Moreover, NAC demonstrates significant otoprotection against combinations of continuous and impulse noise trauma in chinchillas (Bielefeld, Kopke, Jackson, Coleman, Liu, & Henderson, 2007). These studies support the additional role of NAC and glutathione in cochlear otoprotection against toxins and noise that induce harmful reactive oxygen species.

Kopke et al. (2000) studied the otoprotective effects of salicylate (50 mg/kg) and NAC (325 mg/kg) administered 1 hour before noise trauma in chinchillas. The antioxidants were administered via intraperitoneal injection 1hr pre- and 1hr post-exposure to a 6-hour octave band noise centered at 4 kHz (105 dB SPL). In the control group who received no treatment, permanent threshold shifts were significantly reduced to a maximum of 40 dB, and hair cell loss was marked. However, the pretreatment experimental group, treated 1 hour before noise exposure, sustained permanent threshold shift of only 10 dB, and hair cell injury was reduced significantly. The experimental group treated 1hr postnoise-exposure sustained a 23 dB high-frequency hearing loss and no hair cell protection. This study shows that aug-menting the animal's endogenous antioxidant reserve around the time of acoustic stress reduces cochlear injury and preserves hearing, thus strengthening the hypothesis that noise-induced hearing loss is secondary to the generation of ROS. Whether oral administration of otoprotective nutraceuticals affords similar protection in humans exposed to impulse or chronic noise remains under investigation. Combining ear plugs and/or ear muffs with oral antioxidant regimens are preventive medicine options for those at high risk of occupational or recreational noise exposure (Kopke et al., 2000).

A window of opportunity exists for optimum otoprotection depending on the duration and intensity of noise trauma. Evidence of ROS in the cochlea extends for 2 weeks with peak inflammatory activity at 7 to 10 days postacoustic insult (Yamashita, Jiang, Le Prell, Schacht, & Miller, 2005). Usually, patients are subjected to recreational or occupational noise trauma (impulse, chronic, or "acute on chronic") without the potential benefit of adhering to a daily otoprotective supplemental regimen. Sudden hearing loss and tinnitus sustained from noise trauma are rarely viewed as medical emergencies by the lay person, as opposed to other sudden motor and sensory symptoms such as chest pain, dyspnea, vertigo, sudden monocular visual loss, aphasia, limb weakness and numbness, and other symptoms. With the knowledge that research suggests the ability to potentially halt or reverse hearing loss, as well as possibly prevent the onset of tinnitus via outer hair cell preservation, patients and doctors should be more aggressive in exploring novel antioxidant interventions via oral, transtympanic and possibly intravenous routes—in addition to steroids, vasodilators, neuropotectants rheologic agents, and hyperbaric oxygen—within that 2-week window.

At present, intratympanic steroid treatment for idiopathic sudden sensorineural hearing loss in patients who fail oral steroid treatment appears free of serious adverse events and can improve hearing thresholds and speech discrimination (Slattery, Fisher, Iqbal, Friedman, & Liu, 2005). If treatment within a 2-week window remains impractical, new research has shown that 26% of patients with sudden sensorineural hearing loss undergoing intratympanic injection with dexamethasone within 5 *weeks* after sustaining hearing loss can achieve an improvement of 20 dB in threshold or 20% in speech discrimination scores versus 9.1% in an untreated control group (Haynes, O'Malley, Cohen, Watford, & Labadie, 2007). Whether combination treatment approaches of potent antioxidants in conjunction with rescue steroid therapy prove to be safe, synergistic, and effective for the rescue of hearing and prevention of tinnitus remains to be studied prospectively. Optimum dosages, routes of administration, and safety profiles have yet to be determined.

It is encouraging to recognize that NAC is not the only antioxidant with such otoprotective potential available on the market. Recalling that the antioxidants display synergism, optimum otoprotective strategies will likely include a combination approach such as ALA, ALCAR, NAC (or glutathione), Co-Q10, resveratrol, lecithin, d-methionine, green tea, magnolia, and possibly other nutraceuticals that offer novel and diverse neuroprotective mechanisms including, free radical scavenging activity,

inhibition of several inflammatory mediators, mitochondrial DNA protection and even selective, voltage-dependent NMDA antagonism.

The nutraceuticals reviewed in this section on noise-induced hearing loss, with their potent antioxidant and anti-inflammatory capacity, have the potential to satisfy the demands of an ideal otoprotective agent. Namely, they (1) address current known mechanisms of cochlear injury; (2) function as an antioxidant that replenishes glutathione and shields mitochondria; (3) inhibit DNA damage, lipid peroxidation, apoptosis, necrosis, and cell death; (4) are nontoxic, inexpensive, and readily available in stable powder and possibly aqueous solution for oral and/or transtympanic administration; and, most importantly, (5) are clinically effective (Kopke, Jackson, Coleman, Liu, Bielefeld, & Balough, 2007).

N-acetylcysteine is safe for most adults. The safety data derive largely from acetaminophen poisoning studies which show that NAC doses up to 100 grams over 72 hours are safe and effective at reducing hepatic necrosis. NAC is not present in food. Side effects include nausea, vomiting, diarrhea or constipation, and more rarely, rashes, fever, headache, drowsiness, hypotension, and liver problems. Inhalation of NAC may cause oral swelling, rhinitis, drowsiness, diaphoresis, and chest discomfort. Contraindications include pregnancy, breast feeding, allergies to acetylcysteine, and asthma. NAC should not be taken with nitroglycerin as both substances cause vasodilation possibly leading to headache, dizziness, and presyncope. Supplemental dosages ranges from 100–2,500 mg/day (NMCD, http://www.naturaldatabase.com, retrieved December 30, 2008).

Summary

A growing body of scientific work is revealing the ability of nutraceuticals to combat disease in animal and human studies via improved mitochondrial bioenergetics, free radical scavenging, antiinflammatory, and anticancer activity. The diverse mechanisms of nutraceuticals may afford novel protection against ototoxic medications, noise, and the effects of aging by slowing the mitochondrial clock and supporting mtDNA structure and function. Side effects are mild and no deaths from toxicity have been reported. Nutraceuticals offer the potential for synergistic activity among other antioxidants and vitamins and may slow the process of aging in the cochlea as well as assist the cochlea in recovery from acute trauma. They do not interfere with aminoglycoside levels and can limit ototoxic damage. The cochlea can be protected from noise with nutraceutical pretreatment and/or rescue treatment, resulting in possible hearing preservation, limited hair cell injury, and the possible prevention or reduction of tinnitus and hyperacusis. The supplements are readily available at health food stores. Typically, we recommend natural products (not always possible or practical), chelated minerals, and formulae prepared in facilities that meet or exceed these standards: FDA-registered Drug Establishment, certified US Pharmacopeia (USP), or Good Manufacturing Practice (GMP). A healthy diet, moderate exercise, restorative sleep, daily multivitamins, minerals, antioxidants, and essential fatty acids plus select otoprotective nutraceuticals may offer patients the best opportunity for hearing health and overall wellness. Further animal and human research is indicated to increase the amount of data regarding select nutraceutical effectiveness in otolaryngological diseases and disorders, the window of opportunity for otoprotection, dosing and routes of administration, short- and long-term safety and tolerability, and drug and herb interactions.

Acknowledgments

Our sincere gratitude is extended to Veronica Chua, R.N., Alan T. Marty, MD, Mrs. Cristy McAuley, Janene Wandersee, librarian, Sally Harvey, librarian, Lora Robbins, librarian, Kathleen Shepler, Mrs. Marie Moneysmith, Melanie West, the staff at Plural Publishing and to the editors, Jennifer Derebery, MD and William Luxford, MD. Dr. Seidman and Dr. Robb have no financial conflicts of interest to declare.

References

Ahmad, N., Gupta, S., & Mukhtar, H. (2000). Green tea polyphenol epigallocatechin-3-gallate differentially modulates nuclear factor kappaB in cancer cells versus normal cells. *Archives in Biochemistry and Biophysics, 376*, 338–346.

Ahuja J. K., Goldman, J. D., & Moshfegh, A. J. (2004). Current status of vitamin E nutriture. *Annals of New York Academy of Sciences, 1031*, 387–390.

Albanes, D., Heinonen, O. P., Taylor, P. R., Virtamo, J., Edwards, B. K., Rautalahti, M., et al. (1996). Alpha-tocopherol and beta-carotene supplements and lung cancer incidence in the alpha-tocopherol, beta-carotene cancer prevention study: effects of base-line characteristics and study compliance.

Journal of the National Cancer Institute, *88*, 1560-1570.

Alberg, A. (2002). The influence of cigarette smoking on circulating concentrations of antioxidant micronutrients. *Toxicology*, *180*, 121-137.

Alberg, A. J., Chen, J. C., Zhao, H., Hoffman, S. C., Comstock, G. W., & Helzlsouer, K. J. (2000). Household exposure to passive cigarette smoking and serum micronutrient concentrations. *American Journal of Clinical Nutrition*, *72*, 1576-1582.

Ames, B. N. (2006). Low micronutrient intake may accelerate the degenerative diseases of aging through allocation of scarce micronutrients by triage. *Proceedings of the National Academy of Sciences of the United States of America*, *103*, 17589-17594.

Andreassen, O. A., Ferrante, R. J., Dedeoglu, A., & Beal, M. F. (2001). Lipoic acid improves survival in transgenic mouse models of Huntington's disease. *Neuroreport*, *12*, 3371-3373.

Angeli, S. I., Liu, X. Z., Yan, D., Balkany, T., & Telischi, F. (2005). Coenzyme Q-10 treatment of patients with a 7445A-G mitochondrial DNA mutation stops the progression of hearing loss. *Acta Otolaryngologica*, *125*, 510-512.

Avramovich-Tirosh, Y., Reznichenko, L., Mit, T., Zheng, H., Fridkin, M., & Weinreb, O., et al. (2007). Neurorescue activity, APP regulation and amyloid-beta peptide reduction by novel multi-functional brain permeable iron-chelating-antioxidants, M-30 and green tea polyphenol, EGCG. *Current Alzheimer Research*, *4*, 403-411.

Baloh, R. W., & Honrubia, V. (2001). *Clinical neurophysiology of the vestibular system.* Oxford, Oxford University Press.

Basu, A., & Lucas, E. A. (2007). Mechanisms and effects of green tea on cardiovascular health. *Nutrition Review*, *65*, 361-375.

Bielefeld, E. C., Kopke, R. D., Jackson, R. L., Coleman, J. K., Liu, J., & Henderson, D. (2007). Noise protection with N-acetyl-l-cysteine (NAC) using a variety of noise exposures, NAC doses, and routes of administration. *Acta Oto-Laryngologica*, *127*, 914-919.

Black, F. O., Pesznecker, S., & Stallings, V. (2004). Permanent gentamicin vestibulotoxicity. *Otology and Neurotology*, *25*, 559-569.

Boettcher, F. A., & Salvi, R. J. (1991). Salicylate ototoxicity: Review and synthesis. *American Journal of Otolaryngology*, *12*, 33-47.

Boehm, K., Borrelli, F., Ernst, E., Habacher, G., Hung, S. K., Milazzo, S., et al. (2009). Green tea (Camellia sinensis) for the prevention of cancer. *Cochrane Database Systematic Reviews*, *8*, CD005004.

Bonkovsky, H. L. (2006). Hepatotoxicity associated with supplements containing Chinese green tea (Camellia sinensis). *Annals of Internal Medicine*, *144*, 68-71.

Brum, L. F., Elisabetsky, E., & Souza, D. (2001). Effects of linalool on [(3)H]MK801 and [(3)H] muscimol binding in mouse cortical membranes. *Phytotherapy Research*, *15*, 422-425.

Butt, M. S., & Sultan, M. T. (2009). Green tea: nature's defense against malignancies. *Critical Reviews in Food Science and Nutrition*, *49*, 463-473.

Cadoni, G., Scipione, S., Agostino, S., Addolorato, G., Cianfrone, F., Leggio, L., et al. (2007). Coenzyme Q 10 and cardiovascular risk factors in idiopathic sudden sensorineural hearing loss patients. *Otology and Neurotology*, *28*, 878-883.

Campbell, K. C., Larsen, D. L., Meech, R. P., Rybak, L. P., & Hughes, L. F. (2003). Glutathione ester but not glutathione protects against cisplatin-induced ototoxicity in a rat model. *Journal of American Academy of Audiology*, *14*, 124-133.

Campbell, K. C. M., Meech, R. P., Klemens, J. J., Gerberi, M. T., Dyrstad, S. S. W., Larsen, D. L., et al. (2007). Prevention of noise- and drug-induced hearing loss with D-methionine. *Hearing Research*, *226*, 92-103.

Campbell, K. C., Meech, R. P., Rybak, L. P., & Hughes, L. F. (1999). D-Methionine protects against cisplatin damage to the stria vascularis. *Hearing Research*, *138*, 13-28.

Campbell, K. C., Meech, R. P. Rybak, L. P., & Hughes, L. F. (2003). The effect of D-methionine on cochlear oxidative state with and without cisplatin administration: mechanisms of otoprotection. *Journal of American Academy of Audiology, 14,* 144–156.

Campbell, K. C., Rybak, L. P., Meech, R. P., & Hughes, L. (1996). D-methionine provides excellent protection from cisplatin ototoxicity in the rat. *Hearing Research, 102,* 90–98.

Chandra, R. K. (1997) Nutrition and the immune system: An introduction. *American Journal of Clinical Nutrition, 66,* 460–463.

Chen, G. D., Kong, J., Reinhard, K., & Fechter, L. D. (2001). NMDA receptor blockage protects against permanent noise-induced hearing loss but not its potentiation by carbon monoxide. *Hearing Research, 154,* 108–115.

Chen, Y., Huang, W. G., Zha, D. J., Qiu, J. H., Wang, J. L., Sha, S. H., et al. (2007). Aspirin attenuates gentamicin ototoxicity: From the laboratory to the clinic. *Hearing Research, 226,* 178–182.

Cheng, A. G., Cunningham, L. L., & Rubel, E. W. (2005). Mechanisms of hair cell death and protection. *Current Opinions in Otolaryngology Head and Neck Surgery, 13,* 343–348.

Chiou, G. C., Li, B. H., & Wang, M. S. (1994). Facilitation of retinal function recovery by natural products after temporary ischemic occlusion of central retinal artery. *Journal of Ocular Pharmacology, 10,* 493–498.

Chou, C. W., Huang, W. J., Tien, L. T., & Wang, S. J. (2007). (−)-Epigallocatechin gallate, the most active polyphenolic catechin in green tea, presynaptically facilitates Ca2+-dependent glutamate release via activation of protein kinase C in rat cerebral cortex. *Synapse, 11,* 889–902.

Chow, H-H. S., Cai, Y., Hakim, I. A., Crowell, J. A., Shahi, F., Brooks, C. A., et al. (2003). Pharmacokinetics and safety of green tea polyphenols after multiple dose administration of epigallocatechin gallate and polyphenon E in healthy individuals. *Clinical Cancer Research, 9,* 3312–3319.

Cid-Ruzafa, J., Caulfield, L. E., Barron, Y., & West, S. K. (1999). Nutrient intakes and adequacy among an older population of the eastern shore of Maryland: The Salisbury Eye Evaluation. *Journal of the American Dietetic Association, 99,* 564–571.

Coleman, J. K., Kopke, R. D., Liu, J., Ge, X., Harper, E. A., Jones, G. E., et al. (2007). Pharmacological rescue of noise induced hearing loss using N-acetylcysteine and acetyl-l-carnitine. *Hearing Research, 226,* 104–113.

Corral-Debrinski, M., Stepien, G., Shoffner, J. M., Lott, M. T., Kanter, K., & Wallace, D. C. (1991). Hypoxemia is associated with mitochondrial DNA damage and gene induction. Implications for cardiac disease. *Journal of the American Medical Association, 266,* 1812–1816.

Cortopassi, G. A., & Arnheim, N. (1990). Detection of a specific mitochondrial DNA deletion in tissues of older humans. *Nucleic Acids Research, 18,* 6927–6933.

Cucciolla, V., Borriello, A., Oliva, A., Galletti, P., Zappia, V., & Della Ragione, F. (2007). Resveratrol: From basic science to the clinic. *Cell Cycle, 6,* 2495–2510.

Darrat, I., Ahmad, N., Seidman, K., & Seidman, M. D. (2007). Auditory research involving antioxidants. *Current Opinion in Otolaryngology and Head and Neck Surgery, 15,* 358–363.

Das, S., & Das, D. K. (2007). Anti-inflammatory responses of resveratrol. *Inflammation Allergy Drug Targets, 6,* 168–173.

DeFelice, S. L. (2002). *FIM rationale and proposed guidelines for the nutraceutical research and education act—NREA.* Presented at Foundation for Innovation in Medicine's (FIM) 10th Nutraceutical Conference, November 10–11, 2002, New York City. Retrieved April 29, 2009, from http://www.fimdefelice.org/archives/arc.researchact.html

Devika, P. T., & Stanely Mainzen Prince, P. (2008). (−)Epigallocatechingallate protects the mitochondria against the deleterious effects of lipids, calcium and adenosine triphosphate in isoproterenol induced myocardial infracted male Wistar rats. *Journal of Applied Toxicology, 28,* 938–944.

Di Rocco, A., Werner, P., Bottiglieri, T., Godbold, J., Liu, M., Tagliati, M., et al. (2004).

Treatment of AIDS-associated myelopathy with L-methionine: A placebo-controlled study. *Neurology, 63,* 1270-1275.

Dou, Q. P., Landis-Piwowar, K. R., Chen, D., Huo, C., Wan, S. B., & Chan, T. H. (2008). Green tea polyphenols as a natural tumour cell proteasome inhibitor. *Inflammopharmacology, 16,* 208-212.

Draczynska-Lusiak, B., Chen, Y. M. & Sun, A. Y. (1998). Oxidized lipoproteins activate NF-kappaB binding activity and apoptosis in PC12 cells. *Neuroreport, 9,* 527-532.

Duan, M., Qui, J., Laurell, G., Olofsson, A., Counter, S. A., & Borg, E. (2004). Dose and time-dependent protection of the antioxidant N-L-acetylcysteine against impulse noise trauma. *Hearing Research, 192,* 1-9.

Ehrnhoefer, D. E., Duennwald, M., Markovic, P., Wacker, J. L., Engemann, S., Roark, M., et al. (2006). Green tea (−)-epigallocatechin-gallate modulates early events in huntingtin misfolding and reduces toxicity in Huntington's disease models. *Human Molecular Genetics, 15,* 2743-2751.

Fairfield, K. M., & Fletcher, R. H. (2002). Vitamins for chronic disease prevention in adults: scientific review. *Journal of the American Medical Association, 287,* 3116-3126.

Feldman, L., Efrati, S., Eviatar, E., Abramsohn, R., Yaravoy, I., Gersch, E., et al. (2007). Gentamicin-induced ototoxicity in hemodialysis patients is ameliorated by N-acetylcysteine. *Kidney International, 72,* 359-363.

Fletcher, R. H., & Fairfield, K. M. (2002). Vitamins for chronic disease prevention in adults: clinical applications. *Journal of the American Medical Association, 287,* 3127-3129.

Flynn, M., Sciamanna, C., & Vigilante, K. (2003). Inadequate physician knowledge of the effects of diet on blood lipids and lipoproteins. *Nutritional Journal, 2,* 19.

Fu, Y., & Koo, M. W. (2006). EGCG protects HT-22 cells against glutamate-induced oxidative stress. *Neurotoxicological Research, 10,* 23-30.

Fuster, V. (2007). A new perspective on non-prescription statins: An opportunity for patient education and involvement. *American Journal of Cardiology, 100,* 907-910.

Gacek, R. R., & Schuknecht, H. F. (1969). Pathology of presbycusis. *International Journal of Audiology, 8,* 199-209.

Gao, X., Wilde, P. E., Lichtenstein, A. H., Bermudez, O. I., & Tucker, K. L. (2006). The maximal amount of dietary tocopherol intake in U.S. adults (NHANES 2001-2002). *Journal of Nutrition, 136,* 1021-1026.

Garetz, S. L., Altschuler, R. A., & Schacht, J. (1994). Attenuation of gentamicin ototoxicity by glutathione in the guinea pig in vivo. *Hearing Research, 77,* 81-87.

Greenwald, P., Anderson, D., Nelson, S. A., & Taylor, P. R. (2007). Clinical trials of vitamin and mineral supplements for cancer prevention. *American Journal of Clinical Nutrition, 85,* 314S-317S.

Hanisch, F., & Zierz, S. (2003). Only transient increase of serum CoQ subset 10 during long-term CoQ10 therapy in mitochondrial ophthalmoplegia. *European Journal of Medical Research, 8,* 485-491.

Harkins, S. W. (1981). Effects of age and interstimulus interval on brainstem auditory evoked potential. *International Journal of Neuroscience, 15,* 107-118.

Hattori, K., Tanaka, M., Sugiyama, S., Obayashi, T., Ito, T., Satake, T., et al. (1991). Age-dependent increase in deleted mitochondrial DNA in the human heart: Possible contributory factor to presbycardia. *American Heart Journal, 121,* 1735-1742.

Haynes, D. S., O'Malley, M., Cohen, S., Watford, K., & Labadie, R. F. (2007). Intratympanic dexamethasone for sudden sensorineural hearing loss after failure of systemic therapy. *Laryngoscope, 117,* 3-15.

Heinonen, O. P., Huttunen, J. K., & Albanes, D., for the Alpha-Tocopherol Beta-Carotene Cancer Prevention Study Group (1994). The effect of vitamin E and beta-carotene on the incidence of lung cancer and other cancers in male smokers. *New England Journal of Medicine, 330,* 1029-1035.

Henderson, D., Bielefeld, E. C., Harris, K. C., & Hu, B. H. (2006). The role of oxidative stress in noise-induced hearing loss. *Ear and Hearing, 27,* 1-19.

Henderson, D., Hu, B. H., McFadden, S. L., Zheng, X. Y., & Ding, D. (2000). The role of glutathione in carboplatin ototoxicity in the chinchilla. *Noise Health, 3*, 1–10.

Henderson, D., McFadden, S. L., Liu, C. C., Hight, N., & Zheng, X. Y. (1999). The role of antioxidants in protection from impulse noise. *Annals of the New York Academy of Sciences, 884*, 368–380.

Hiyama, K., Hirai, Y., Kyoizumi, S., Akiyama, M., Hiyama, E., Piatyszek, M. A., et al. (1995). Activation of telomerase in human lymphocytes and hematopoietic progenitor cells. *Journal of Immunology, 155*, 3711–3715.

Ho, Y. C., Yang, S. F., Peng, C. Y., Chou, M. Y., & Chang, Y. C. (2007). Epigallocatechin-3-gallate inhibits the invasion of human oral cancer cells and decreases the productions of matrix metalloproteinases and urokinase-plasminogen activator. *Journal of Oral Pathological Medicine, 36*, 588–593.

Hockenberry, D. M., Oltvai, Z. N., Yin, X. M., Milliman, C.L., & Korsmeyer, S. J. (1993). Bcl-2 functions in an antioxidant pathway to prevent apoptosis. *Cell, 75*, 241–252.

Hoeffding, V., & Feldman, M. L (1988). Changes with age in the morphology of the cochlear nerve in rats: Light microscopy. *Journal of Comparative Neurology, 276*, 537–546.

Holick, M. F., & Chen, T. C. (2008). Vitamin D deficiency: A worldwide problem with health consequences. *American Journal of Clinical Nutrition, 87*, 1080S–1086S.

Honda, K., Tominaga, S., Oshikata, T., Kamiya, K., Hamamura, M., Kawasaki, T., et al. (2007). Thirteen-week repeated dose oral toxicity study of coenzyme Q10 in rats. *Journal of Toxicological Sciences, 32*, 437–448.

Hou, Y. C., Chao, P. D., & Chen, S. Y. (2000). Honokiol and magnolol increased hippocampal acetylcholine release in freely-moving rats. *American Journal of Chinese Medicine, 28*, 379–384.

Houston, D. K., Johnson, M. A., Nozza, R. J., Gunter, E. W., Shea, K. J., Cutler, G. M., et al. (1999). Age-related hearing loss, vitamin B-12, and folate in elderly women. *American Journal of Clinical Nutrition, 69*, 564–571.

Hyppolito, M. A., de Oliveira, J. A., & Rossato, M. (2006). Cisplatin ototoxicity and oto-protection with sodium salicylate. *European Archives of Otorhinolaryngology, 263*, 798–803.

The Independent Budget for the Department of Veterans Affairs—Fiscal year 2009. (2009). Retrieved August 27, 2009, from http://es3.pva.org/independentb udget .

Isbrucker, R. A., Bausch, J., Edwards, J. A., & Wolz, E. (2006). Safety studies on epigallocatechin gallate (EGCG) preparation. Part 1: Genotoxicity. *Food and Chemical Toxicology, 44*, 626–635.

Isbrucker, R. A., Edwards, J. A., Wolz, E., Davidovich, A., & Bausch, J. (2006). Safety studies on epigallocatechin gallate (EGCG) preparations. Part 2: dermal, acute and short-term toxicity studies. *Food and Chemical Toxicology, 44*, 636–650.

Jager, W., Goiny, M., Herrera-Marschitz, M., Brundin, L., Fransson, A., & Canlon, B. (2000). Noise-induced aspartate and glutamate efflux in the guinea pig cochlea and hearing loss. *Experimental Brain Research, 134*, 426–434.

Jiang, H., Talaska, A. E., Schacht, J., & Sha, S. H. (2007). Oxidative imbalance in the aging inner ear. *Neurobiology of Aging, 28*, 1605–1612.

Jiang, H., Zhang, L., Kuo, J., Kuo, K., Gautam, S. C., Groc, L., et al. (2005). Resveratrol-induced apoptotic death in human U251 glioma cells. *Molecular Cancer Therapeutics, 4*, 554–561.

Jung, J. Y., Han, C. R., Jeong, Y. J., Kim, H. J., Lim, H. S., Lee, K. H., et al. (2007). Epigallocatechin gallate inhibits nitric oxide-induced apoptosis in rat PC12 cells. *Neuroscience Letters, 411*, 222–227.

Kalra, E. K. (2003). Nutraceutical—definition and introduction. *American Association of Pharmaceutical Scientists (AAPS) Pharmaceutical Science, 5*, E25.

Kane, D. J., Sarafian, T. A., Anton, R., Hahn, H., Gralla, E. B., Valentine, J. S., et al. (1993). Bcl-2 inhibition of neural cell death: decreased generation of reactive oxygen species. *Science, 262*, 1274–1277.

Khan, M. J., Seidman, M. D., Quirk, W. S., & Shivapuia, B. G. (2000). Effects of kynurenic acid as a glutamate receptor antagonist in the guinea pig. *European Archives of Otorhinolaryngology*, *257*, 177–181.

Kitano, M., Watanabe, D., Oda, S., Kubo, H., Kishida, H., Fujii, K., et al. (2008). Subchronic oral toxicity of ubiquinol in rats and dogs. *International Journal of Toxicology*, *27*, 189–215.

Klemens, J. J., Meech, R. P., Hughes, L. F., Somani, S., & Campbell, K. C. (2003). Antioxidant enzyme levels inversely covary with hearing loss after amikacin treatment. *Journal of American Academy of Audiology*, *14*, 134–143.

Kopke, R., Bielefeld, E., Liu, J., Zheng, J., Jackson, R., Henderson, D., et al. (2005). Prevention of impulse noise-induced hearing loss with antioxidants. *Acta Otolaryngologica*, *125*, 235–243.

Kopke, R. D., Coleman, J. K., Liu, J., Campbell, K. C., & Riffenburgh, R. H. (2002). Candidate's thesis: Enhancing intrinsic cochlear stress defenses to reduce noise-induced hearing loss. *Laryngoscope*, *112*, 1515–1532.

Kopke, R. D., Jackson, R. L., Coleman, J. K. M., Liu, J., Bielefeld, E. C. & Balough, B. J. (2007). NAC for noise: From the bench top to the clinic. *Hearing Research*, *226*, 114–125.

Kopke, R. D., Weisskopf, P. A., Boone, J. L., Jackson, R. L., Wester, D. C., Hoffer, M.E., et al. (2000). Reduction of noise-induced hearing loss using L-NAC and salicylate in the chinchilla. *Hearing Research*, *149*, 138–146.

Korsmeyer, S. J., Yin, X. M., Oltvai, Z. N., Veis-Novack, D. J., & Linette, G. P. (1995). Reactive oxygen species and regulation of cell death by the Bcl-2 gene family. *Biochimica et Biophysica Acta*, *1271*, 63–66.

Korver, K. D., Rybak, L. P. Whitworth, C., & Campbell, K. M. (2002). Round window application of D-methionine provides complete cisplatin otoprotection. *Otolaryngology Head and Neck Surgery*, *126*, 683–689.

Kris-Etherton, P. M., Taylor, D. S., Yu-Poth, S., Huth, P., Moriarty, K., Fishell, V., et al. (2000). Polyunsaturated fatty acids in the food chain in the United States. *American Journal of Clinical Nutrition*, *71*, 179S–188S.

Langsjoen, P. H., & Langsjoen, A. M. (1999). Overview of the use of CoQ10 in cardiovascular disease. *Biofactors*, *9*, 273–284.

Langsjoen, P. H., & Langsjoen, A. M. (2008). Supplemental ubiquinol in patients with advanced congestive heart failure. *Biofactors*, *32*, 119–128.

Langsjoen, P. H., Langsjoen, J. O., Langsjoen, A. M., & Lucas, L. A. (2005). Treatment of statin adverse effects with supplemental Coenzyme Q10 and statin drug discontinuation. *Biofactors*, *25*, 147–152.

Langsjoen, H., Langsjoen, P., Langsjoen, P., Willis, R., & Folkers, K. (1994). Usefulness of coenzyme Q10 in clinical cardiology: A long term study. *Molecular Aspects in Medicine*, *15*, 165–175.

Le, T., & Keithley, E. M. (2007). Effects of antioxidants on the aging inner ear. *Hearing Research*, *226*, 194–202.

Le Prell, C. G., Hughes, L. F., & Miller, J. M. (2007). Free radical scavengers vitamins A, C, and E plus magnesium reduce noise trauma. *Free Radical Biology and Medicine*, *42*(9), 1454–1463.

Le Prell, C. G., Yamashita, D., Minami, S. B., Yamasoba, T., & Miller, J. M. (2007). Mechanisms of noise-induced hearing loss indicate multiple methods of prevention. *Hearing Research, 226*, 22–43.

Lin, Y. R., Chen, H. H., Ko, C. H., & Chan, M. H. (2005). Differential inhibitory effects of honokiol and magnolol on excitatory amino acid-evoked cation signals and NMDA-induced seizures. *Neuropharmacology*, *49*, 542–550.

Lin, Y. R., Chen, H. H., Ko, C. H., & Chan, M. H. (2006). Neuroprotective activity of honokiol and magnolol in cerebellar granule cell damage. *European Journal of Pharmacology*, *537*, 64–69.

Littarru, G. P., & Langsjoen, P. (2007). Coenzyme Q10 and statins: Biochemical and clinical applications. *Mitochondrion*, 7, S168-S174.

Liu, J. (2008). The effects and mechanisms of mitochondrial nutrient alpha-lipoic acid on improving age-associated mitochondrial and cognitive dysfunction: An overview. *Neurochemical Research*, 33, 194-203.

Lo, Y. C., Teng, C. M., Chen, C. F., Chen, C. C., & Hong, C. Y. (1994). Magnolol and honokiol isolated from Magnolia officinalis protect rat heart mitochondria against lipid peroxidation. *Biochemical Pharmacology*, 47, 549-553.

Low, B., Liang, M., & Fu, J. (2007). P38 mitogen-activated protein kinase mediates sidestream cigarette smoke-induced endothelial permeability. *Journal of Pharmacological Science*, 104, 225-231.

Maras J. E., Bermudez, O. I., Qiao, N., Bakun, P. J., Boody-Alter, E. L., & Tucker, K. L. (2004). Intake of alpha-tocopherol is limited among US adults. *Journal of the American Dietetic Association*, 104, 567-575.

Markaryan, A., Nelson, E. G., & Hinojosa, R. (2008). Detection of mitochondrial DNA deletions in the cochlea and its structural elements from archival human temporal bone tissue. *Mutation Research*, 640, 38-45.

Maroon, J. C., & Bost, J. (2006). *Fish oil: The natural anti-inflammatory.* Laguna Beach, CA: Basic Health Publications.

Marrades, R. M., Roca, J., Barbera, J. A., de Jover, L., MacNee, W., & Rodriguez-Roisin, R. (1997). Nebulized glutathione induces bronchoconstriction in patients with mild asthma. *American Journal of Respiratory and Critical Care Medicine*, 156, 425-430.

Masuda, M., Suzui, M., Lim, J. T. E., & Weinstein, I. B. (2003). Epigallocatechin-3-gallate inhibits activation of HER-2/neu and downstream signaling pathways in human head and neck and breast carcinoma cells. *Clinical Cancer Research*, 9, 3486-3491.

McFadden, S. L., Ohlemiller, K. K., Ding, D., Shero, M., & Salvi, R. J. (2001). The influence of superoxide dismutase and glutathione peroxidase deficiencies on noise-induced hearing loss in mice. *Noise Health*, 3, 49-64.

Miller, J. M., Brown, J. N., & Schacht, J. (2003). 8-iso-prostaglandin F(2 alpha), a product of noise exposure, reduces inner ear blood flow. *Audiology and Neurotology*, 8, 207-221.

Moon, H., Baek, D., Lee, B., Prasad, D. T., Lee, S. Y., Cho, M. J., et al. (2002). Soybean ascorbate peroxidase suppresses Bax-induced apoptosis in yeast by inhibiting oxygen radical generation. *Biochemical and Biophysical Research Communications*, 290, 457-462.

Muthukumaran, S., Sudheer, A. R., Menon, V. P., & Nalini, N. (2008). Protective effect of quercetin on nicotine-induced prooxidant and antioxidant imbalance and DNA damage in Wistar rats. *Toxicology*, 243, 207-215.

Natural Medicines Comprehensive Database. Retrieved January 30, 2008, from http://www.naturaldatabase.com

Nelson, D. I., Nelson, R. Y., Concha-Barrientos, M., & Fingerhut, M. (2005). The global burden of occupational noise-induced hearing loss. *American Journal of Industrial Medicine*, 48, 446-458.

Nelson, E. G., & Hinojosa, R. (2006). Presbycusis: A human temporal bone study of individuals with downward sloping audiometric patterns of hearing loss and review of the literature. *Laryngoscope*, 116, 1-12.

Newman, D. J., Cragg, G. M., & Snader, K. M. (2003). Natural products as sources of new drugs over the period 1981-2002. *Journal of Natural Products*, 66, 1022-1037.

Ohinata, Y., Yamasoba, T., Schacht, J., & Miller, J. M. (2000). Glutathione limits noise-induced hearing loss. *Hearing Research*, 146, 28-34.

Okamoto, T. (2005). Safety of quercetin for clinical application (review). *International Journal of Molecular Medicine*, 16, 275-278.

Oltvai, Z. N., Milliman, C. L., & Korsmeyer, S. J. (1993). Bcl-2 heterodimerizes in vivo with a conserved homolog, Bax, that accelerates programmed cell death. *Cell*, *74*, 609-619.

Packer, L., Tritschler, H. J., & Wessel, K. (1997). Neuroprotection by the metabolic antioxidant alpha-lipoic acid. *Free Radical Biological Medicine*, *22*, 359-378.

Packer, L., Witt, E. H., & Tritschler, H. J. (1995). alpha-lipoic acid as a biological antioxidant. *Free Radical Biological Medicine*, *19*, 227-250.

Pommier, J. P., Lebeau, J., Ducray, C., & Sabatier, L. (1995). Chromosomal instability and alteration of telomere repeat sequences. *Biochimie*, *77*, 817-825.

Pouryaghoub, G., Mehrdad, R., & Mohammadi, S. (2007). Interaction of smoking and occupational noise exposure loss: A cross-sectional study. *BMC Public Health*, *7*, 137.

Pouyatos, B., Gearhart, C., Nelson-Miller, A., Fulton, S., & Fechter, L. (2007). Oxidative stress pathways in the potentiation of noise-induced hearing loss by acrylonitrile. *Hearing Research*, *224*, 61-74.

Prazma, J., Carrasco, V. N., Butler, B., Waters, G., Anderson, T., & Pillsbury, H. C. (1990). Cochlear microcirculation in young and old gerbils. *Archives of Otolaryngology-Head and Neck Surgery*, *116*, 932-936.

Puel, J. L., Pujol, R., Tribillac, F., Ladrech, S., & Eybalin, M. (1994). Excitatory amino acid antagonists protect cochlear auditory neurons from excitotoxicity. *Journal of Comparative Neurology*, *341*(2), 241-256.

Pujol, R., & Puel, J. L. (1999). Excitotoxicity, synaptic repair, and functional recovery in the mammalian cochlea: A review of recent findings. *Annals of the New York Academy of Sciences*, *884*, 249-254.

Qu, J., Kaufman, Y., & Washington, I. (2009). Coenzyme Q10 in the human retina. *Investigative Ophthalmology and Visual Science*, *50*, 1814-1818.

Raper, N. R., Cronin, F. J., & Exler, J. (1992). Omega-3 fatty acid content of the US food supply. *Journal of American College of Nutrition*, *11*, 304-308.

Reagan-Shaw, S., Nihal, M., & Ahmad, N. (2008). Dose translation from animal to human studies revisited. *FASEB Journal*, *22*, 659-661.

Reagan-Shaw, S., Mukhtar, H., & Ahmad, N. (2008). Resveratrol imparts photoprotection of normal cells and enhances the efficacy of radiation therapy in cancer cells. *Photochemical Photobiology*, *84*, 415-421.

Rezk, Y. A., Balulad, S. S., Keller, R. S., & Bennett, J. A. (2006). Use of resveratrol to improve the effectiveness of cisplatin and doxorubicin: study in human gynecologic cancer cell lines and in rodent heart. *American Journal of Obstetrics and Gynecology*, *194*, 23-26.

Rohdewald, P. (2002). A review of the French maritime pine bark extract (Pycnogenol), a herbal medication with a diverse clinical pharmacology. *International Journal of Clinical Pharmacological Therapeutics*, *40*, 158-168.

Rosenhall, U., Pederson, K., Dotevall, M. (1986). Effects of presbyacusis and other types of hearing loss on auditory brain stem responses. *Scandanavian Audiology*, *15*, 179-185.

Rundek, T., Naini, A., Sacco, R., Coates, K., & DiMauro, S. (2004). Atorvastatin decreases the coenzyme Q10 level in the blood of patients at risk for cardiovascular disease and stroke. *Archives of Neurology*, *61*, 889-892.

Rybak, L. P. (2007). Mechanisms of cisplatin ototoxicity and progress in otoprotection. *Current Opinions in Otolaryngology Head and Neck Surgery*, *15*, 364-369.

Rybak, L. P., & Ramkumar, V. (2007). Ototoxicity. *Kidney International*, *72*, 931-935.

Saiko, P., Szakmary, A., Jaeger, W., & Szekeres, T. (2008). Resveratrol and its analogs: Defense against cancer, coronary disease and neurodegenerative maladies or just a fad? *Mutation Research*, *658*, 68-94.

Sanders, L. M., & Zeisel, S. H. (2007). Choline dietary requirements and role in brain development. *Nutrition Today*, *42*, 181-186.

Schilling, G., Coonfield, M. L., Ross, C. A., & Borchelt, D. R. (2001). Coenzyme Q10 and remacemide hydrochloride ameliorate motor deficits in a Huntington's disease transgenic mouse model. *Neuroscience Letters, 315,* 149-153.

Schuknecht, H. F. (1964). Further observations on the pathology of presbycusis. *Archives of Otolaryngology, 80,* 369-382.

Schuknecht, H. F., & Gacek, M. R. (1993). Cochlear pathology in presbycusis. *Annals of Otology, Rhinology and Laryngology, 102,* 1-16.

Seaman, D. R. (2002). The diet-induced proinflammatory state: A cause of chronic pain and other degenerative diseases? *Journal of Manipulative and Physiological Therapeutics, 25,* 168-179.

Segal, J. A., Harris, B. D., Kustova, Y., Basile, A., & Skolnick, P. (1999). Aminoglycoside neurotoxicity involves NMDA receptor activation. *Brain Research, 815,* 270-277.

Seidman, M., Babu, S., Tang, W., Emad, N., & Quirk, W. S. (2003). Effects of resveratrol on acoustic trauma. *Otolaryngology-Head and Neck Surgery, 129,* 463-470.

Seidman, M. D. *Resveratrol, an extract from grapes and red wine, reduces bioinflammation, DNA damage, age-related hearing loss and improves cognitive abilities.* In preparation.

Seidman, M. D. (1998). Glutamate antagonists, steroids, and antioxidants as therapeutic options for hearing loss and tinnitus and the use of an inner ear drug delivery system. *International Tinnitus Journal, 4,* 148-154.

Seidman, M. D. (2000). Effects of dietary restriction and antioxidants on presbyacusis. *Laryngoscope, 110,* 727-738.

Seidman, M. D., Ahmad, N., Joshi, D., Seidman, J., Thawani, S., & Quirk, W. S. (2004). Age-related hearing loss and its association with reactive oxygen species and mitochondrial DNA damage. *Acta Otolaryngological Supplement, 552,* 16-24.

Seidman, M. D., Khan, M. J., Bai, U., Shirwany, N., & Quirk, W. S. (2000). Biologic activity of mitochondrial metabolites on aging and age-related hearing loss. *American Journal of Otology, 21,* 161-167.

Seidman, M. D., Khan, M. J., Dolan, D. F., & Quirk, W. S. (1996). Age-related differences in cochlear microcirculation and auditory brain stem response. *Archives in Otolaryngology-Head and Neck Surgery, 122,* 1221-1226.

Seidman, M. D., Khan, M. J., Tang, W. X., & Quirk, W. S. (2002). Influence of lecithin on mitochondrial DNA and age-related hearing loss. *Otolaryngology-Head and Neck Surgery Journal, 3,* 138-144.

Seidman, M. D., & Moneysmith, M. (2006). *Save your hearing now: The revolutionary program that can prevent and may even reverse hearing loss.* New York: Warner Wellness.

Seidman, M. D., Quirk, W. S., Nuttall, A. L., & Schweitzer, V. G. (1991). The protective effects of allopurinol and superoxide dismutase-polyethylene glycol on ischemic and reperfusion-induced cochlear damage. *Otolaryngology-Head and Neck Surgery, 105,* 457-463.

Shankar, S., Singh, G., & Srivastava, R. K. (2007). Chemoprevention by resveratrol: molecular mechanisms and therapeutic potential. *Frontiers in Bioscience, 12,* 4839-4854.

Sha, S. H., & Schacht, J. (2000). Antioxidants attenuate gentamicin-induced free radical formation in vitro and ototoxicity in vivo: D-methionine is a potential protectant. *Hearing Research, 142*(1-2), 34-40.

Shay, J. W., & Wright, W. E. (1996). Telomerase activity in human cancer. *Current Opinions in Oncology, 8,* 66-71.

Shults, C. W., Flint Beal, M., Song, D., & Fontaine, D. (2004). Pilot trial of high dosages of coenzyme Q10 in patients with Parkinson's disease. *Experimental Neurology, 188,* 491-494.

Shults, C. W., Haas, R. H., Passov, D., & Beal, M. F. (1997). Coenzyme Q10 levels correlate with the activities of complexes I and II/III in mitochondria from parkinsonian and nonparkinsonian subjects. *Annals of Neurology, 42,* 261-264.

Shults, C. W., Oakes, D., Kieburtz, K., Beal, M. F., Haas, R., Plumb, S., et al. (2002). Effects of coenzyme Q10 in early Parkinson disease: Evidence of slowing of the functional decline. *Archives of Neurology, 59,* 1541-1550.

Sima, A. A. (2007). Acetyl-L-carnitine in diabetic polyneuropathy: Experimental and clinical data. *CNS Drugs, 21*, 13–23.

Sima, A. A., Calvani, M., Mehra, M., Amato, A., & Acetyl-L-Carnitine Study Group (2005). Acetyl-L-carnitine improves pain, nerve regeneration, and vibratory perception in patients with chronic diabetic neuropathy: an analysis of two randomized placebo-controlled trials. *Diabetes Care, 28*, 89–94.

Singh, U., & Jialal, I. (2008). Alpha-lipoic acid supplementation and diabetes. *Nutrition Reviews, 66*, 646–657.

Slattery, W. H., Fisher, L. M., Iqbal, Z., Friedman R. A., & Liu, N. (2005). Intratympanic steroid injection for treatment of idiopathic sudden hearing loss. *Otolaryngology-Head and Neck Surgery, 133*, 251–259.

Smith, K. M., Matson, S., Matson, W. R., Cormier, K., Del Signore, S. J., Hagerty, S. W., et al. (2006). Dose ranging and efficacy study of high-dose coenzyme Q10 formulations in Huntington's disease mice. *Biochimica et Biophysica Acta, 1762*, 616–626.

Sohal, R. S., & Allen, R. G. (1985). Relationship between metabolic rate, free radicals, differentiation and aging: A unified theory. *Basic Life Sciences, 35*, 75–104.

Soleas, G. J., Diamandis, E. P. & Goldberg, D. M. (1997). Wine as a biological fluid: History, production, and role in disease prevention. *Journal of Clinical Lab Analysis, 11*, 287–313.

Southorn, P. A., & Powis, G. (1988). Free radicals in medicine, I: Chemical nature and biologic reactions. *Mayo Clinic Proceedings, 63*, 381–389.

Storch, A., Jost, W. H., Vieregge, P., Spiegel, J., Greulich, W., Durner, J., et al. (2007). Randomized, double-blind, placebo-controlled trial on symptomatic effects of coenzyme Q(10) in Parkinson disease. *Archives of Neurology, 64*, 938–944.

Su, L. J., & Arab, L. (2006). Salad and raw vegetable consumption and nutritional status in the adult US population: Results from the Third National Health and Nutrition Examination Survey. *Journal of the American Dietetic Association, 106*, 1394–1404.

Syed D. N., Afaq, F., Kweon, M. H., Hadi, N., Bhatia, N. Spiegelman, V. S., et al. (2007). Green tea polyphenol EGCG suppresses cigarette smoke condensate-induced NF-kappaB activation in normal human bronchial epithelial cells. *Oncogene, 26*, 673–682.

Thangapazham, R. L., Singh, A. K., Sharma, A., Warren, J., Gaddipati, J. P., & Maheshwari, R. K. (2007). Green tea polyphenols and its constituent epigallocatechin gallate inhibits proliferation of human breast cancer cells in vitro and in vivo. *Cancer Letters, 245*, 232–241.

Tima, L., & Keithley, E. M. (2007). Effects of antioxidants on the aging inner ear. *Hearing Research, 226*, 194–202.

Tipoe, G. L., Leung, T. M., Hung, M. W., & Fung, M. L. (2007). Green tea polyphenols as an anti-oxidant and anti-inflammatory agent for cardiovascular protection. *Cardiovascular Hematological Disorders Drug Targets, 7*, 135–144.

Tse, A. K., Wan, C. K., Shen, X. L., Yang, M. & Fong, W. F. (2005). Honokiol inhibits TNF-alpha-stimulated NF-kappaB activation and NF-kappaB-regulated gene expression through suppression of IKK activation. *Biochemical Pharmacology, 70*, 1443–1457.

Tse, A. K., Wan, C. K., Zhu, G. Y., Shen, X. L., Cheung, H. Y., Yang, M., et al. (2007). Magnolol suppresses NF-kappaB activation and NF-kappaB regulated gene expression through inhibition of IkappaB kinase activation. *Molecular Immunology, 44*, 2647–2658.

Ullmann, U., Haller, J., Decourt, J. P., Girault, N., Girault, J., Richard-Caudron, A. S., et al. (2003). A single ascending dose study of epigallocatechin gallate in healthy volunteers. *Journal of Internal Medicine Research, 31*, 88–101.

Ullmann, U., Haller, J., Decourt, J. D., Girault, J., Spitzer, V. & Weber, P. (2004). Plasma-kinetic characteristics of purified and isolated green tea catechin epigallocatechin gallate (EGCG) after 10 days repeated dosing in healthy volunteers. *International*

Journal of Vitamin and Nutritional Research, 74, 269-278.

van Ginkel, P. R., Sareen, D., Subramanian, L., Walker, Q., Darjatmoko, S. R., Lindstrom, M. J., et al. (2007). Resveratrol inhibits tumor growth of human neuroblastoma and mediates apoptosis by directly targeting mitochondria. *Clinical Cancer Research, 13,* 5162-5169.

Vignes, M., Maurice, T., Lante, F., Nedjar, M., Thethi, K., Guiramand, J., et al. (2006). Anxiolytic properties of green tea polyphenol (−)-epigallocatechin gallate (EGCG). *Brain Research, 1110,* 102-115.

Wallace, D. C. (1992). Diseases of the mitochondrial DNA. *Annual Review of Biochemistry, 61,* 1175-1212.

Xie, D., Liu, G., Zhu, G., Wu, W., Ge, S. (2004). (−)-Epigallocatechin-3-gallate protects cultured spiral ganglion cells from H_2O_2-induced oxidizing damage. *Acta Otolaryngologica, 124,* 464-470.

Yamashita D., Jiang, H. Y., Le Prell, C. G., Schacht, J., & Miller, J. M. (2005). Postexposure treatment attenuates noise-induced hearing loss. *Neuroscience, 134,* 633-642.

Yang, S. W., Lee, B. R., & Koh, J. W. (2007). Protective effects of epigallocatechin gallate after UV irradiation in cultured human retinal pigment epithelial cells. *Korean Journal of Ophthalmology, 12,* 232-237.

Zhang, B., & Osborne, N. N. (2006). Oxidative-induced retinal degeneration is attenuated by epigallocatechin gallate. *Brain Research, 1124,* 176-187.

Zhang, B., Safa, R., Rusciano, D., & Osborne, N. N. (2007). Epigallocatechin gallate, an active ingredient from green tea, attenuates damaging influences to the retina caused by ischemic/reperfusion. *Brain Research, 1159,* 40-53.

Zhang, D., Tao, Y., Gao, J., Zhang, C., Wan, S., Chen, Y., et al. (2002). Pycnogenol in cigarette filters scavenges free radicals and reduces mutagenicity and toxicity of tobacco smoke in vivo. *Toxicological Industrial Health, 18,* 215-224.

Zhang, W. J., & Frei, B. (2001). A-Lipoic acid inhibits TNF-alpha-induced NF-kappaB activation and adhesion molecule expression in human aortic endothelial cells. *FASEB Journal, 15,* 2423-2432.

Zs-Nagy, I., Cutler, R. G., & Semsei, I. (1988). Dysdifferentiation hypothesis of aging and cancer: A comparison with the membrane hypothesis of aging. *Annals of the New York Academy of Sciences, 521,* 215-225.

Zs-Nagy, I., & Semsei, I. (1984). Centrophenoxine increases the rates of total and mRNA synthesis in the brain cortex of old rats: An explanation of its action in terms of the membrane hypothesis of aging. *Experimental Gerontology, 19,* 171-178.

12

Implantable Hearing Devices

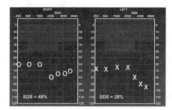

WILLIAM H. SLATTERY, III, M.D.

It is estimated that 32 million Americans have a hearing loss severe enough to cause problems with communication. The severity of this loss ranges from mild, in which the individual may have difficulty only when significant background noise is present, to a profound loss in which even in the quietest situation the patient is unable to understand and communicate. Most hearing loss is sensorineural in nature. Less than 10% of the hearing-impaired population has losses correctable by medical or surgical means. Although hearing loss may affect all frequencies, it is most common for individuals to have some component of high-frequency sensorineural hearing loss. Patients with a mild loss may receive no treatment other than instructions on modifying their acoustic environment to

diminish background noise when selecting seating arrangements to allow improved listening conditions. Individuals with conductive losses usually have the opportunity to undergo surgical therapy to have the loss corrected. However, in some cases, due to congenital abnormalities or infection, surgical correction is not an option. Individuals with profound sensorineural loss may receive cochlear implants, which provide electrical stimulation directly to the cochlear nerve.

Most of the population with sensorineural hearing loss must rely on amplification to provide a better means of improving communication. This is most commonly accomplished with conventional air-conduction hearing aids. In recent years, hearing aids have decreased in size, and improved microchips have been developed, resulting in improved signal processing capabilities. Hearing aids have become easier to program with digital processors; thus they are able to provide much better individualization of amplification according to each patient's needs. Despite the improvement in conventional hearing aid technology, only approximately 20% of the hearing-impaired population who could receive benefit from amplification actually uses these devices. (Fredrickson, Coticchia, & Khosla, 1996)

There are many reasons why patients do not wear a hearing aid. One of the most common reasons is that conventional air-conduction hearing aids do not provide enough amplification of the sounds that the individual actually wishes to hear. In addition, they produce troubling amplification of unwanted sounds, especially when background noise is present. Another major problem with conventional hearing aids is the limited high-frequency response. High-frequency output is limited by high-frequency feedback, which occurs when the microphone and receiver of conventional air-conduction hearing aids are in close proximity. Although new circuitry (feedback cancellation) has diminished some of these complaints, some conventional air-conduction hearing aid users still complain of feedback problems. Poor fit can result when the ear canal enlarges due to long-term use of the device causing feedback problems. As microchip technology has allowed hearing aids to become smaller to improve their cosmetic acceptance, it can result in greater problems with feedback as the microphone and speaker are placed closer together. Limited frequency output may produce problems with distortion, and, in particular, limited high-frequency amplification restricts sound localization abilities.

Cosmesis is still a major complaint of conventional air-conduction hearing aids. Many patients believe that wearing such a device indicates a disability and/or carries a stigma of old age. Earmolds may cause an occlusive effect in blocking residual hearing as well as producing discomfort, skin irritation, and the potential for increased infections of the ear canal (EAC). Discomfort is especially noted with smaller devices that fit more medially in the EAC. The occlusion effect, in addition to being uncomfortable, can result in loss of low-frequency information. There is a significant breakdown rate in conventional hearing aids due to wax in the receiver. Cerumen can not only occlude the receiver of the hearing aid, but also may cause wax impaction by the medial displacement of wax in the EAC.

Implantable hearing devices have become a viable alternative to conventional hearing aids. There are two main types of implantable devices. The more commonly used device is the bone-anchored hearing aid, or BAHA. Used in Europe since 1977, the BAHA received FDA clearance in 1996 as a treatment for conductive and mixed hearing losses. In 2002, it was also approved for treatment of unilateral sensorineural hearing loss or single-sided deafness. The other class of implantable devices is the middle ear implant, in which stimulation of the ossicular chain or direct stimulation to the cochlea is performed. This chapter reviews both devices.

Requirements of Implantable Devices

The goal of the middle-ear implant is to improve the efficiency of the device by improving *gain*, sound quality, hearing in noise, and eliminate acoustic feedback. It should improve the quality of life. The ideal implantable hearing device should be easy to implant. Additionally, it should cause no trauma or damage to the normal auditory system. It is extremely important that the auditory system remain intact in case of device failure. Experience with cochlear implants has demonstrated both the reliability of devices implanted in the postauricular and mastoid area, as well as revealed potential complications. Potential risks of implantation include further sensorineural hearing loss, damage to the dura or CSF leak, as well as the possibility of cholesteatoma or skin implantation into the middle ear or mastoid area. Skin complications can occur with any type of implant, and infection of the device is always a risk. Additionally, difficulties arising from coupling of the device to the ossicular chain or inner ear may directly damage these structures. The facial nerve and chorda tympani also may be at risk with surgical approaches for implantation, resulting in facial paralysis or weakness, or taste disturbance. Increased stiffness of the ossicular chain resulting from device fixation to the ossicles may impede low-frequency response, whereas those implants that increase the mass effect on the ossicular chain reduce the high-frequency response.

The ideal device must prove to be safe over a long period of time. Batteries are required for these fully implantable devices; changes should be able to be easily performed in the office or on an outpatient basis. It is to be expected that these devices, worn for years, will require future upgrades. The devices should allow technology that is easily upgradable allowing better speech processing strategies to be programmed when made available.

Theoretically, a device that worked 24/7 would offer a significant advantage over conventional air-conduction hearing aids. The ability to use a device in all normal daily activities such as water exposure during bathing or swimming is also a significant benefit. While wearing conventional air-conduction hearing aids, patients are unable to use them while sleeping or during water exposure. The ideal implant offers significant cosmetic benefit by being as invisible as possible. The lack of maintenance or need to clean the EAC is a significant advantage to the hearing impaired patient. A long battery life is essential to reduce the need for additional surgical procedures to change the battery.

Conventional Versus Implantable Hearing Aids

Gain is the amount of acoustic energy a device is able to deliver above the incoming signal. An implantable hearing aid must provide better *gain* than conventional air-conduction devices or some other real benefit to justify its use in an individual patient. Amplification of high frequencies is expected, and *gain* must be significant enough to provide real benefit to the patient. Most patients with significant hearing loss require significant *gain* levels in the high frequencies to receive any benefit from a device. If the device does not provide enough amplification in the high frequencies, then the amount of benefit the patient receives will be reduced. The maximum level of output in decibels SPL required to accommodate various levels of hearing loss is approximately 50 dB above the hearing threshold. To provide benefit to patients with moderate to moderate-to-severe hearing loss, a hearing aid must provide a maximum output level equivalent to 90 to 115 dB SPL, whereas a flat frequency response up to 8 kHz is desirable for maximum speech comprehension (Miller & Fredrickson, 2000).

Conventional air-conduction hearing aids amplify sound before it reaches the middle ear. A microphone converts the incoming acoustic signal into an electrical signal, while the amplifier and signal processor modify the electrical signal to increase its strength. The receiver then converts the amplified electrical signal into an acoustic signal for presentation to the tympanic membrane for transmission via the middle ear to the inner ear in the normal physiologic manner.

In contrast, the implantable devices provide acoustic energy to the middle ear or inner ear, bypassing the external ear canal, and in some cases the middle ear space. The microphone converts the incoming acoustic signal into an electrical signal. The amplifier and signal processor modify the electrical signal to increase its strength. The receiver converts the amplified electrical signal into a vibratory signal for presentation to the ossicular chain or to the cochlea directly, bypassing the tympanic membrane. Middle ear implants take advantage of the direct vibration of the middle ear ossicles to drive the ossicular chain.

Middle ear implants may be totally or partially implantable. The partially implantable device consists of a microphone and a speech processor connected to a transmitter fitted with an external coil that transmits electrical energy transcutaneously to the internal device. An internal receiving coil connected to a receiver provides electrical energy to a transducer connected to the ossicular chain. The external device also has a battery to power the system.

A fully implantable device contains essentially all of the elements of a par-

tially implantable device with the exception of a transducer coil and receiver. A microphone is placed under the skin, or is attached to the middle ear space and is connected to the internal speech processor. The entire system is powered by a rechargeable battery.

The middle ear implantable devices all stimulate the ossicular chain or cochlear fluids; however, they differ primarily by the type of transducer used to connect to the ossicular chain or cochlea. These devices provide a broad frequency response with low linear and nonlinear distortion. They are able to amplify high frequencies without the problem of acoustic feedback seen in conventional hearing aids, allowing the potential for better hearing in background noise with a more natural sound quality. A fully implantable device can also eliminate the perceived social stigma of visible conventional hearing aids.

Types of Middle Ear Implants

The definition of an implantable hearing device is any surgically implanted device that converts acoustic energy to mechanical energy and then delivers vibratory, stimulation to the inner ear. A transducer is a device that converts one form of energy to another. There are essentially two types of transducers currently used in middle ear implants: piezoelectric and electromagnetic. Each type has its advantages and disadvantages related to power, efficiency, frequency response, and reliability (Miller & Fredrickson, 2000).

Piezoelectric devices make use of ceramic crystals that change shape when voltage is applied. This change in shape can provide mechanical energy to stimulate the ossicular chain or inner ear. The change in the shape of the ceramic is not permanent; the ceramic reverts to its original shape when the electric current is no longer applied. There are two types of piezoelectric ceramic crystals: monomorph and bimorph. The monomorph piezoelectric crystal consists of a single layer, which expands and contracts to directly create the vibrations. The bimorph consists of two bonded ceramic layers, which are arranged in opposing electrical polarities. When the current is passed through the bonded layers; the entire structure bends, creating the vibration. Anatomic size restrictions limits piezoelectric ceramic materials use, as the amount of bending is proportional to the length of the crystal, reducing the amount of transductive power available.

The electromagnetic transduction of sound involves the creation of mechanical vibration by passing a current through a coil proximal to a magnet. As the electricity passes through the coil, an electromagnetic field is created, vibrating the magnet, which by direct or indirect contact will cause movement of the middle ear structures and/or cochlear fluids. The magnet may be attached directly to the middle ear vibratory pathway; the tympanic membrane, incus, or stapes. A fluctuating magnetic field is generated when the coil is energized by electrical signals that correspond to the acoustic input. The magnetic field causes the magnet to vibrate, inducing vibration of the ossicular chain or the cochlear fluids directly. The force generated by this system is directly proportional to the proximity of the magnet with the induction coil.

One method to produce electromagnetic stimulation is to separate the magnet from the induction coil. The coil is housed in a separate device, usually within the external ear canal while the magnet is attached to the ossicular chain. However, it sometimes can be challenging to control the spatial relationship of the magnet and the coil when the magnet is attached to one part of the ear and the coil is located within the ear canal, which may result in a wide variation in device performance. This can manifest as varying frequency responses, or fluctuation of output levels if the distance between the alignment of the coil and magnet changes.

Another method of electromechanical stimulation is to house the coil and magnet together, often in a single assembly. If the magnet and coil are housed together, a probe extending from this assembly must be in contact with the ossicular chain. As current is passed through the assembly, vibrations from the probe are sent directly to the ossicular chain. This form of electromechanical stimulation optimizes the spatial and geometric relationships to avoid the problem of changing alignment that may occur between the coil and magnet. The major limitation of this type of housing both the magnet and coil together is the attachment of the stimulating device, or coupler, to the ossicle or inner ear. If the device shifts relative to the position of the ossicles or inner ear, there may be a reduction in the optimal transmission of auditory stimulus.

History of Middle Ear Implants

The use of a magnetic field to stimulate the ossicles is not new. This concept can be traced back to 1935, when Wilska placed iron particles directly on the tympanic membrane (Wilska, 1935). A magnetic field was generated by an electromagnetic coil inside an ear phone, which caused the iron fillings to vibrate in synchrony with the magnetic field, producing vibration of the tympanic membrane, simulating hearing. Later, Rutschmann glued 10-mg magnets onto the umbo, causing it to vibrate via the application of a modified magnetic field with an electromagnetic coil. The resulting vibration of the ossicles produced hearing sensation (Rutschmann, 1959). Attachment of devices into the middle ear space did not occur until the 1970s with the RION device, to be discussed later in this chapter. Frederickson et al. developed the first mechanical device at Washington University in St. Louis, Missouri, in 1973 (Fredrickson, Tomlinson, Davis, & Odkuist, 1973). This device utilized a multichannel digital signal processor that transmitted power to the implanted coil via a transcutaneous link. It was implanted in 12 rhesus monkeys. After 2 years of implantation, no damage was found to the cochlea or peripheral auditory system. Frederickson found that the results from mechanical stimulation were similar to those produced by acoustic stimulation, and that high-intensity signals could be delivered to the inner ear effectively (Fredrickson, Coticchiam, & Khosla, 1995).

Maniglia at Case Western Reserve University in Cleveland, Ohio, demonstrated the use of an electromagnetic device in the cat (Maniglia et al., 1997). This group utilized the malleus as the microphone for a totally implantable device, which was implanted in cats for approximately 9 months. As with Frederickson's experiments, the results demonstrated thresholds from mechanical stimulation that were comparable to acoustic stimulation with no adverse effects on the middle or inner ear. Dumon, in Bordeaux, France, worked on piezoelectric devices placed in contact with the round window membrane (Dumon, Zennro, Aran, & Bebear,

1995). Twelve guinea pigs were stimulated over a 7-month period. This group attached the piezoelectric devices to the round window without removal of any other component of the ossicular chain.

Specific Devices

A variety of implantable devices have been investigated. This chapter reviews those that are currently approved and that have been implanted into humans. Patient selection criteria, depends on the type of transducer and the method by which the sound is stimulated (Table 12–1).

RION

The RION, developed at Ehime University and Teikyo University in Japan in collaboration with the Rion Company by Dr. Yanagihara and colleagues, was first implanted in 1984 (Figure 12–1) (Yanagihara, Aritomo, Yamanaka, & Gyo, 1987). This is a partially implantable middle ear device that uses a piezoelectric transducer approach. The device itself consists of a microphone, speech processor, and battery that are contained in an external behind-the-ear-unit. The internal component consists of an ossicular vibrator and internal coil, which are coupled. The essential component is the vibratory element consisting of a bimorph, or two piezoelectric ceramic elements pasted together with opposite polarity, that have been coated with layers of biocompatible material. The free end of the bimorph is attached to the stapes, and is also attached to a housing unit screwed into the mastoid cortex providing fixation. The bimorph vibrates in response to applied electrical current.

Table 12–1. Middle Ear Implantable Devices

Company	Transducer	Semi/Fully Implantable	Comments
RION	Piezoelectric	Semi-implantable	Only in Japan
Implex/TICA	Piezoelectric	Fully implantable	Bankrupt
Envoy	Piezoelectric	Fully implantable	Esteem I approved in Europe Esteem II Phase 2 in US
SoundTec	Magnet implant	Semi-implantable	FDA Approved September 01
Otologics/MET	Electromagnetic	Fully implantable	Approved in Europe Fully Implantable Phase 2
Soundbridge	Electromagnetic	Semi-implantable	Approved in Europe FDA Approved July 00

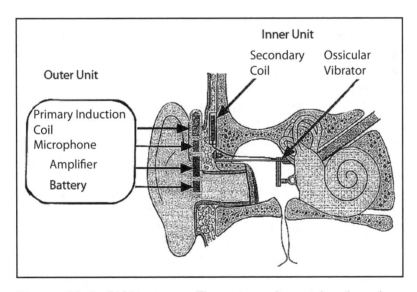

Figure 12–1. RION system. The outer unit contains the microphone, amplifier, and battery. The internal component contains the ossicular vibrator.

The indications for this device are mixed hearing loss, or in patients with significant mastoid disease. Its primary use has been in patients with conductive hearing loss from chronic otitis media. Patient selection criteria are listed in Table 12-2. Frequency responses are attenuated after approximately 5000 kHz,

Table 12–2. RION Device Patient Selection Criteria

- Average bone-conduction speech frequency hearing level (500, 1000, 2000 Hz), do not exceed 50 dB.
- There is a moderate-to-severe deafness in the contralateral ear.
- An intraoperative vibratory hearing test demonstrates the effectiveness of the unit.

---

so those, patients with significant sensorineural hearing loss above this frequency may not receive as much benefit as those with pure conductive hearing loss. The Rion has been implanted in Japan, but is not currently available in the United States.

The device may be placed in the postauricular area during a canal wall down mastoidectomy for treatment of chronic ear disease or through a transmastoid facial recess approach. The housing unit fits in the mastoid with a tip that extends to the stapes. The open mastoid cavity is the preferred approach, because it allows adequate exposure to the ossicles, but this requires the ear canal to be closed off. The device is fixed to the mastoid cortex and the bimorph container is placed over the stapes. A seat is then surgically created for the internal coil and electric unit.

The device has been worn by some patients for more than 10 years (Yanagihara, Sato, Hinohira, Gyo, & Hori, 2001). Implanted patients report natural sound quality without feedback or discomfort, which is very close to perceived normal hearing. Long-term sensorineural hearing loss has not occurred with the use of this device. There have been no complications during implantation in more than 39 patients in Japan.

TICA Implex

The totally implantable communication assistance (TICA) device was developed at the University of Tubingen, Germany, in collaboration with Implex Corporation in Munich in the mid-1990s (Figure 12–2). Unfortunately, the company went bankrupt and the device is no longer available for use. The TICA device is reviewed for historical purposes, as it represents the first fully implantable device that was utilized in humans and allowed the development of some important concepts that have been used elsewhere. The TICA was a fully implantable device that used a piezoelectric transducer to stimulate the ossicular chain. In addition, it used a microphone implanted in the ear canal, which picked up sound. This sensor provided an electrical input into the fully implanted unit or can, which was implanted subcutaneously in the mastoid area. The can was a hermetically sealed titanium container that included the speech processor, battery, and a receiving coil. The actuator attached to the body of the incus, causing vibration of the ossicular chain. The induction coil within the titanium can was used to receive electrical impulses to permit recharging of the battery. The patient would recharge the battery by wearing a small headband that could also be used for programming the device. A wireless remote control could be used by the patient to select four programs, adjust the volume, as well as switch the device on and off. The battery life was 50 hours, whereas recharging took approximately 2 hours. The speech processor consisted of a digitally programmable three-channel audioprocessor. The induction coil could be used to receive input similar to cochlear implants for processing. Also, similar to cochlear im-

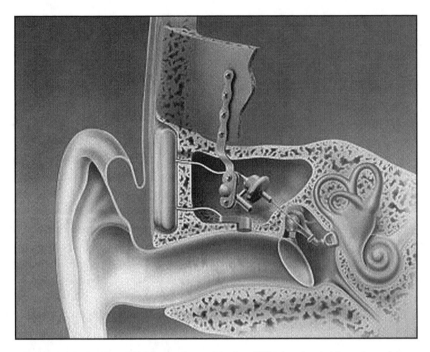

Figure 12–2. The TICA device with the fully implantable microphone in the ear canal. The speech processor battery unit is housed in a subcutaneous pocket in the postauricular area. The stimulator attaches to the incus to vibrate the ossicles.

plants, fitting would start about 8 weeks postoperatively, and several programming sessions were usually required.

There were several advantages to the TICA, such as having no external components as well as being MRI-compatible. It had a wide frequency range from 100 Hz to 10,000 KHz. The battery life was estimated to be 3 to 5 years before a replacement was needed.

Approximately 20 patients were implanted with the TICA device (Zenner & Leysieffer, 2001). All patients had bilateral moderate to severe sensorineural hearing loss and the patients had not benefitted from hearing aids. One problem that arose after implantation of the TICA was feedback. The incus was stimulated by the actuator. The feedback occurred as sound was generated by the stimulation of the ossicular chain and picked up by the microphone implanted in the ear canal. The stimulation of the ossicular chair caused sound vibration to be transported to the cochlea, but this also resulted in the eardrum acting as a speaker; generating sound into the ear canal. This necessitated disarticulation of the ossicular chain between the malleus and incus. To avoid feedback or sound coming out the ear canal from vibration of the malleus and eardrum, the neck of the malleus was removed.

Implanted patients described their hearing as being distortion-free and transparent. They reported excellent speech intelligibility, as well as an improved ability to listen to music, especially in the presence of background noise. Patients were also able to use the device during sporting events, including swimming, as well as in the shower. Unfortunately, the company did not stay in business. The experience of the TICA implant demonstrated that a fully implantable device was possible, and allowed the development of many of the components, now utilized in other subsequently developed devices.

Vibrant Soundbridge

The Vibrant Soundbridge is the first FDA-approved implantable middle ear hearing device to treat sensorineural hearing loss, and has been implanted in thousands of patients worldwide (Figure 12–3). It is a partially implantable middle ear hearing device initially developed by Symphonics Devices, Inc., of San Jose, California. Subse-quently Med-El Corporation of Innsbruck, Austria has taken over the production and distribution of the device. The Vibrant Soundbridge is a semi-implantable hearing aid consisting of two parts: the speech processor worn externally, and the implantable vibrating ossicular prosthesis (VORP). The VORP is surgically placed subcutaneously in the postauricular area. The floating mass transducer (FMT) is connected to the internal receiver, and is attached to the stapes. The FMT is a unique electromagnetic transducer that contains a magnet of inertial mass within two electromagnetic coils. When activated, the magnet mass vibrates within the FMT between the two coils causing the entire unit to vibrate. Titanium strips are attached around the long process of the incus to hold the device in place. The

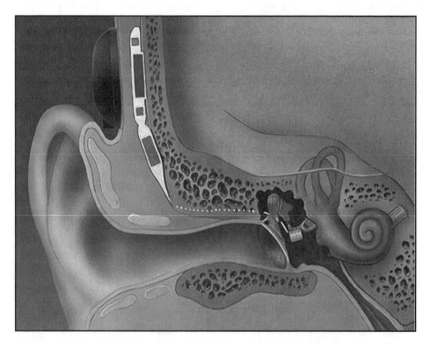

Figure 12–3. The Vibrant Soundbridge with the external microphone, with the coil for transcutaneous stimulation of the internal device. The internal device connects to the floating mass transducer, which attaches to the incus.

floating mass transducer is oriented in the direction of the stapes so vibration of the device will be directly into the inner ear, parallel to the plain of the stapes. The external auditory processor is held in place over the internal receiver by a magnet.

The auditory processor contains a microphone that picks up sound from the environment and converts it into an electrical signal. The auditory processor is contained within the external unit, which also contains an induction coil to transmit the electrical signal to the internal VORP. A receiving coil picks up the signal and transmits it to the floating mass transducer, causing it to vibrate, which then stimulates the cochlea.

Placement of the internal device requires an outpatient mastoidectomy similar to cochlear implantation. The facial recess is widely opened to visualize the incudostapedial joint, and to allow the FMT to pass through easily. The FMT is crimped onto the incus after the VORP is imbedded in the cortical bone in a seat behind the mastoid posterior to the sigmoid sinus. The external processor is attached six weeks after surgery, at which time the device is programmed. Current indications for the Vibrant Soundbridge are found in Table 12–3.

Table 12–3. Vibrant Soundbridge Patient Selection Criteria

- Adult, 18 or over
- Word recognition score, 50% or better
- Normal middle ear function
- Realistic expectations
- Pure tone air conduction thresholds within the following table

Clinical trials for this device began in 1996, and the device was approved by the FDA in 2000. The FDA trials demonstrated over 94% of patients reported improvement in their signal quality satisfaction rating with the Vibrant Soundbridge compared to their previous conventional air conduction hearing aids. Ninety-seven percent of patients who had complained of feedback problems with their presurgery air-conduction hearing aids reported no feedback with the Vibrant Soundbridge. Eighty-eight percent of patients reported improved sound quality satisfaction rating of their own voice. Ninety-eight percent of subjects reported satisfaction with the overall fit and comfit of the Vibrant Soundbridge (Luetje et al., 2002). The Vibrant Soundbridge has recently been implanted over the round window membrane as a means to directly stimulate the cochlear fluid. Colletti implanted seven patients with atresia or chronic otitis media in which the stapes was not available to be stimulated. The classic transmastoid approach was utilized; however, the bony lip of the round window was drilled out to allow the floating transducer to fit over this area (Colletti, Soli, Carner, & Colletti, 2006). Thresholds in the normal range were accomplished for all patients implanted with the floating mass transducer placed over the round window. Long-term affects of this type of stimulation are not known; however, additional studies are currently being performed to investigate this mode of stimulation.

SoundTec

The SoundTec DDHS system was developed by Jack Hough of Oklahoma City, Oklahoma (Figure 12–4). Although new

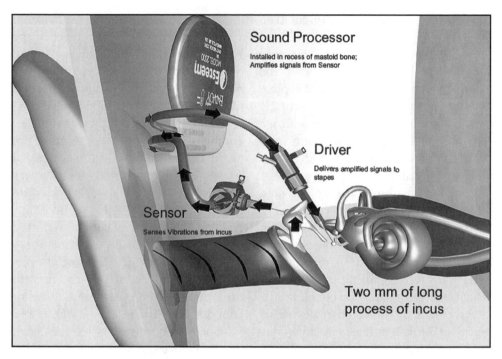

Figure 12–4. The SoundTec device: The magnet is attached to the incus between the incus and stapes joint.

devices are no longer available, it is reviewed for historical purposes, as many patients in the United States have this device. The SoundTec used an electromagnetic approach that separated the magnet and the induction coil. A tiny magnet, approximately the size of a grain of rice, was attached to the incudostapedial joint. The magnetic coil, which would drive the magnet, was located in the ear canal in a conventional in-the-ear mold. The sound processor, microphone, and battery were located in a behind-the-ear external unit and were linked to the coil in the external ear canal. The magnet was placed during an outpatient procedure via the transcanal approach, with the tympanic membrane elevated to attach the magnet to the incudostapedial joint. A deep-seated ear canal fitting was required for the ITE (in the ear) unit after complete healing occurred.

One hundred and three patients were implanted at 10 sites for the FDA trial before approval was given in 2001 for treatment of sensorineural hearing loss. The SoundTec direct system gave an average of 7.9 dB increase in functional gain over optimally fitted air-conduction hearing aids. Patients' AFAB and speech discrimination scores were much higher for the SoundTec direct system compared to their optimally fitted air conduction hearing aids (Hough, Dyer, Matthews, & Wood, 2001). Unfortunately, this device is no longer available for implantation.

Envoy Esteem

The Envoy Esteem has been developed by St. Croix Medical, Inc., of Minneapolis, Minnesota (Figure 12–5). This is a fully implantable system that utilizes a piezo-

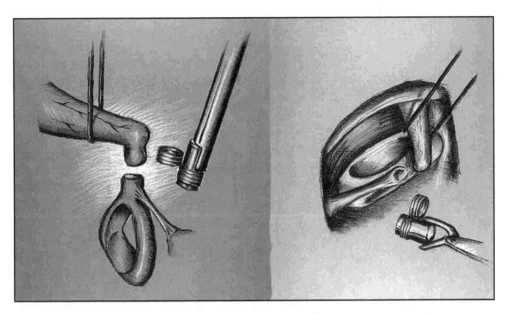

Figure 12–5. The Envoy fully implantable system. The eardrum is used as a microphone to pick up sound via a transducer attached to the malleus head. The internal component consists of a battery and speech processor. There is an internal coil for programming the device. The stimulation of the ossicles occurs via attachment to the stapes.

electric transducer for reception and transduction. The transducer consists of two internal plates separated by a thin conduction material. The first transducer (sensor) detects movement of the malleus in response to sound stimulation. This sensor acts as a microphone sending signals to the processor. The second piezoelectric transducer (the driver) is placed on the stapes. The piezoelectric units use the bimorph design for the sensor and driver. One of the sensors is fixed to the malleus to detect vibration and stabilized by fixation to the cortical skull bone. A small amplifier in the base increases the gain. The fully implantable device also contains a speech processor powered by a lithium iodine battery.

The Esteem device is implanted through a postauricular mastoidectomy, with the attic area opened widely to allow adequate room for placement of the sensor and driver. A bed is created in the cortical bone to attach the sound processor/battery unit. The facial recess is opened up to allow adequate visualization of the chorda tympani, facial nerve, and stapes and to allow adequate space for the piezoelectric driver to be positioned in contact with the stapes. The bone of the posterior ear canal must also be thinned carefully to allow adequate visualization. The incudostapedial joint is separated and a 2-mm section of the long process of the incus is resected. Disarticulation is required in order to separate the vibrating malleus from the stapes, which will be stimulated. In some cases, full removal of the incus may be necessary, with the sensor attached to the malleus head (Envoy-Voices, March 2000).

The Envoy has gone through two generation of devices. The first device, the Esteem 1, had a battery life of 2.5 to

5 years, and no recharging of the battery was required. The Esteem 2, or second generation device, has recently being utilized in clinical trials. This device has a longer battery life, extended to 5 to 8 years without the need to recharge. There is also a broader fitting range resulting in improved gain of 10 to 20 dB over the Esteem 1.

The first devices were implanted in Europe in March of 2000. Phase I trial (Safety study) for the Esteem 1 began in March of 2002. The Esteem 1 is currently approved with its CE mark for European implantation (The CE Mark is the U.S. FDA equivalent). The Esteem 2 should be approved for CE mark in 2008. Phase II clinical trials for the Esteem 2 are scheduled to begin in 2008. At this time neither device is approved by the FDA in the United States.

MET

The Otologics MET is a fully implantable ossicular stimulator produced by Otologics of Boulder, Colorado (Figure 12–6). The initial device tested was a partially implantable device that consisted of an external digital speech processor and an implanted unit. The external components consisted of a microphone, speech processor, battery, and transmitter housed in a disc. The external unit is held in place with magnets that align it to the

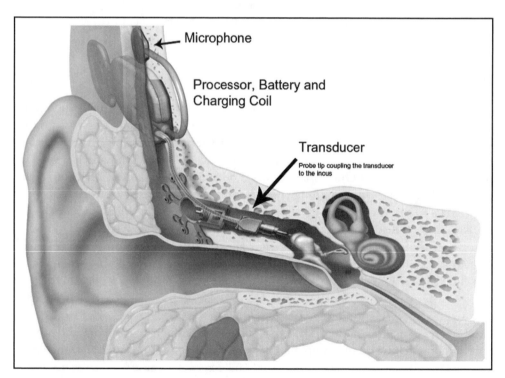

Figure 12–6. Otologic Met. The microphone is placed in the subcutaneous pocket behind the ear. The internal device consists of a speech processor, battery, and coil. The electromechanical stimulator is attached to the body of the incus. The ossicular chain is kept intact.

internal unit, similar to a cochlear implant. The implanted components consist of a subcutaneous electrical package containing a transcutaneous receiver and a transducer motor in a hermetically sealed case. The electromagnetic motor drives a biocompatible probe tip, which is placed in a hole in the body of the incus. Activation of the device causes mechanical motion of the probe tip, which in turn vibrates the ossicular chain.

The transducer was found to have a linear input/output curve to beyond 1000 dynes at 1 kHz with low distortion. The frequency response is relatively flat, varying only about 10 dB up from 1 kHz to 10,000 kHz.

The device is placed during an outpatient surgical procedure through a postauricular transmastoid approach. A mounting device is placed into the mastoid cortex that secures the electrical mechanical motor, while a seat is created to place the electronic housing container. A laser hole is created in the incus body for the probe tip to rest. Six to eight weeks postoperatively, the device can be activated and programmed.

The partially implantable device is currently available in Europe. FDA trials for the partially implantable device were not completed in the United States, as the fully implantable device has subsequently become available. The fully implantable device is currently undergoing both European and U.S. FDA trials at the time of this writing for the treatment of conductive and mixed hearing loss and congenital atresia.

The fully implantable device consists of the same transducer stimulator as the partially implantable device. In addition, the internal case contains the battery, speech processor, receiving coil for programming and battery recharging, and a separate microphone, which is attached to the receiving coil. The microphone is placed in the postauricular area subcutaneously. It is anticipated that the battery will last approximately 12 years. The battery requires daily recharging that takes less than 1 hour, during which time the patient can still use the device. The induction coil in the internal receiver receives a transcutaneous charge from a battery charger, which is also the method by which the device will be programmed. The MET has a remote control that is used for volume control and turning the device on and off. A copy of the Otologics MET criteria is given in (Table 12–4).

The Otologic MET has several different attachments which may be used on the transducer for stimulation. The classic or original device was designed to attach to the incus. Subsequently, additional adapters have been created, allowing the device to attach to the stapes,

Table 12–4. Otologic Met Patient Selection Criteria

Frequency response					
	Frequencies				
	500	**1000**	**2000**	**3000**	**4000**
Upper limits	65	75	80	85	85

oval window, or round window, for direct stimulation. Clinical trials of these new attachments have not yet begun.

BAHA Device

The BAHA, or bone anchored hearing aid device, was first pioneered in 1977 (Figure 12–7). Originally brought to market by Entific Corporation, the BAHA was recently acquired by Cochlear Corporation. The BAHA consists of an implantable titanium percutaneous screw abutment that fits into the skull, and a separate external device. The external device contains the microphone, speech processor, battery, and vibratory unit. The percutaneous plug is utilized only for transmission of the vibratory signal to the skull. Essentially, the BAHA works as a direct connect bone-conduction hearing aid.

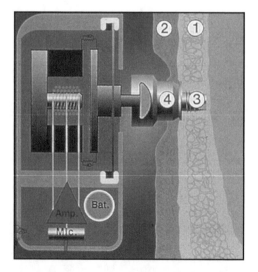

Figure 12–7. The BAHA device. 1. Skull bone. 2. Skin and subcutaneous tissue. 3. Implanted titanium fixture. 4. Titanium abutment. The external processor consists of the microphone, amplifier, and battery unit.

Conventional bone conduction hearing aids put pressure against skin to cause vibration; in contrast, the percutaneous screw of the BAHA allows direct bone stimulation, allowing much better bone conduction as the soft tissue of the skull is avoided. The major disadvantage of the system is the cosmetic appearance of the percutaneous pedestal. However, patients report this device is much more comfortable than traditional bone-conduction devices, as well as providing better sound quality without the need of wearing a headband to keep the aid in place.

The device is placed in an outpatient procedure usually performed under local anesthesia. The pedestal is placed in the postauricular area approximately 5.5 cm from the external ear canal. The skin tissue around the device is thinned, and the subcutaneous soft tissue is removed down to the periosteum to allow placement of the device. A small hole is made in the periosteum, followed by a 3- to 4-mm hole in the skull, into which the self tapping pedestal is placed. The skin is then closed around the device. There is usually a 2- to 3-cm area surrounding the device where the skin has been thinned and the soft tissue removed, which may result in a bald spot around the pedestal. Newer implantation techniques that have been developed allow the hair follicles to be preserved while still thinning the skin. Osseointegration, or the direct contact between living bone and the loaded implant surface, must take place before the BAHA can be used, which usually requires 3 to 4 months.

The area around the abutment usually heals within 1 to 2 weeks after implantation. Special care must be utilized for hygiene around the pericutaneous pedestal to avoid undue trauma. A soft toothbrush is given to patients to clean around the pedestal, with brushing of the implant being performed during hair washing. Occasionally, small areas of granulation tissue may present at the skin- titanium junction. These usually resolve by treatment with an antibiotic ointment and topical cleaning with hydrogen peroxide. Occasionally, the skin will become thickened around the device, requiring topically applied steroid ointment to thin the skin.

A major advantage of the BAHA system is that patients are able to test the sound quality prior to implantation. A headband with the external processor/vibrator can be used to simulate the results one would receive if the device was implanted. Although the results from implantation are better than those given by the headband simulator, patients are able to get an idea preoperatively of the sound quality and benefit that they may receive. In cases of congenital atresia, the BAHA may be placed bilaterally. The device has been placed in children as young as 2 years of age. In these young patients, the device is placed more posterior, permitting future reconstructive surgery if the patient decides to proceed with this when they become older.

There are two indications for the BAHA: treatment of patients with conductive hearing loss, and those with single-sided deafness. Patients with normal bone-conduction thresholds and only a conductive hearing loss are the ideal candidates for the device Patients with a history of a chronic ear surgery, or chronic otitis media, congenital atresia, conductive hearing loss not amenable to surgery, or external otitis are included in the conductive hearing loss group. The BAHA has been found to be especially useful in those cases of congenital atresia cases in which reconstructive surgery cannot be performed. Patients with draining ears or ears that drain when occluded with an earmold are also suitable candidates. Although the better the bone thresholds, the better the results, those patients with sensorineural hearing loss whose bone conduction thresholds between 500 to 3000 Hz are less than 45 dB with a speech discrimination score of 60% or better are also candidates. Additionally, a more powerful external unit can provide additional amplification for those patients who have bone conduction thresholds up to 60 dB at those frequencies (Hakansson et al., 1990).

The other approved indication for the BAHA is the treatment of single-sided deafness, which was approved by the FDA in September of 2002 (Wazen et al., 2003). As with patients treated for conductive hearing loss, preoperative testing with the headband is recommended to improve patient acceptance. A total unilateral hearing loss may occur as a result of surgery, infection, trauma, or conditions such as sudden sensorineural hearing loss. Although CROS (contralateral routing of sound) hearing aid devices traditionally have been utilized for this group of patients, they have not been widely accepted, leaving most patients with single-sided deafness without any viable solution for their condition. The BAHA has found a nitch with good acceptance in this patient group. In the past, the handicap to patients with unilateral deafness was underestimated by physicians. Patients with unilateral deafness often complain of difficulty hearing in background noise, difficulty hearing when sound is presented in the deaf side, as well as trouble localizing sound. The BAHA device has been shown to help patients with unilateral deafness improve their speech intelligibility in noise. This is done by allowing some release from the head shadow effect, and has provided a greater benefit to the wearer when compared to a traditional CROS hearing aid system. One of the most common indications for the BAHA is in patients undergoing acoustic neuroma removal when deafness is the known outcome. The buttress is placed at the same time as the acoustic neuroma removal. However, patient acceptance in this group is not as successful as in other cases of single-sided deafness, as they have not had the opportunity to try the test band preoperatively

Conclusion

Much work has been done over the past several decades to develop implantable hearing devices. Although there have been many successes, this field must be considered still in its infancy, with virtually all of these devices undergoing modification. Although development is rapid, and the outcomes from current devices are encouraging, patients must be informed that the long-term results are presently not known. At the time of this writing, the field appears to be moving toward the use of these devices for conductive or mixed losses, as opposed to pure sensorineural hearing loss. Further clinical trials will need to be conducted in order to learn more about this emerging field.

Experience has taught that clinical trials for implantable devices always take longer and cost more than originally estimated. Additionally, many manufacturers have had difficulty in the mass production of reliable products. In addition to manufacturing problems, cost has been a major issue, as many government agencies and insurance carriers have not routinely paid for these devices. However, as outcome studies demonstrate real improvement by the use of implantable devices, the trend is beginning to turn for coverage of the cost of surgery and the device.

It is of interest that subjects describe the results from these devices as being better than their conventional air-conduction hearing aids. The patient's subjective assessment of improvement far outweighs the objective measures that have been utilized in clinical trials. It appears that the benefit described by patients is not measured by functional gain alone. Although the exact rationale for this perceived improvement is not known, better amplification of high frequencies than conventional air conduction hearing aids is theorized to be responsible for much of this benefit. Perhaps the development of new measurement tools will be necessary to adequately measure the device's benefit as this area of otology continues to grow.

References

Colletti, V., Soli, S. D., Carner, M., & Colletti, L. (2006) Treatment of mixed hearing losses via implantation of a vibratory transducer on the round window. *International Journal of Audiology*, *45*(10), 600–608.

Dumon, T., Zennaro, O., Aran, J. M., & Bebear, J. P. (1995b). Piezoelectric middle ear implant preserving the ossicular chain. *Otolaryngology Clinics of North America*, *28*(1), 173–187.

Envoy–Voices. (2000, March). *First chronic implant performed*. Minneapolis, MN: St. Croix Medical.

Fredrickson, J. M., Coticchia, J. M., & Khosla, S. (1995). Ongoing investigations into an implantable electromagnetic hearing aid for moderate to severe sensorineural hearing loss. *Otolaryngology Clinics of North America, 28*(1), 107–120.

Fredrickson, J. M., Coticchia, J. M., & Khosla, S. (1996). Current status in the development of implantable middle ear hearing aids. In *Advances in otolaryngology* (Vol. 10, pp. 189–204). St. Louis, MO: Mosby.

Fredrickson, J. M., Tomlinson, D. R., Davis, E. R., & Odkuist, L. M. (1973) Evaluation of an electromagnetic implantable hearing aid. *Canadian Journal of Otolaryngology, 2,* 53–62.

Hakansson, B., Liden, G., Tjellstrom, A., Ringdahl, A., Jacobsson, M., Carlsson, P., et al. (1990). Ten years of experience of the Swedish bone anchored hearing system. *Annals of Otology, Rhinology and Laryngology, 99*(Suppl.), 1–16.

Hough, J., Dyer, R., Matthews, P., & Wood, M. (2001). Early clinical results: SOUNDTEC Implantable Hearing Device phase II study. *Laryngoscope, 111,* 1–8.

Luetje, C. M., Brackman, D., Balkany, T. J., Maw, J., Baker, R. S., Kelsall, D., et al. (2002). Phase III clinical trial results with the Vibrant Soundbridge implantable middle ear hearing device: A prospective controlled multicenter study. *Otolarygology Head and Neck Surgery, 126*(2), 97–107.

Maniglia, A. J., Ko, W. H., Garverick, S. L., Abbass, H., Kane, M., Rosenbaum, M., et al. (1997). Semi-implantable middle ear electromagnetic hearing device for sensorineural hearing loss. *Ear, Nose, and Throat Journal, 76*(5), 333–338, 340–341.

Miller, D. A., & Fredrickson, J. M. (2000). Implantable hearing aids. In M. Valente (Ed.), *Audiology treatment* (pp 489–510). New York: Thieme.

Rutschmann, J. (1959). Magnetic audition: Auditory stimulation by means of alternating magnetic fields acting on a permanent magnet fixed to the eardrum. *IRE Transactions Med Electron, 6,* 22–23.

Wazen, J. J., Spitzer, J. B., Ghossaini, S. N., Fayad, J. N., Niparko, J. K., Cox, K., et al. (2003). Transcranial contralateral cochlear stimulation in unilateral deafness. *Otolaryngology-Head and Neck Surgery, 129*(3), 248–254.

Wilska, A. (1935). Einmethode zur bestimmung der horsch wellanamplituden des trommelfells bei verscheiden frequenzen. *Skandinavisches Archives of Physiology, 72,* 161–165.

Yanagihara, N., Aritomo, H., Yamanaka, E., & Gyo, K. (1987). Implantable hearing aid: Report of the first human applications. *Archives of Otolaryngology, Head and Neck Surgery, 113*(8), 869–872.

Yanagihara, N., Sato, H., Hinohira, Y., Gyo, K., & Hori, K. (2001). Long-term results using a piezoelectric semi-implantable middle ear hearing device: The RION device E-type. *Otolaryngology Clinics of North America, 34*(2), 389–400.

Zenner, H. P., & Leysieffer, H. (2001). Total implantation of the Implex TICA hearing amplifier implant for high frequency sensorineural hearing loss: The Tubingen University experience. *Otolarygology Clinics of North America, 34*(2), 417–446.

13

Assistive Listening Devices

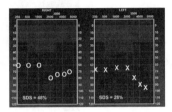

RANDY DRULLINGER

ALDs and the Modern Practice

Assistive listening devices (ALDs) have been an overlooked and underused tool in many practices. The hassle of deciding which items to carry, where to display them, and how to manage excess inventory has kept many practitioners from recognizing the benefits that ALDs can bring. Increasingly today, products in this category are being recognized as another component in treating hearing loss, along with hearing aids and aural rehabilitation, allowing us to address the hearing-impaired patient's entire communication needs within their own listening environment.

In this chapter, we explore the importance to the practitioner of offering ALDs to their hearing-impaired patients, and how best to implement adding them to an existing practice.

What Is an ALD?

Assistive listening devices in the past consisted mainly of niche products such as flashing door bell ringers, smoke alarms that strobe, and telephone signaling systems. These were unglamorous and utilitarian in nature, and geared more toward the deaf or severely hearing-impaired communities. In contrast, today's modern ALDs are much more suited to the majority of the population that suffers from mild to moderately severe hearing loss, in addition to those with profound loss, and include technologies such as Bluetooth and FM systems to create products that enhance active lifestyles. Most are now designed to work in conjunction with digital hearing aids to provide or extend benefits the wearer already receives from their hearing aids.

An example of this is the Oticon Streamer™, a Bluetooth device that allows users of the Oticon Epoq family of hearing aids to connect wirelessly to their cell phone or MP3 player. This and other such products have brought a whole new world of connectivity to hearing aid users who, up until this point, were unable to use a cell phone without taking out their hearing aids.

Another such product is Jitterbug™ cellphone, which has an ear piece that works well with in-the-ear (ITE) hearing aids. Additionally, there are other cell phones designed to use with hearing aids, but they are not widely available. The author's research has indicated that the trend is leaning toward middleware products, such as the Oticon Streamer or the Starkey Eli, which can connect to any Bluetooth device (Figure 13-1).

This new generation of products is helping people stay active and connected despite their hearing loss, and has made it more profitable for the hearing health care practice to carry these products, as the margins are much better and the appeal much broader.

Categories of ALDs

Assistive listening devices come in three main categories today: Personal listening systems, Alerting devices, and telephone systems including, cellular and Bluetooth devices.

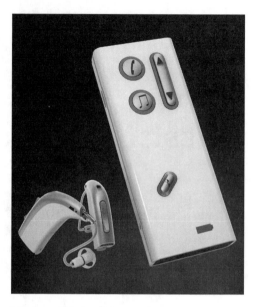

Figure 13–1. Oticon streamer.

Personal Listening Systems

Products in this category include television amplification (Sennhieser Set 100J™, Clearsounds 2000™), and personal FM systems (Phonak SmartLink System™, Williams Pocket Talker™). The Phonak SmartLink™, to illustrate one such device, provides users with a wireless microphone/transmitter that can be placed near the desired audio source and focused to allow the source to wirelessly feed audio directly into the users hearing device. For example, if the user was attending a meeting or lecture, the wireless transmitter could be placed on the lectern and transmit audio directly to the hearing device worn by the hearing impaired user in the audience (Figure 13-2).

In the same manner, the TV amplification devices offer a similar wireless experience as the SmartLink™, with the audio source being the television set.

The TV amplification devices offer an integrated headset so they can be used

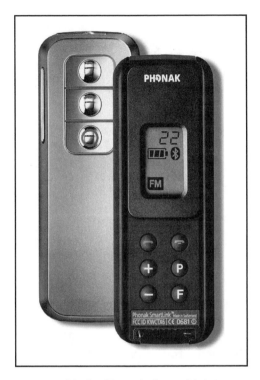

Figure 13–2. Phonak SmartLink transmitter.

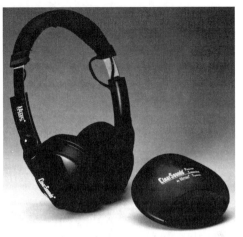

Figure 13–3. Clearsounds TV amplifier.

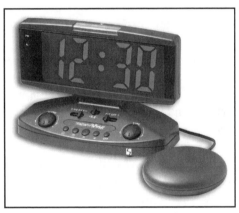

Figure 13–4. Clearsounds Wake and Shake alarm clock.

with or without a hearing aid. In addition to the hearing impaired individual, family members and friends who watch TV in the same room have appreciated that these systems allow those with normal hearing to listen comfortably at their usual volumes (Figure 13-3).

Alerting Devices

Products in this category include doorbell signalers, telephone ringer alerts, alarm clocks with a feature that shakes the bed to awaken the sleeper, and smoke alarms that strobe when activated.

These signals, which seem mundane in the hearing world, can have a big and sometimes life-saving impact on those who are hearing impaired (Figure 13-4).

Telephone Systems

This category, by far, offers products that are attractive to the widest variety of people. The telephone is the number one communication device in use today, whether hearing impaired or not. In the not too distant past, those who were deaf required a special TTY/TTD hooked up to a land line in order to communicate by phone. Today, they can simply purchase an inexpensive cell phone and use the texting feature, which is available on most cell phones.

The telephone has also become a de facto "testing" device for those who have recently purchased hearing aids. More often than not the "test" fails as the user experiences feedback and lack of clarity. This then becomes an issue for the patient who may have spent thousands of dollars on a sophisticated digital hearing device, only to have it not work well on a $100 phone! Providing a telephone with the delivery of a new hearing aid, or encouraging the patient to purchase a phone that has been demonstrated to be compatible with the new hearing aids, can go a long way to both increasing overall patient satisfaction, as well as lowering the return rates on hearing aids.

Telephones like the Clearsounds A55™ provide sound-shaping technology to enhance clarity rather than simply amplifying sound. The design of the earpiece lends itself to use with hearing aids, and the cordless feature is also a plus.

Another phone by the same manufacturer, the Clearsounds Emergency Connect™ phone, offers a separate remote feature that can be worn, like a wristwatch, by the user. In the event the wearer cannot physically reach the phone itself to dial out in case of an emergency, he or she can control the phone with the wrist remote. This device can be useful for any individual at risk, such as an elderly person living alone or a patient with impaired balance, whether or not they have hearing impairment (Figures 13-5 and 13-6).

Cellular telephone technology is also catching up to the needs of the hearing impaired. Most of the early cell phones were incompatible with digital hearing aids. Today, major manufacturers such as Sony/Ericsson are offering cell phones that are compatible with hearing aids. In

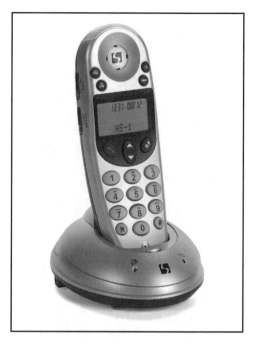

Figure 13–5. Clearsounds Amplifies cordless phone.

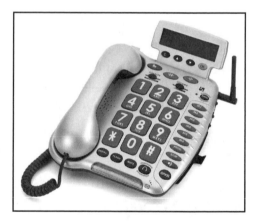

Figure 13–6. Clearsounds Emergency Connect phone.

addition, the proliferation of Bluetooth technology has also led to products such as the Starkey Eli™ and the Oticon Streamer™ that allow the user with a hearing aid to connect wirelessly to a cell phone, MP3 player or other Bluetooth device (Figure 13-7).

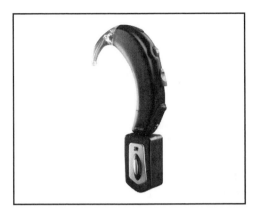

Figure 13–7. Starkey Eli.

Should ALDs Be a Part of the Practice?

In the opening paragraph, we alluded to concerns such as inventory that are arguments against selling ALDs in the clinical setting. In response, there are three main reasons that should compel most practices to add an ALD strategy to their mix.

Additional Revenue Stream

The ability to add an additional revenue stream within the existing infrastructure of a practice with no additional personnel needed should be very attractive to the practitioner.

The front office staff can be trained and incentivized financially to recommend and show products such as telephones or alerting devices, while the audiologist and/or dispenser can demonstrate the more sophisticated Bluetooth and personal FM systems.

Completeness of Care

As we have discussed, hearing aids do not always work in certain listening situ-

ations, despite the wearer's expectations. When a user encounters a problem talking on the phone, or in some other situation such as listening to television with background noise, he or she may start doubting his or her decision to purchase a hearing aid in the first place. This can lead to higher returns that will negatively impact the practice revenue and create an unhappy patient. Managing expectations at the beginning, as well as suggesting the appropriate ancillary devices for the patient's lifestyle, may go a long way to solving the individual needs of the hearing impaired, and increase overall patient satisfaction. Not only will lower returns improve the practice bottom line, but happy patients refer their friends and family to your practice, which will also have a positive impact on revenues and the clinic reputation.

The "Searcher"

Anyone who works with the hearing impaired population understands the difficulty many patients have in, first, accepting the hearing loss, and then taking steps to correct it. According to the Better Hearing Institute, many hearing impaired patients wait years, even decades, before getting treatment for their loss (http://www.betterhearing.org).

The term "Searcher" has been coined to describe these people and the journey they undertake from the onset of hearing loss, through acceptance, and finally culminating in the successful treatment of that hearing loss. ALDs may provide a first step for these people by allowing them to accept a solution that allows them to communicate more effectively in certain situations, while not requiring them to wear a hearing aid. Once patients start to experience success using ALDs, they may seek more permanent solutions such as hearing aids. ALDs can also be of help to those who may only have a mild hearing loss, where hearing aids are not an option. This will allow them to function more successfully in their environments.

Starting an ALD Program

Once the determination has been made to add ALDs to a practice, three steps need to be undertaken in order to have a successful launch. The first is: What products should be selected?

Product Selection

Although there are many ALD products available to choose from, care must be taken in selecting the ones that best fit into the existing practice environs, and are likely to be interesting to one's patient base. There are several major distributors of ALDs that provide a wide selection of products, making it easier since one will only have a couple of vendors to deal with. A small amount of inventory should be held at any given time, but most products can be shipped overnight from the distributor to the clinic or directly to the patient. Once the selection has been made and the distributor selected, a demo kit should be ordered for each audiologist or/provider to have in their office. A training session should be scheduled with the distributor to go over the features of each product and key selling points. Front staff and reception should be included, as many of these products can be recommended and shown in the reception area.

Pricing

Pricing of ALDs is largely straightforward. The typical retail pricing practice is to charge twice what you paid for the unit from the wholesale distributor. For example: if the phone wholesales for $107.95, the retail price point should be $215.90. If desired, the price may be rounded up or down to reflect a more common price point, such as $219.95. It would also be advisable to check pricing online at various other retailers to make sure you are competitive.

Price lists should be distributed to all who will be recommending these products, and prices should be prominently featured on displayed products.

Marketing

Marketing of these products is essential in creating awareness for the products carried. Two distinct types of marketing should be done: internal marketing and external marketing

Internal Marketing

This type of marketing includes items such as, counter cards placed on the reception desk featuring different products and specials; brochures or catalogues outlining the benefits of the products, carried; or delivery kit cards that feature several products and are included in hearing aid delivery kits.

External Marketing

ALD products can be featured in patient newsletters, on your company website, or through direct mail campaigns throughout the year. As with any marketing effort, the look and the feel should reflect positively on the practice and clearly spell out the features of the product as well as how to order it, and the price.

Conclusion

As we have discussed, ALDs can serve as much more than a profit center in the modern practice. They can and should be an extension of the totality of services that are offered to the hearing impaired patient. Strategically implemented, they not only will create an alternative revenue stream, but, more importantly, increase patient satisfaction at the same time.

14

Hearing Aid Dispensing for the Otolaryngologist

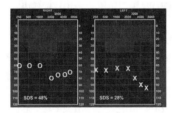

NEIL GIDDINGS, M.D.

"Marketing is what we do so we don't have to advertise."

Marketing and advertising may be foreign concepts to the practitioner. Although beneficial to most business owners, it is the rare otolaryngology residency that devotes time to teaching the "business" of running a practice. In order to expand beyond simply servicing those patients noted in the office setting who require amplification, the shift from "marketing" to advertising services in mailers, print, or televised media is often necessary.

This chapter reviews the transition from marketing to actually advertising a dispensing practice. Examples and profit/loss statements from real life are included and analyzed.

Marketing

In every otolaryngology practice, marketing opportunities abound. The relationship that the practice has with the community, as well as the goodwill that is engendered by the physician, office staff, and audiologists, is probably the best source of referrals to the hearing aid practice. The trust that patients have in the physician can be easily transferred to the competent dispensing staff, while the large number of patients who normally are seen in the office comprise a pool of individuals with possible hearing difficulties, some of whom may benefit from amplification. Many practices develop a successful business model by marketing directly to those patients seen within the medical otolaryngology practice, resulting in a productive hearing aid business.

It is important to distinguish between the concepts of "marketing" versus "advertising." Marketing techniques include word of mouth recommendations by patients and referring physicians. One could argue that marketing one's practice is inherent in activities such as serving on a hospital or school board committee. Common "marketing" techniques directed toward referring physicians; such as the inherent value of a "Thank you summary letter," are discussed in previous chapters.

If marketing directly to one's hearing-impaired patients theoretically provides an adequate business model for a hearing aid business in the physician's office, why contemplate advertising to individuals who are not yet established patients?

The simple answer is advertising has the potential to reach an even larger number of patients who may benefit from hearing aid services. That being said, there are a large number of potential complications and pitfalls that may befall the practice that becomes interested in advertising. Frequent questions that arise include the following:

Is it ethical for a physician to advertise externally?

Is it cost-effective?

Is new business wanted, or needed?

Can the dispensing staff handle a greater patient volume than the practice usually generates?

Is the advertising message appropriate for the greater practice?

How does an otolaryngology practice make the transition from marketing, to advertising both philosophically as well as practically?

Let us address some of these questions individually.

Is It Ethical?

Only recently have physicians have begun to advertise their medical practices as a business much as other professionals have long done. Despite the growing acceptance of advertising, many medical practices have steered clear of this, feeling it was somehow less than professional. Each practice must make its own philosophical decision as to whether advertising and openly competing with hearing aid dispensers and dispensing audiology practices is appropriate for the community in which they live. With very few exceptions, virtually all states allow physician practices to dispense hearing aids, and there is no question that advertising a hearing aid business is legal. The American Medical Association has stated that it is ethical and appropriate for physicians to advertise elective products, such as cosmetic surgical procedures or products that may be purchased through their offices. The American Academy of Otolaryngology encourages physicians to dispense hearing aids as an appropriate treatment for many types of hearing loss, and has published a position paper that dispensing is within the scope of practice for an otolaryngologist.

Dispensing hearing aids is a business model that is different from that of the medical office practice "selling" physician services. It involves selling a product, that must be competitively priced, and may involve competing against other hearing aid dispensers in the community. The physician needs to understand that external advertising for hearing aid sales always has been, and will continue to be, a large component of the hearing aid retail community. The physician, through appropriate and tasteful advertising, can offer these patients better medical service at a competitive price, in a setting where objective information is provided, allowing the hearing impaired patient to make an informed decision concerning amplification. The physician practice is not "dependent" strictly on hearing aid sales for income, and can allow the patient some objectivity that may be lacking in some other dispensing sites.

Is It Cost-Effective?

Well-done advertising is cost-effective for the hearing aid industry and the individual dispenser. If it were not, hearing aid dealers would not be running full-page ads in their local newspaper on a regular basis to get patients into their office! Those advertisements are expensive, as well as requiring time and effort to develop. Frequently, the costs of direct advertising are supported or shared with the manufacturer of the hearing aid being advertised. The physician practice can determine the number of hearing aids that are necessary to be sold to recoup the practice out-of-pocket expense for advertising. Although direct advertising in newspapers may be cost effective, it may not be the most appropriate, or tasteful way, to increase patient visits to your hearing aid business. Other examples of direct advertising by mail to potential patients are discussed later in this chapter.

Is New Business Wanted, or Needed?

Although advertising may lead to greater sales and income potential, not every practice wants to expand their hearing aid services, nor is it prepared for the additional staffing required to handle a larger volume of patients or front the start-up costs that may be necessary to increase the volume of business that advertising generates.

Hearing aid sales provide income to a practice that is not physician dependent. This is an attractive model, in an era where reimbursement for medical services continues to decline even as overhead increases. Increased revenue from hearing aid sales may be beneficial to offset decreased reimbursement for medical and surgical services and allow expansion for additional new services in the otolaryngology practice. However, increasing unit sales, although providing revenue, does involve the possible need to hire more employees, increase office space requirements and inventory, as well as increase the complexity of employee benefits. Each practice must weigh the advantages and disadvantages of dispensing, as well as determine if their physical settings are appropriate for the potential increased burdens associated with greater employee and patient volumes.

Is the Message Appropriate for the Greater Practice?

Each otolaryngology practice has a unique patient population and some practice opportunities are not heavily engaged in audiologic or otologic services. The work involved in managing a hearing aid business is not to be taken lightly. If the practice specializes in head and neck cancer, or voice disorders, running a separate hearing aid dispensing business may not fit with the practice mission, or long-term goals. A practice does not have to be a subspecialty otologic practice nor specialize in hearing disorders to recognize the benefits that a well-run hearing aid business may offer the owners. There is also the potential of the hearing aid business generating increased patient visits to the medical practice. The alert audiologist or dispenser may note a conductive or unilateral hearing loss for appropriate medical or surgical referral. The professionals performing a hearing aid evaluation may also ask screening questions including general questions about head and neck health, sleep disorders, recurrent infections, or swallowing problems that may appropriately require referral to an otolaryngologist in the medical practice.

How Does an Otolaryngology Practice Make the Transition from Marketing to Advertising?

Marketing occurs, good or bad, on a daily basis at every provider's office. The interactions that each patient has with the physician, the front desk staff, scheduling and billing staff are direct opportunities to market the expertise of the provider, as well as the support staff, to patients who may benefit from amplification. Relationships with other physicians, community service organizations, and involvement with local hospitals, community activities, or service organizations, are all marketing opportunities that, although real, are not discussed here as we consider advertising for the hearing aid business. The transition from marketing to advertising, including examples, are the basis for the remainder of this chapter.

Advertising the Practice

Before any attempt is made at advertising, it is essential to have processes in place to track the success, or failure of that particular venture It is not useful in one's hearing aid or any other medical practice, to advertise with no mechanism to assess the outcome on patient volume, business expansion, or the resulting net profit (or loss) to the business. The real costs, including time, effort, and supplies versus the revenue that is generated from this advertisement must be defined and measured to assess the success of an individual campaign. Both new and return patients arriving in your office will need to be queried and recorded as to how and why they made an appointment in order to determine whether a given advertising campaign is successful. In our office, each patient is questioned, when they are seen for a hearing aid evaluation, as to where they heard about our office, who referred them, and whether they have seen, or heard, our recent advertisements (Figure 14–1). This information is then recorded and reviewed regularly.

PATIENT INFORMATION

Last Name:_____ First:_____
Middle:_____

Birthdate:_____ Social Security Number:_____-_____-_____

Address:_____ _____ _____
_____
       Street   City   State   Zip

Home Phone:_____ Work (other)
Phone:_____

Primary Care Dr.:_____
 Referring Dr.:_____

How did you hear of Columbia Hearing Centers?
       Friend   Doctor   Radio   TV   Other

For Minor Patients

Parent/Guardian's Name:_____

Address:_____ _____ _____
_____
       Street   City   State   Zip

Home Phone:_____ Work (other)
Phone:_____

Insurance Information

| Name of Insurance | Policy Holder | Policy |
Number
1.   _____   _____
      _____

2.   _____   _____
      _____
Is this a State Industrial Claim? YES   NO

       If Yes – Claim # _____ Date of Injury _____

I certify that I am the patient or duly authorized general agent of the patient able to furnish the information requested. I acknowledge that the charges incurred by my dependent(s) or me are my responsibility. I acknowledge the 1.5-% per month finance charge if my account is not paid in full after 60 days. I also request assignment of insurance benefits to Columbia Hearing Centers.

I give permission for Columbia Hearing Centers to leave pertinent messages on my answering machine at home and leave messages at my place of employment limited to requests to return the phone call.

I hereby authorize Columbia Hearing Centers to contact my primary care physician regarding my hearing and related information.

Figure 14–1. Columbia Hearing Centers intake form.

There are three main media opportunities available for advertising:

Direct mailings

Newspaper or magazine advertisements

TV and radio

We review them individually.

Direct Mailings

Direct mailings are the easiest way of contacting a large group of individuals, who potentially may be interested in hearing aid services. Lists of current and former patients may be obtained from the medical practice's database, either by screening for patients above a certain age, or by limiting the search to patients who have been seen previously for audiologic, otologic, or hearing aid services through the office. Lists also may be available for purchase commercially from multiple services, which prescreen those listed based on supplied demographic information. The more accurately the demographic information is defined, the more valuable the list may be for contacting potential new customers. Our experience suggests that selectively directed mailings are often effective in developing new business.

HIPPA regulations prevent direct advertising to patients for services based on their medical records or diagnosis. However, it is not illegal to send informational mailings or "newsletters" to patient populations to educate patients about amplification or other treatments to improve hearing.

Our first attempt at direct mailing involved notification of an "open house," by mailing a letter to 2000 patients over 65 years of age, who had previously been seen at our office. A small advertisement was also placed in the local newspaper, announcing the open house at our hearing aid office (Figure 14–2).

The expense breakdown was as follows:

Total costs for this mailing, and small advertisement in the paper	$15,000
Total gross revenues for this mailing and advertisement in the paper	$17,600
Gross profit	$2,600

Whereas this might appear at first glance to have been a modest success, after subtracting out cost of goods, as well as incentive paid to our audiologist and dispensers, this advertising experience resulted in a net loss.

Our second attempt at direct mail as an advertising medium involved purchasing a mailing list to 37,000 local individuals based on demographics and compatible age (Figure 14–3).

The revenue breakdown was as follows:

Total payment for a 37,000 postcard mailing	$16,000
Gross revenues from hearing aid sales	$3,200
Contribution from hearing aid manufacturer	$8,000
Net loss	$4,800

What we learned (the hard way) from this advertising experience was twofold and invaluable. First, a purchased mailing list may not accurately delineate individuals who are actively considering amplification despite being in an "appropriate" age and because of the proximity to the

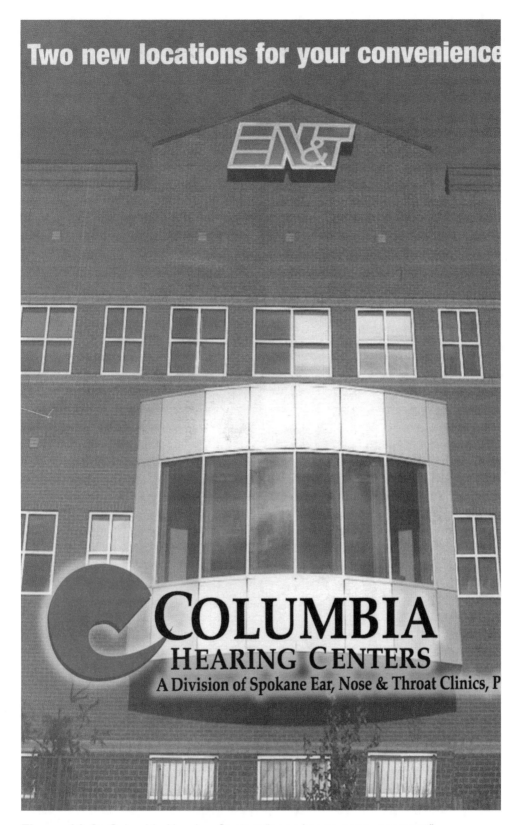

Figure 14–2. Columbia Hearing Centers "open house announcement."

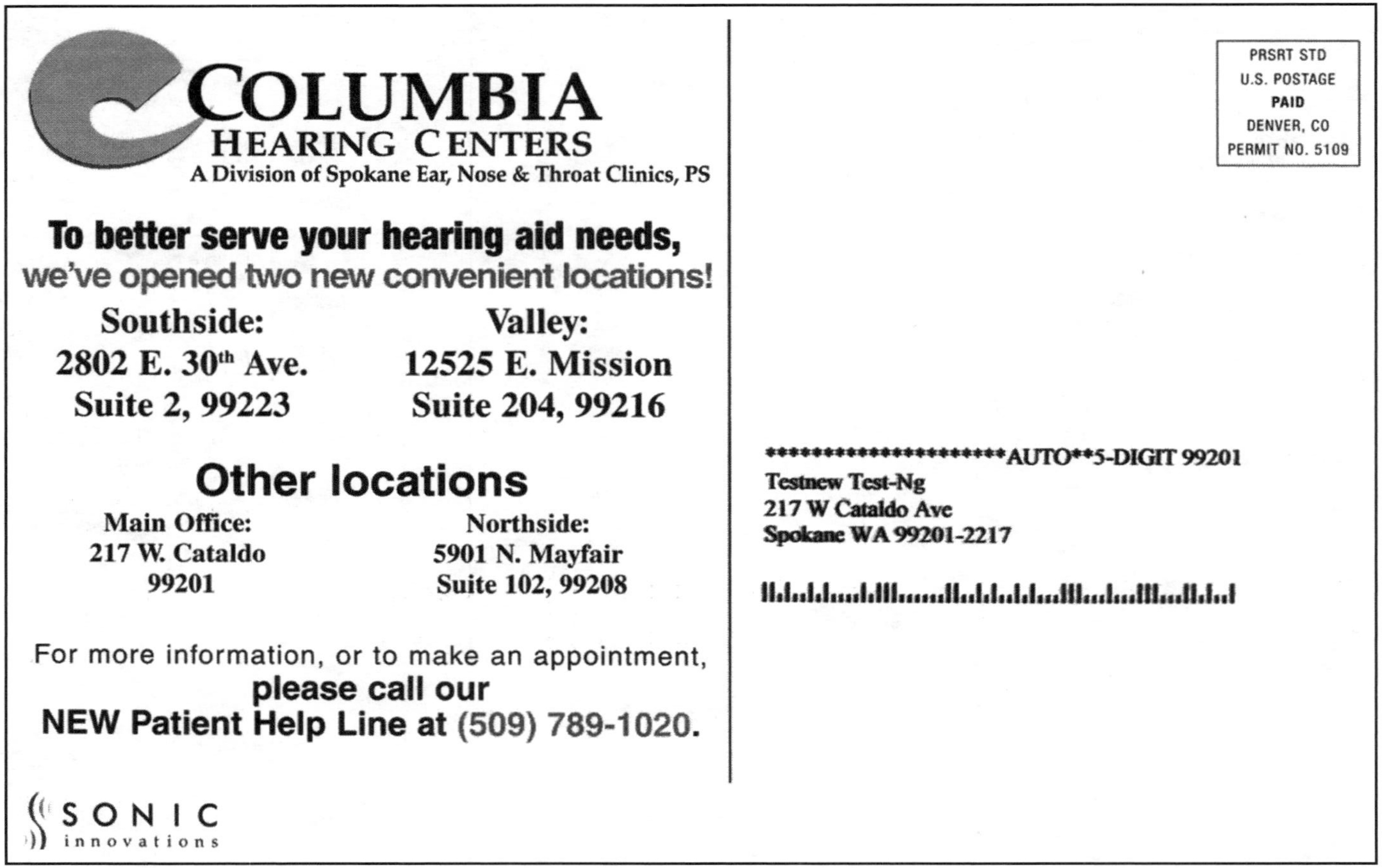
COLUMBIA
HEARING CENTERS
A Division of Spokane Ear, Nose & Throat Clinics, PS
To better serve your hearing aid needs,
we've opened two new convenient locations!
Southside:
2802 E. 30th Ave.
Suite 2, 99223
Valley:
12525 E. Mission
Suite 204, 99216
Other locations
Main Office:
217 W. Cataldo
99201
Northside:
5901 N. Mayfair
Suite 102, 99208
For more information, or to make an appointment,
please call our
NEW Patient Help Line at (509) 789-1020.
SONIC
innovations
PRSRT STD
U.S. POSTAGE
PAID
DENVER, CO
PERMIT NO. 5109
*********************AUTO**5-DIGIT 99201
Testnew Test-Ng
217 W Cataldo Ave
Spokane WA 99201-2217

Figure 14–3. Columbia Hearing Center post card.

practice. Second, major hearing aid manufacturers, are more than happy to offset some advertising costs because of the obvious direct benefit to them of increased hearing aid sales. We have found hearing aid manufacturers to be good partners, and they remain a reliable source to offset some of our direct hearing aid advertising costs. Almost all major manufacturers have programs for local advertising on a regular basis, and should be approached, especially when new technology or features appear on the market, that may require education of either established patients, or potential new hearing aid users as to their benefits.

Newspaper or Magazine Advertisement

Newspaper or magazine advertisements are less accurately directed at the patient population that may benefit from amplification, but they offer the availability of your product to a much larger group of individuals, and also may help to build brand recognition. Direct advertising may result in direct sales, but having your or your practice's name in front of large groups of people over long periods of time is also a well-established advertising tool to build brand recognition for any product. It may be more difficult to quantify these benefits over a long period of time, but short-term success in hearing aid sales may still be measured by querying patients in the dispensary as to the source of their finding the practice following newspaper or magazine advertisements.

Our medical group did not feel that large full-page ads in the newspaper were compatible with its mission, but did decide to produce selective advertisements in the newspaper medium, which are felt to be both informative as well as aligned with our long-term medical goals. An example is found in Figure 14–4.

This advertisement was our first attempt at direct newspaper advertising, and reaches approximately 250,000 people on a daily basis. The income/revenue breakdown is as follows:

Total costs newspaper ad, plus dessert and refreshments	$4,470
Contribution by manufacturer	$2,500
Net profit, including employee costs	$9,500

Other possible benefits from this campaign included a large number of patients who came through our office, who may purchase hearing aids at a future date, as well as the realization that those who did purchase a hearing aid, if serviced properly, also will likely continue to purchase hearing aids every 3 to 7 years, on a regular basis, as new technologies become available, or their current hearing aids become unrepairable.

We analyzed two possible reasons this advertisement had been more successful than previous advertisements, including providing food, so that there was some benefit to a patient who came who did not elect to purchase a hearing aid, as well as the stated appeal of new, as opposed to older technology, being discussed at this informational session.

Following the success of this newspaper advertisement, a second newspaper ad was developed in conjunction with one of the hearing aid manufacturers, as

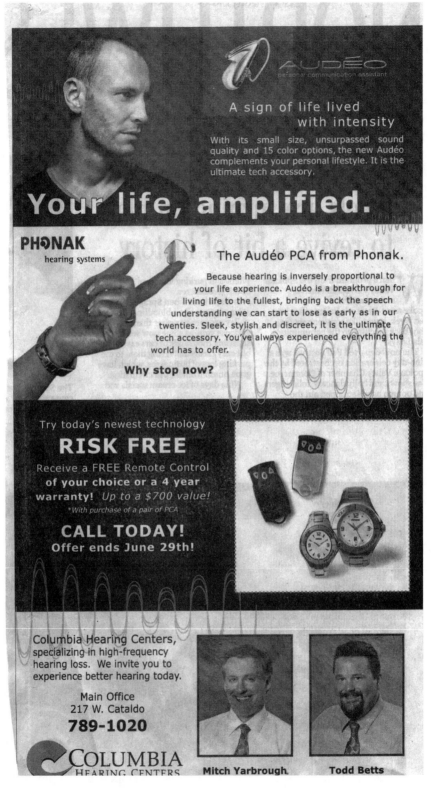

Figure 14–4. Newspaper advertisement.

well as a letter being sent to a select group of patients in our own database who had not purchased a new hearing aid in approximately 5 years (Figure 14-5).

Mailing costs for 800 letters $2,400

Newspaper advertisement
costs (*paid by manufacturer*) $0

Net profits $42,500

This general newspaper advertisement was coupled with a direct mailing to our own patients who were most likely to be interested in new technology, as well as, based on the age of their current hearing aid, were most likely to be in need of a new hearing aid. Once again, food was provided as an incentive to patients for the information session. The combination of a large number of people seeing the advertisement, plus tightly focused identification of patients from our own database, resulted in a very successful advertising campaign.

TV and Radio Advertising

Television and radio advertising is more expensive than either newspaper advertisements or direct mailings. Most otolaryngology practices do not have the available revenue to advertise on major networks, but cable-television and radio stations are able to provide very eco-nomical opportunities to advertise to large groups of people. These advertising options also can very accurately provide demographic information about potential listeners or viewers of these mediums.

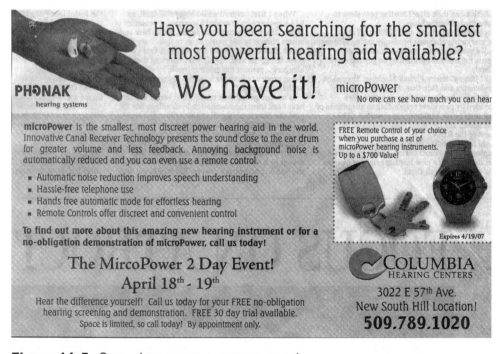

Figure 14–5. Second newspaper announcement.

Media consultants are available to help identify potential opportunities through these channels, and the net costs to the practice is zero dollars, because most media consultants buy large blocks of TV or radio time, at a discount, and then resell the time to the purchaser (i.e., the hearing aid practice) at their full value. The difference between the discount and the full value is the income that the media consultant recognizes. Because the hearing aid practice would not be able to purchase comparably large blocks of time, the actual costs of the media consultant is transparent to the practice.

Media consultants have a large database of accurate information concerning the demographics of who is listening or watching these outlets, during any specified block of time, as seen in the example below (Figure 14-6).

An example of the profit/loss statement from one such campaign in our own office is as follows:

TV advertising campaign cost	$10,500
Offset by manufacturer	$7,000
Total costs	$3,500
Net revenues	$53,000

Based on this experience we continue to run TV advertisements because of demonstrated benefit, and as well as the development of brand recognition. The TV advertisements are professionally produced at a national level, sometimes involving hearing aid manufacturers, and have been deemed appropriate by members of out physician practice, as well as other members of the community who reviewed them and found them both informative as well as entertaining.

Developing Brand Recognition

Although the goal of any advertising campaign is to increase business, it also is important to track the success of that campaign for comparison and other purposes. Developing brand recognition is a more difficult concept to track, but probably is equally important in the long run for generating ongoing business. As our hearing aid business has matured, we have entered into some relationships with manufacturers that benefit their product more in the long run by the development of brand recognition, than is recognized by any short-term increases in product sales.

A perfect illustration of this would be a small, colorful car, which we obtained for transportation by one of our hearing aid dispensers, who services five outreach clinics. The car is on the road over 200 miles per week, and when not in use, sits in front of our main office, as another reminder about our hearing aid business. Many patients make comments about the car, and people frequently stop to talk with the hearing aid dispenser, at stoplights or a stop sign concerning the brightly painted car and its message (Figure 14-7).

Cost breakdown for the car:

Purchase price for car	$10,000
Graphics	$586
Total costs	$10,586

Maintenance costs at this time have been minimal, whereas operation of the car by the employee has been less expensive than reimbursing the employee per mile for use of their own vehicle. Also, the expected life of the vehicle is 5 to 7 years,

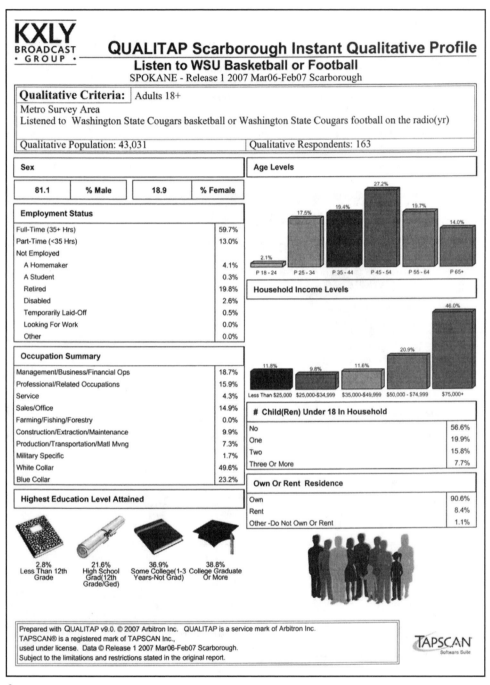

KXLY BROADCAST · GROUP ·

QUALITAP Scarborough Instant Qualitative Profile
Listen to WSU Basketball or Football
SPOKANE - Release 1 2007 Mar06-Feb07 Scarborough

Qualitative Criteria: Adults 18+

Metro Survey Area
Listened to Washington State Cougars basketball or Washington State Cougars football on the radio(yr)

Qualitative Population: 43,031 | Qualitative Respondents: 163

Sex

| 81.1 | % Male | 18.9 | % Female |

Age Levels

27.2%
17.5% 19.4% 19.7% 14.0%
2.1%

P 18 - 24   P 25 - 34   P 35 - 44   P 45 - 54   P 55 - 64   P 65+

Employment Status

Full-Time (35+ Hrs)	59.7%
Part-Time (<35 Hrs)	13.0%
Not Employed	
A Homemaker	4.1%
A Student	0.3%
Retired	19.8%
Disabled	2.6%
Temporarily Laid-Off	0.5%
Looking For Work	0.0%
Other	0.0%

Household Income Levels

46.0%
20.9%
11.8% 9.8% 11.6%

Less Than $25,000 $25,000-$34,999 $35,000-$49,999 $50,000 - $74,999 $75,000+

Occupation Summary

Management/Business/Financial Ops	18.7%
Professional/Related Occupations	15.9%
Service	4.3%
Sales/Office	14.9%
Farming/Fishing/Forestry	0.0%
Construction/Extraction/Maintenance	9.9%
Production/Transportation/Matl Mvng	7.3%
Military Specific	1.7%
White Collar	49.6%
Blue Collar	23.2%

 # Child(Ren) Under 18 In Household

No	56.6%
One	19.9%
Two	15.8%
Three Or More	7.7%

Own Or Rent Residence

Own	90.6%
Rent	8.4%
Other -Do Not Own Or Rent	1.1%

Highest Education Level Attained

2.8% Less Than 12th Grade | 21.6% High School Grad(12th Grade/Ged) | 36.9% Some College(1-3 Years-Not Grad) | 38.8% College Graduate Or More

A

Figure 14–6. Examples of demographic information available to purchasers of radio and TV advertising time to better target intended sales audience. *continues*

QUALITAP™ Rank Report

Qualitative Criteria: Adults 18 +

Metro Survey Area
Listened to Washington State Cougars basketball or Washington State Cougars football on the radio(yr)

Stations ranked by cume persons.

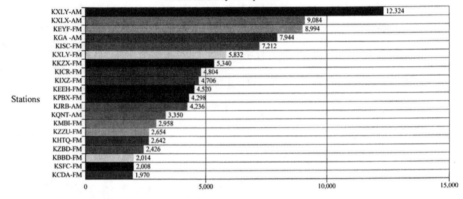

Station	Value
KXLY-AM	12,324
KXLX-AM	9,084
KEYF-FM	8,994
KGA -AM	7,944
KISC-FM	7,212
KXLY-FM	5,832
KKZX-FM	5,340
KICR-FM	4,804
KIXZ-FM	4,706
KEEH-FM	4,520
KPBX-FM	4,298
KJRB-AM	4,236
KQNT-AM	3,350
KMBI-FM	2,958
KZZU-FM	2,654
KHTQ-FM	2,642
KZBD-FM	2,426
KBBD-FM	2,014
KSFC-FM	2,008
KCDA-FM	1,970

Population Information:		Survey Respondent Information:	
Adults 18 +:	442,696	Adults 18 +:	829
Qualitative Population:	47,904	Qualitative Respondents:	90
% of Adults 18 +:	10.8%		

How to read this report:

KXLY-AM reaches 12,324 Adults 18 + who meet the qualitative criteria described above, during Mon-Sun 6am-12m, which is equal to 25.7% of the qualitative population. Compared to the market composition of 10.8%, KXLY-AM's listeners are 138% more concentrated in the qualitative criteria than the average adult in the market. In Mon-Sun 6am-12m, 746 target adults are listening during an average quarter hour, which is equal to 1.6% of the qualitative population.

B

Figure 14–6. *continued*

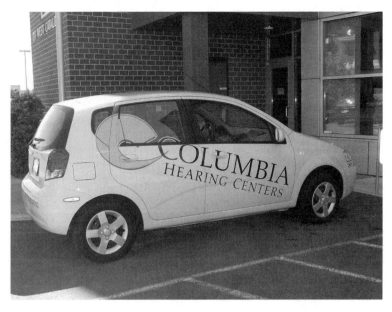

Figure 14–7. Marketing car.

so we consider that its benefit will continue for a number of years.

Summary

The transition from general marketing to direct advertising can be done in a tasteful, appropriate fashion that is compatible with a general medical model for dispensing hearing aids. Effective targeting of the audience requires ongoing assessment for outcomes of any advertising campaign. The physician owner has other professional sources to assist in his or her marketing and sales of hearing aids. Hearing aid manufacturers are interested in providing money, as well as their advertising expertise to offset direct marketing costs that benefit the sales of their product. Media consultants are available at little or no charge, when considering television, or radio advertisement. Long-term advertisement costs for development of brand recognition may be more difficult to quantify, but have long-term benefit.

15

Economics of Hearing Aid Dispensing

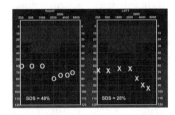

BRAD VOLKMER, M.B.A.

Hearing aid dispensing can be a great business addition to the otolaryngology practice. A considered and thoughtful approach to the components required to successfully dispense hearing aids and the development of an operational model are critical to the successful undertaking of hearing aid dispensing. It is important for the otolaryngologist to understand all of the operational requirements and the related costs. Establishing up front the performance expectations for a dispensing component to the office practice will facilitate the management and administration of the program as an individual cost center and profit center.

The individual operational components of a hearing aid dispensary include the appropriate staffing and personnel; all equipment including test equipment, office equipment, and computer equipment; and the appropriate layout and allocation of space. The availability of these components in the existing office space and within the current scope of practice will determine the initial and incremental costs necessary to establish a hearing aid dispensary. Within each of these operational components, there are multiple options and no single absolute choice.

Personnel and Staffing

In order to dispense hearing aids, the practice must hire and retain personnel licensed and certified to dispense hearing aids. There are two alternatives for providing this technical expertise: an audiologist or hearing instrument specialist (hearing aid technician). In most instances, it is appropriate to hire an additional office person for the clerical and front desk duties to maximize the time of the dispensing individual with the patients.

An audiologist provides the practice with flexibility in the application of its personnel. Audiologists can not only dispense hearing aids, but also can fulfill the necessary roles in the office of diagnostic testing, balance and other special testing, and rehabilitation. The hearing instrument specialist, although not trained nor licensed to provide the full array of diagnostic testing and other services, can be very proficient at the dispensing of hearing aids. In some practices, it may be appropriate to incorporate both an audiologist and hearing instrument specialist to maximize patient service and skill levels. The audiologist may perform the diagnostic testing and set the initial expectations for hearing amplification with the patient. The hearing instrument specialist completes the process by dispensing the hearing aid. The audiologist also may supervise the total operations.

The front office person, or hearing aid clerk, relieves the dispensing individual from the tasks not directly related to patient activity. These typically include setting initial appointments and follow-up sessions; the shipping and handling of earmolds and other related dispensary items; telephone questions; and learning to perform hearing aid checks and cleanings as part of his or her routine support activities.

The otolaryngologist can maximize the efficiency of his or her practice by establishing an appropriate order of patient management dependent on the type of personnel, and by setting this intraoffice referral expectation with each patient. In so doing, the physician extends his or her professional seal of approval to the dispensing individuals providing those services (Kochkin & MarkeTrak, 2007). The dispensing personnel should provide continuity of care in the process of hearing aid selection, programming and fitting, follow-up, and outcome measurement. Additionally, the otolaryngologist should expect the dispensing individual to be the technical and professional resource as it relates to hearing aid technology and its application to any specific hearing loss.

The dilemma of appropriate compensation for these dispensing individuals is a persistent question whether in the development of a hearing aid dispensing practice or in the ongoing dispensary. First, salary and compensation information for audiology as a profession is available in a variety of sources. The American Academy of Audiology and the American Speech-Language-Hearing Association regularly publish compensation surveys. Additionally, state and government institutions such as universities and large clinics establish regular salary and pay scales, and by virtue of their public nature must make available their compensation data. A final resource may be simply to contact colleagues who have successfully attracted and retained dispensing personnel.

There are at least three basic models under which dispensing personnel may be compensated. These include straight salary, a base salary plus commission, or a straight commission-based compensation structure. There are pros and cons to each of these structures, and they are somewhat dependent on the expectations and requirements of the individuals within each practice.

First, a word about incentives or commissions. Webster's dictionary defines incentive as "something exciting one to action or effort." Therefore, any commission or incentive must be perceived as incrementally rewarding. Any incentive or commission must work and be rewarding for both the practice and the individual. The incentive or commission must be clearly defined and seen as attainable. And in most cases, simple is the best model to follow. Any incentive or commission formula that requires substantial manipulation to calculate is likely to be unclear, and therefore unrewarding.

Table 15-1 provides an example of three different models for three different expectation levels in otolaryngology practices. In each model the assumption is made that the percent of time devoted to diagnostics is not within the control or purview of the audiologist or hearing technician, but rather driven by the needs of the otolaryngologist in the practice. Therefore, any incentive based on required effort that is out of the control of the individual may not be perceived as "incentive." Model 1 supposes equal

allocations of effort between diagnostics and dispensing. In Model 2, effort is allocated substantially to hearing aid dispensing, and in Model 3 the practice requires substantially more time committed to diagnostics and other test services. The annual gross margin line is the net of the cost of goods for the hearing devices, and represents the difference between average sales price and average cost of goods (a very conservative and realistic unit margin of $1200 is utilized). The monthly units are average numbers and are taken from surveys published through *The Hearing Journal*. The percentage commissions are paid directly on gross net dollars (total revenue less any return for credits), and maintain a very simple approach. The net on gross line provides the annual marginal gross revenues less any commissions, whereas the net overall line provides the additional marginal gross revenues to the practice net of total compensation, commissions, and the base salary. In these models, one can see that hearing aid dispensing adds incremental

Table 15–1. Incentive/Commissions Examples

	Model 1	Model 2	Model 3
% Diagnostics	50%	25%	75%
% Dispensing	50%	75%	25%
Base Salary	$60,000	$48,000	$72,000
Commissions	10%	20%	0%
Mo. Units/Pts	15/9	20+/12+	7/4
Annual Gross Margin	$216,000	$316,800	$100,800
Annual Commissions	$21,600	$63,360	$0
Total Annual Pay	$81,600	$111,360	$72,000
Net on Gross	$194,400	$253,440	$100,800
Net Overall	$134,400	$205,440	$28,800

revenues to the practice, and commission payment structures may provide sufficient incentive to reward both the individual and the practice. Please note that these marginal gross revenue numbers do not include the full operating costs of hearing aid dispensing as they only incorporate the cost of goods and personnel expenses.

These models do not presume to present the definitive structure for any practice. There are a multitude of variations on these payment and compensation structures. Again, one great resource might be colleagues who have successfully implemented a program within their practices.

Hearing Aid Dispensing Equipment

Hearing aid dispensing requires a commitment to test equipment, and office and computer equipment, and related supplies in order to fulfill rehabilitation and dispensing of hearing aids. There are many sources from which this equipment and these products may be acquired, and some of the test equipment may be shared with your diagnostic applications. However, dispensing hearing aids will require access to or the investment in at least the items discussed herein.

In Tables 15–2 and 15–3, all the equipment and materials necessary to dispense hearing aids are listed. In many cases, there may be a manufacturer or model name associated with this description. These references do not suggest that these are the only products or manufacturers providing these items; however, years of implementation and application experience suggest that these will more than suffice, and are appropriate to each need. The cost figures associated with each item represent those available on January 1, 2008.

The high-cost items are substantially represented in the equipment and software categories. The practice may already have an audiometer available, and to the extent that it is not utilized full-time and available for dispensing might eliminate this cost. The availability of the sound booth may be consistent with that of an audiometer. The other large cost item is either the real-ear measurement system or the HI PRO Real-Ear Hearing Aid test box. These systems allow the selection, fitting, and modifications of performance in the process of hearing aid dispensary. Finally, a dedicated computer with sufficient memory and capability to operate several different hearing aid fitting and dispensing programs is required. Basically, as of 2008, almost all hearing aids manufactured are digital in nature, and require computer-based software to program them to any specific hearing loss.

The direct dispensary space and any support space also will have to be outfitted with appropriate furniture. The dispensing room typically will require a desk and chair, and appropriate side chairs for the patients. If the hearing aid dispensary is separate from the office practice, there may be a need to outfit a small waiting room also. And as the dispensary will be a distinct business component of the practice, there will be a need for storage and filing cabinets, as well as a work room with countertops or a worktable.

The total investment in equipment and related supplies therefore will depend substantially on what exists currently within the practice. Adding dispensing to an existing diagnostic practice may run as little as $10,000, or may go as high as $45,000 in an independent setting or in a completely new dispensing practice.

Table 15–2. Hearing Aid Dispensary Start-Up Equipment

Equipment & Software	Estimated Cost
No Need to purchase new Audiometer and Sound Booth if already have one for your office	
InterAcoustics Audiometer (**If Applicable**) (2 Channel) insert earphones and headphones	$2,500–6,000
Sound booth (Dependent on size) (**If Applicable**)	$3,500–10,000
Speaker system	
NOAH software 3.0 1-2 user license	$850.00
Hi Pro Box /NOAH Link	$650.00
Sound field speakers	$525.00
Equipment Suggestions	
****Real Ear available in complete system or in smaller packages depending on your office needs***	
Real Ear Measurement, Hearing Instrument Test & Fitting System with Built-In Hi Pro OR Fonix System	$12,240.20
Real Ear/Hearing Aid Test Box/HI PRO, NOAH	$6,855.10
PC Computer 2 Ghz or above processor required, Pentium 4 or above, minimum 1 Gb RAM, Intel/NVidia Video card with DDR video memory and a USB 2.0 Hub. Recommended Belkin USB-Serial Adaptor (F-5U409 -for HI PRO box) *Must have Windows XP Pro for operating system.*	Up to $1000.00
Printer	
Hearing Aid Software & Cables through Manufacturers	
TOTAL	

Marketing and Management Tools	Cost
Marketing Kit, Assistive Listening Device Brochures	$0.00
HearForm Software: practice management, database marketing, measure & evaluate productivity, sales, inventory tracking	
Care Credit-Patient financing (credit card terminal provided at no charge)	$0.00
Hearing Aid Style Information Brochure	
Office Brochures (from EPIC, AAO-HNS, Manufacturers)	$0.00
TOTAL	

Table 15–3. Hearing Aid Dispensary Start-Up Supplies

Impression Material & Supplies:	Estimated Cost
Silicone Impression Material, Matrics Start-Up Kit 4 cartridges 18 mixers & SILG Impression gun	$50.00
Foam Ear Dams (Mini, S, M, L—1 bag of 50 each size)	$4.47
Cotton Ear Dams (Mini, S, M, L—1 bag of 50 each size)	$4.89
Cotton balls and Alcohol	
Glue	
Otoprobe Penlight with Eartip Assortment	$7.93
Welch Allyn Otoscope with rechargable handle complete set	$97.85
Tubing Double Bend—12 Std., 13 Std., 13 Thick (1 pack of 25)	$4.75
Tubing Double Bend—13 Super Thick (1 pack of 25)	$4.75
Tubing Scissors 3.5"	$3.50
Tubing Ear Blower (without box)	$3.56
Tubing Puller (Fishline)	$5.22
Reamer	$5.22
Needle nose pliers	$28.45
Hearing Aid Stethoscope with ITE & BTE Adapters	$15.68
ITE Probe Listening Tip	$1.52
Ear Plugs (Box 200) Uncorded	$42.75
Modular Storage System for Small Hearing Aid Parts	$76.00
Hooks or tie rack to hang cables	$15–40.00
Hearing Aid Batteries	**Cost**
Display Rack with 5 packs of each size 10, 13, 312, 675 5 Cartons of each size 10, 13, 312, 675—Recommend Power One, Energizer, or Private label with Company Name & Logo	Varies
Activair Battery Tester	$8.50
Hearing Aid Maintenance Supplies	**Cost**
Redwing Grinding and Polishing Kit	$346.75
Deluxe Screwdriver Set (6 piece)	$3.23

Table 15–3. *continued*

Hearing Aid Maintenance Supplies	Cost
Hearing Aid & Earmold Cleaning Tools (Nelson Tool Set)	$28.50
Bransonic Ultrasonic Cleaner Machine	$94.05
Audiologists Choice Ultrasonic Disinfectant	$8.08
Audiologists Choice Hearing Aid & Disinfectant Cleaner	$2.80
Otoease Earmold Lubricant (per Dozen)	$20.43
Audiowipes Disinfectant Towelettes - Canister	$7.17
The Complete Care Kit Bags	Free
DriAid Kit Audiologist's Choice®	$5.00

There may be additional costs for remodeling and/or space build out depending on the location of the hearing aid dispensary.

Space and Facilities

The most successful hearing aid dispensing operations within otolaryngology practices are when the hearing aid program is established as a unique enterprise within the practice. This includes the definition and assignment of space unique to hearing aid dispensing. The minimum requirements for space will depend on whether the dispensing practice is being established within the shared confines of an existing office, or whether it is being established as an independent enterprise.

If an established office practice is developing hearing aid dispensing within its current office quarters, the minimum amount of space required is approximately 300 sq. ft. This consist of 100 sq. ft. for a sound booth; a 100 sq. ft. fitting office and staff space; and a 100 sq. ft.

work area for supplies and inventory, grinding and reworking hearing aids, and inspection and repairs. It is assumed in this type of practice, that the necessary functions of reception and waiting, business and management, appointments, and filing will be shared with the medical practice.

To establish an independent and separate hearing aid dispensary, the minimum space requirement is approximately 750 sq. ft. That 750 sq. ft. must accommodate the individual and unique spaces mentioned in the previous paragraph as well as accommodate the activities and needs present above in these shared functions of the combined dispensary/medical practice model.

Business and Operational Considerations

Beyond skilled dispensing, the most important considerations and decisions to be made to establish a successful dispensary are the business policies and practices, and the management plan. These include cash management protocols, pricing, and establishing management expectations and metrics. Some of these models will require more information initially, and other models are independent of the ability to reasonably estimate the number of hearing aid patients and hearing aids on an annual basis.

Cash Management Policies

Hearing aid dispensing, in general, is a different model than the provision of medical and surgical services within the otolaryngology practice. Medical and surgical services are generally covered by insurance and therefore there is relatively little cash management. Services generally are billed to insurance companies, and it is expected that they will be paid some 60 to 180 days later. Additionally, although these services are provided uniquely, they are not necessarily custom, and do not carry a significant cost of goods. Hearing aids are substantially customized to each patient, and with each order there is a significant cost of goods billed to the practice. Hearing aids also are more consistent with a "cash and carry" business model. Because of these tendencies, it is necessary to establish business practices that managed the cash flow process. It is appropriate to collect the full amount from the patient at the time the hearing aid is ordered. This accomplishes two important factors: (1) the practice is not carrying an accounts receivable for which it has not received any cash or payment; and (2) it eliminates the need to reopen the conversation with the patient regard-

ing payment for services and technology. The overall psychological impact is to move the process from one of a pricing and cost discussion to one of successful treatment and better hearing.

Pricing

There are many approaches to pricing hearing aids and related services within an individual practice. These pricing methodologies are dependent on the amount of relatively accurate information that is available upfront, and the desired position of the practice within the marketplace. One of the most common pricing methodologies is competitive pricing. This simply involves a review of the competitive marketplace to determine the relative pricing levels of competitors for each type of technology. The decision then is where to place the individual practice's pricing in relationship to its competitors. Does one wish to be higher priced (implying greater professional value), priced the same (providing one's own patients the same value), or priced more competitively (price is competitive focus)? This approach ignores the cost structure of this practice and is not related to an internal financial model.

Standard markup pricing is used when one wishes to be assured of making the same gross margin on every hearing aid unit. A decision is made initially to add either a fixed dollar amount or a fixed percentage to the cost of the hearing aid in order to establish the price. This ensures a preset, nominal dollar return on all hearing aid units. Potentially, this methodology has the disadvantage of ignoring the pricing structure of the competitive marketplace, and perhaps the overall cost of providing the hearing aid dispensing services within the practice.

Average cost pricing is a methodology that simplifies the pricing presentation to patients and customers. This process generally requires the development of a cost matrix grouping the technologies in distinct categories or levels, and then across all models in each category developing the weighted average cost per unit. Once this average cost is calculated, standard and/or competitive pricing techniques are used to finalize prices. Average cost pricing generally reduces the number of price points, and thereby reduces the confusion of presenting the patient with a multitude of technology options and costs.

Cost-oriented pricing requires the use of a bookkeeper or accountant to perform the function of cost accounting and cost allocation within the office to assure that the hearing aid dispensing section is carrying its fair and appropriate share of overhead for the offices. These cost data are then spread across the anticipated or desired unit volumes; the unit or model costs are added to this, and the desired profit margin is added to this total. This methodology has the advantage of assuring complete coverage of all costs related to hearing aid dispensing and guaranteeing a specific return to the practice. It has the disadvantage of generally requiring the greatest amount of initial effort.

A relatively new approach within the hearing aid dispensing industry is unbundled pricing. This approach is more consistent with the standard delivery of medical and surgical services within an office practice. It requires the delineation of each component part of service, by code, and then adds to that bill of service the cost of the hearing aid plus a handling fee. This approach generally emphasizes the importance of professional services over products; it differentiates the audiologist or hearing instrument specialist from a retail salesperson. This approach also may allow for more flexibility to identify and bill those difficult patients who require more office visits and time, as well as substantiate the level of service and billing to all patients. Finally, in most states and with a well thought-out hearing aid patient agreement form, it allows for return for credit on the product only, and not on the portion paid for professional services.

Management and Measurement

In general, the average otolaryngologist does not have a significant amount of time to devote to the management of a hearing aid dispensing enterprise. There are, however, five lines of critical data which should be monitored on a regular basis, and several key business driver ratios which can readily indicate problem areas within the dispensing practice. The following are the five critical data components which should be monitored each month or cycle of business:

- Units dispensed
- Average selling price/unit
- Average cost/unit
- Receipts/deposits
- Payables/obligations

The number of units dispensed each month should provide a direct correlation to both the business model originally outlined, and to the number of patients seen by the physicians of the practice and referred to the hearing aid dispensary for hearing aid evaluations. The average selling price for all units that month or cycle will indicate consistency with both the pricing methodology incorporated into the business plan, and whether there are inconsistencies in product selection as reflected by price. The average unit cost for all hearing aids in any particular cycle should be consistent with the data used in the business plan, and over time will reflect variations or inconsistencies with the plan. A review of the monthly receipts and/or deposits related to the hearing aid dispensary will ensure cash flow to cover all costs of the enterprise, and should be consistent with the data used in calculating the average selling price. The last individual financial metric is to review the total accounts payables that have accumulated for that regular month or cycle. Comparing this information with receipts generates the gross return to the practice for that time frame, and should be consistent with the data used in calculating the average unit cost.

Three additional key business driver ratios that may be important to review regularly include the following:

1. Fitting ratio (are you successfully dispensing to those people who need hearing aids): The number of customer's sold/total number of potential customers (85% to 90%)
2. Binaural dispensing rate (percent of patients receiving two hearing aids): Number of binaural sets sold/total customers sold (70%—the national average)
3. Return for credit rate (indicates time/money losses to the return of hearing aids): 1 minus [units sold/units ordered] (less than 10%)

Certainly, more information is available than the management data mentioned above. Most of these indicators can be further sorted by individual dispenser, type and style of hearing aids, and manufacturers. However, by reviewing these data, practice administrators and otolaryngologists can readily track any changes within the hearing aid dispensing business and request further information or analysis.

Legal and Structural Considerations

At the point in the planning process where it becomes evident that it is appropriate to proceed with the establishment of a hearing a dispensary, it will be important to contact legal counsel to obtain a review of the structure and process under which hearing aids will be dispensed. There are several overriding federal regulations, primarily Stark and Stark II legislation, which must be considered. At this time, and throughout the country, the dispensing of hearing aids is a safe harbor exception under Stark II. Hearing aid dispensing is not regulated overall by federal jurisdiction. Hearing aid dispensing is governed individually by each state's legislation and requirements. Dispensing licensure is also regulated individually by state. Therefore, it will be necessary and appropriate to obtain a legal opinion regarding the structure and format of the proposed hearing aid dispensary within the otolaryngology practice unique to its geographic location (Portman, 2001) (The Federal Social Security Act, Anti-Kickback Statute).

Business Expectations and Modeling

As with any business enterprise, hearing aid dispensing is affected by a number of variables that differ within each practice. These include pricing philosophy, resource sharing within the office, patient demographics, overall area demographics, product and technology selection, and compensation and pay practices. There is not necessarily a set of perfect or specific answers to these variables. The final choices simply must accommodate and agree with the overall practice philosophy, the marketplace environment, and be of sound financial basis.

There are a couple of methods of evaluating and estimating the activity a hearing aid dispensary would generate within the otolaryngology practice. If the current patient business within the practice is anticipated to generate referrals to the hearing aid dispensary then the following considerations can be made. The otolaryngology practice should review the past 6 to 12 months of patient activity and calculate the number of patients seen with ICD-9 diagnosis codes 387.20, 388.01, 388.12, 388.31, and 389.11. Approximately 17 to 20% of individuals within these codes are candidates for hearing aid evaluations. Based on review of existing practice data, 85 to 90% of those individuals receiving hearing aid evaluations purchase hearing aids; and 70% of those individuals receive two hearing aids and are fit binaurally (Kochkin & Marke-Trak, 2005). Applying these statistics to the individual practice data will yield at least one set of potential business numbers with which to model the hearing aid practice.

The practice also should review all patients greater than 50 years of age who present to the office with balance disorders or complaints. As part of the general workup for these individuals it may be appropriate to perform hearing testing as there is a high correlation in this demographic and within this complaint. This is not a suggested diagnosis or treatment for balance disorders, but simply a suggestion for complete assessment of patients in these categories.

A second, and higher level consideration, is to review the demographics of the patients seen in the office within the past 6 to 12 months. For those patients age 55 years and older, there is a statistical probability of hearing loss of 30% (Radcliffe, 2000). Current data from the hearing aid marketplace suggest that there is a 22% market penetration, and therefore roughly 6% (30% × 22%) of all patients in this age demographic are likely to have hearing loss and may be candidates for hearing aids (Radcliffe, 2000).

A further consideration, after reviewing the existing patient demographics, is the availability of dispensing time for the audiologist or hearing aid specialist within the practice. Published surveys in *The Hearing Journal* suggest that the average monthly units dispensed in an otolaryngology practice approximate 12 to 15 units per month per dispensing individual. This number is directly driven by the amount of time available for dispensing versus other diagnostic testing requirements within the practice. A busy and proficient dispensing audiologist with little distraction by other services within the practice can average 20 to 24 units per month.

Once the potential business volume is established, one can apply a basic overall economic model to determine the financial impact and contribution to the practice. Figure 15–1 suggests ranges as percent of gross sales. Again, each of these categories will vary based on many of the philosophical and business decisions and assumptions applied to the hearing aid dispensary.

Along with the dispensing of hearing aids comes additional sales and retention opportunities for those patients. The complete hearing aid dispensary not only provides hearing aids, but also will be counted on for hearing aid repairs, battery sales, earmold sales, and periodic adjustments and reprogramming. Each of these components should also be priced based on time allocations and or outside costs. Additionally, there is an opportunity to support the hearing-impaired individual and his or her family with a variety of assistive listening devices (ALDs), which will help out in various listening situations, and ease the burden for both the family and the patient. Although the incremental unit revenues from these devices are relatively small, they can be demonstrated and sold by the front desk support staff as opposed to the professional dispensing staff. In the busy dispensing practice, these revenues can be significant.

Category	% of Gross Sales
Cost of Goods	35%–50%
Direct Labor	33%–22%
Overhead	20%–10%
Gross Profit	12%–18%

Figure 15–1. Cost as present table.

pensary, and then addresses the overall definition of a marketing plan.

There are several distinct methods for establishing market position for the hearing aid dispensary. First and harkening to the old adage, a satisfied customer or patient is the best form of marketing or advertising any practice could desire. Word-of-mouth will be the best testimonial for quality services and appreciated outcomes (Kochkin & Rogin, 2000). And it is true that a satisfied customer or patient will tell one to three people, whereas a dissatisfied or disgruntled the patient will tell 10 or 12 people. Good and quality work is its own best advertisement and reward.

One should consider forming strategic relationships and partnerships that position the otolaryngology practice and its hearing aid dispensary as the preferred choice within the community. This involves education and awareness of referral sources, primary care physicians, and other entities within the community who may have access to people of the hearing impaired demographic. Statistics demonstrate that only 15 to 17% of primary care physician screen or test for hearing loss in their patient populations who are most likely to have some form of hearing loss. It is incumbent on the otolaryngologist and his or her practice

Marketing and Promotion of the Hearing Aid Dispensing Program

There are a variety of opportunities and programs to market the hearing aid dispensary component of the otolaryngology practice. This discussion first addresses methods by which market position may be established for a new hearing aid dis-

audiologists to educate and inform this segment of the professional medical community regarding the potential for hearing loss and hearing rehabilitation.

Careful thought should be given to the choice of manufacturers and products offered in the hearing aid dispensary. It is essential to select several manufacturers who offer the full line of technology, at all price points, so that flexibility is maintained on behalf of the patients. Additionally, one should coordinate technology and price points to meet the demographics of those patients within the practice service area. It is inappropriate to expect a relatively less affluent population to purchase expensive, high-end hearing products. Most of the top-tier manufacturers will have products and technology at all price points and can accommodate your patients' needs.

It is appropriate to consider up front a plan for marketing the hearing aid dispensing component of the practice. It is important that this plan take on a written format such that it can be reviewed, disseminated, and regularly referred to during the course of each cycle of the marketing plan's life. A written plan allows consistency both in message and in cost management. It generally prevents being easily sidetracked or impulsive. Committing the plan to writing, allows all participants in the process to dive in and understand the positioning of the hearing aid dispensary within the practice in the service

community. Figure 15–2 is an example of the components of a marketing calendar.

The marketing calendar defines three distinct approaches for planning, advertising, and marketing. Patient acquisition is directed toward education and promotional activities within the marketplace to draw in new patients to hearing aid dispensing the practice. Retention marketing is geared toward existing patients of the practice, many of whom may already have purchased hearing aids, with the eye toward retaining them both for interim services as well as new hearing aids eventually. Free media is directed toward the cost-effective dissemination of hearing issues, hearing services, and technology that generally is best distributed through local and community newspapers and other media. These local outlets generally are thirsty for newsworthy and novel information within their communities. The marketing calendar is a combination of these three approaches performed in a rotating and consistent fashion during the course of any 12 month cycle (Hosford-Dunn, Dunn, & Harford, 1995).

Summary

The hearing aid dispensary can be an important and contributing component to the otolaryngology practice. Careful

Example of Marketing Calendar

Patient Acquisition	Retention Marketing	Free Media
Consumer Education Seminars	Patient Newsletter	Staff Highlight (New People)
Advertising and Promotions	Retention letter, Batteries, etc.	New Technology or Diagnostics
Direct Mail Programs	Regular Check-up; Birthdays, etc.	Service Organizations

Figure 15–2. Example of marketing calendar.

consideration should be given to the business and operational planning and implementation of the hearing aid dispensary prior to committing substantial dollars to equipment or outside consultants.

References

The Federal Social Security Act, Anti-Kickback Statute, §1128B(b).

Hosford-Dunn H., Dunn, D. R., & Harford, E. R. (1995). *Audiology business and practice management.* San Diego, CA: Singular.

Kochkin, S., & MarkeTrak VII. (2005). Hearing loss population tops 31 million people. *Hearing Review, 12*(7), 16–29.

Kochkin, S., & MarkeTrak VII. (2007). Obstacles to adult non-user adoption of hearing aids. *Hearing Journal, 60*(4), 24–50.

Kochkin, S., & Rogin, C. M. (2000). Quantifying the obvious: The impact of hearing instruments on quality of life. *Hearing Review, 7*(1), 6–34.

Portman, R. M. (2001). HHS Issues Phase I of Final Stark Rules. *AAO-HNS Bulletin, 20,* 32–33.

Radcliffe, D. (2000). Is hearing loss increasing at younger ages? Many think so, but it's hard to prove. *Hearing Journal, 53*(5), 23–29.

16

Lessons from the Real World

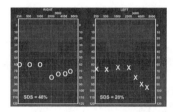

MICHAEL VALENTE, Ph.D.

Introduction

Directing a professionally and financially successful Audiology practice in the current medical environment can present significant obstacles and challenges. Unlike a private practice where much of the energy may be focused on a profitable hearing aid segment, services provided in a medical environment include both rehabilitative (including hearing aid dispensing) and diagnostic procedures. Unfortunately, reimbursement for many audiologic diagnostic procedures continues to decline while expenses (salary; fringe benefits; invoice costs for hearing aids, earmolds, and assistive technology; office supplies; postage, etc.) continue to rise. This dys-synchrony between falling income for diagnostic procedures and rising expenses simply makes the ability to achieve and maintain profitability more challenging. The diligent director of an audiology practice must keep a close eye on the monthly and annual profit/loss (P/L) statements so he or she is aware of the possible need to adjust the expenses and activities of the division.

Audiology, unlike most other professional services in a medical school environment, has the means to overcome these financial obstacles primarily through a successful hearing aid dispensing practice. If established appropriately, the reimbursement rate for all hearing aid related services should be 100% of billable charges. Collection of nearly 100% of billable charges allows many audiologic practices in medical environments to overcome the insufficient income paid for most diagnostic audiology procedures. What follows in this chapter is a broad description of the required key elements that must be in place in order for hearing aid dispensing to help an audiology practice survive in a medical school environment. Many, if not most, of the recommendations here also are applicable to the private practice setting.

Elements Required for a Successful Dispensing Practice

The major ingredients required for a successful hearing aid dispensing program within in a large medical school include:

1. Strong support of the chairperson
2. Competent and professional audiologists who engage in lifelong learning and provide quality patient care
3. State of the art and appropriate equipment
4. Otolaryngology and other referring physician specialists
5. Competent, knowledgeable, and professional support staff
6. Additional resources such as business office, human resources, billing, and collections, scheduling, accounting, telecommunications, computer support, and maintenance.
7. Appropriate billing for hearing aid related services
8. Ability and resources to negotiate hearing aid agreements
9. Ability and resources to negotiate contracts with insurance companies
10. Tracking invoices and credits
11. Appropriate charges for services
12. Successful marketing tools

It is important to note that these factors may or may not be required in other audiology environments (i.e., private practice, community speech and hearing center, private ENT office, nonmedical school hospital environment, not-for-profit clinic, etc.) or in other audiology programs at other large medical schools. Equally important is that *all* these elements need to be operating in an atmosphere of synchrony and harmony because the whole is only as great as the sum of its parts.

Support of the Chairperson

The audiology practice in most medical schools resides within the Department of Otolaryngology-Head and Neck Surgery. Typically, in this environment, the chairperson is either an otolaryngologist specializing in head and neck surgery or, less commonly, an otologist. The first author has been fortunate to have past experiences whereby one chairperson specialized in head and neck surgery while, recently, a second individual specialized in otology. In both cases, the chairperson offered full support and the author was extremely fortunate to direct the audiology program with minimal interference and micromanaging. Both chairpersons had the philosophy of hiring competent professionals and allowing those professionals to do what they were trained to do. Their philosophy was to place faith in the audiology director's decisions and not interfere unless there was evidence to support the need to do so. It is the author's belief that having the full support of the chairperson is *critical* for the success of an audiology program. Literally, success starts from the top!

Competent and Professional Audiologists

Employing professional and highly trained audiologists is equally as important as having a supportive chairperson. Audiologists must be intelligent, demonstrate initiative and self-motivation, and have a bent toward critical thinking. They should not be intimidated by teaching or speaking at conferences, should engage in research and evidence-based principles (EBP), and should enjoy participating in bringing cutting-edge technology to the clinic. These factors are essential in such an environment, as is understanding the relationship of the business-side of clinical audiology and the financial success of the division. Obviously, the success of any audiology program begins with the skills and sensitivity of those providing direct patient care. Audiologists within this environment must:

1. Provide a level of direct patient care that is second to none and strive to provide care that would be the same as provided to members of their own family
2. Enjoy the challenge of the introduction of new cutting-edge diagnostic and treatment technology
3. Be capable of functioning as a team member, welcoming the challenge of daily interactions with physicians, residents, and students
4. Desire the intellectual stimulation afforded by attending continuing

education opportunities and involvement in research.
5. Possess high ethical standards that are aimed at providing patients with hearing technology based on its appropriateness without being influenced by any other factors.

Sufficient and Appropriate Equipment

The services provided by an audiologist can only be as good as the equipment he or she uses to provide clinical services. Where appropriate, each piece of state of the art equipment should be checked regularly and calibrated at least annually. In addition to the sound-treated test suites, audiometers, CD players for speech audiometry, loudspeakers for sound-field testing, high-frequency audiometers, portable audiometers, immittance units, and various pieces of equipment for electrophysiologic testing, a dispensing practice must have the following minimal list of equipment:

1. *Coupler and real-ear measuring systems:* are an essential component of hearing aid dispensing. Dispensing of hearing aids without verification using real-ear measures is unethical, does not adhere to best practice standards, and does not provide quality patient care. All new and repaired hearing aids arriving to the clinic must be electroacoustically tested using coupler measures to assure that the performance adheres to the manufacturer's specifications and/or that the aid has been repaired correctly.

2. *Current computer(s) technology* for storing patient information and programming hearing aids via NOAH and interface devices. At our facility, each audiologist has his or her own computer for E-mail, accessing the World Wide Web, as well as the university patient database system, for storing presentations and reports. In addition, each dispensing room has a computer that communicates to a programming interface and to a central server dedicated specifically to audiology. In this way, any patient may be seen by any audiologist at any of our three clinical sites and his or her records can be accessed for hearing aid programming. In addition, each counseling and test suite has a computer and monitor to access patient databases to provide excellent patient care.

3. *Electronic dehumidifier:* this piece of equipment is essential for in-office hearing aid repairs related to moisture and buildup of debris.

4. *Telephone:* an operational telephone is placed within each dispensing room for programming the memory in the hearing aid dedicated for use with the telephone. In this manner, adjustments to the telecoil response of the hearing aid can be made in real time allowing a higher probability of success.

5. *Ultrasonic cleaner:* this piece of equipment is necessary for cleaning earmolds when behind-the-ear aids are dispensed.

6. *Microscope, grinder/buffer, drill:* these and other smaller pieces of equipment are essential for making small in-house repairs of hearing aids and earmolds.

Otolaryngologist and Other Referring Physicians

At the authors' facility, there are 23 attending physicians and approximately 28 resident physicians within the Department of Otolaryngology. These physicians provide daily clinical services to a vast array of patients, many of whom are sent to Audiology Division for evaluation. Our facility also receives referrals from physicians within the outpatient clinics at the medical school, inpatients from within the hospital, and additional referrals from private practitioners within the community. *Our division has a system in place where all referrals are noted on a special form. This form is sent to the Director of Audiology who in turn prepares a personal letter of appreciation to every physician or other professional who was identified as referring a patient.* The authors strongly feel some type of program should be instituted in every audiology program because it establishes a referral database and open communication to outside referring professionals in a positive light.

The audiology and otolaryngology staff at this medical school work as a wonderful team to improve the hearing ability of patients via medicine, surgery, amplification, and/or hearing assistive technology. This strong atmosphere of teamwork came about due to mutual respect for the unique skills of each specialty, interaction in educational events (Otolaryngology Grand Rounds, Otology/Audiology Grand Rounds, research presentations, etc.); collaborative research, and the leadership of the chairperson. In the area of amplification, attending physicians and residents do not counsel a patient seen by one of the staff audiologists who recommended amplification.

That is, patients do not hear, for example, hearing aids do not help "nerve deafness," "you only need one hearing aid," or "in-the-ear hearing aids are better than behind-the-ear hearing aids." By the same token, audiologists do not counsel patients as to candidacy for otologic surgery or medications. This should not be viewed as a "turf" issue, but rather an acknowledgment of the differing skills and training unique to each profession. The two professions must work strongly *together* to develop a treatment plan that is in the best interests of their patients to ensure that patients do not receive conflicting advice. In the rare instance where differences of opinion may arise, these professionals need to come together for discussion, and jointly arrive at a best treatment plan for their patient. Audiologists and otolaryngologists need to work as partners and not adversaries in the treatment of hearing impairment. This philosophy works well in the authors' environment and we are confident that it can work in other environments.

Competent, Knowledgeable, and Professional Support Staff

Every audiologist knows that the successful performance of an audiology practice is directly related to the skills and dedication of the support staff. The authors are referring to the secretaries or receptionists who schedule both patient appointments and staff meetings, as well as contact patients for other issues in addition to scheduling. These other issues may include informing patients that their hearing aids or earmolds have arrived, mailing batteries and other assistive and amplification related items, and creating and processing purchase orders for sup-

plies. Supporting staff arrange the Division "Master Schedule" so the purpose of the patient visit (hearing evaluation, impression, hearing aid evaluation (HAE), hearing aid fitting, pick up a hearing aid, etc.) is placed into the proper time slot and for the correct audiologist, schedule conferences and meetings, and determine when to direct a call to an audiologist or answer the patient's question themselves. There are the endless daily tasks of faxing, copying, E-mailing reminders to the staff, and effectively communicating with patients in the waiting room or on the telephone who are hearing impaired. As this person often is the patient's first contact with the department, his or her possession of a cheerful, professional, and helpful demeanor is as crucial as a conscientious work ethic. Without a competent, knowledgeable and professional support staff, the audiology practice cannot function in a patient-centered way.

Additional Resources

Audiologists are professionals trained to diagnose and treat patients with hearing loss within their scope of practice. Their full attention needs to be focused on direct patient care, teaching, and research. Audiologists should not have to address issues related to billing and collection, computer maintenance, and other areas outside their realm of expertise or training. A successful practice requires *other* professionals to be in place who are equally trained and dedicated to providing services such as:

1. *Business office* personal to take care of invoices for hearing aids, earmolds, hearing assistive technology, and office supplies. These

professionals also keep records of vacation and sick time, process all issues related to payroll, post job offerings for Audiology within the university, process all new hires, update personnel records, coordinate parking for staff, process purchase orders for computers, process key and telecommunication requests, track payment of dues to professional organizations and licensing agencies, handle mail, tag inventory, handle pagers, process billing for inpatient care, and create vendor blanket orders so individual purchase orders are not required for each hearing aid or earmold that is ordered.

2. *Human resources* personnel to take care of all issues related to hiring of professional and support staff orientation, fringe benefits, personnel issues, HIPPA compliance, and others.

3. *Billing and collection* personnel to ensure that each fee ticket is billed correctly and to the appropriate payer, payment is received and the payment amount for the provided service is correct. These professionals must also maintain expertise related to insurance and other third-party payment issues.

4. *Scheduling staff* who have the responsibility of being sure that all patients are correctly scheduled (time, date, office and clinic) and of handling scheduling if warranted (i.e., an audiologist calls in sick). These people also work with the Division secretaries to create the "master schedule" for each audiologist. This "master schedule" includes the day and times the audiologist sees patients, and the amount of time allotted for each type of procedure (audiologic evaluation, earmold impression, counseling, auditory brainstem response (ABR), hearing aid evaluation, hearing aid fittings, hearing aid repair, annual recheck, etc.) This staff is also responsible for scheduling meetings, conferences, research, and calibration of equipment or gathering norms for new equipment, as well as teaching schedules, and many other duties of the audiologist. This staff member also has the important function of calling patients the day prior to the scheduled appointment, to minimize the number of "no shows."

5. *The accounting office* monitors the activity of the Division to help determine profit/loss, staff productivity, and comparative data across months and years.

6. *Telecommunications* personnel take care of the phone, fax, and E-mail services.

7. *Computer support services* maintain staff computers as well as insure the computers that communicate with equipment are functioning properly. These are the professionals called when issues of incompatibility or software upgrades come into play. The efforts of the computer staff are invaluable because their skills assure that any patient can be seen at any of the three clinical sites at any computer and their records can be accessed.

8. The skills of the *maintenance staff* are critical so the patient waiting rooms, examination rooms, and staff offices are clean. The first thing patients notice when visiting

a clinic is the waiting room; it is essential for that area to look clean and neat. All these professionals, and others, are necessary if the practice is to be professionally and financially successful.

Billing for Hearing Aid Related Services

In a section below entitled "Ability to Negotiate Contracts with Insurance Companies," the author provides suggestions for negotiating contracts with insurance companies for hearing aid coverage. This particular section relates to some guidelines established over the years at our facility related to billing for hearing aid services.

When earmolds are ordered for a behind-the-ear fitting, our facility requires the patient to pay for the earmolds at the time they are ordered. This policy was enacted because, after earmolds were ordered, numerous patients decided either not to pursue amplification or simply to not show for the next appointment. The Division was left paying for the cost of the earmolds. It is important to remember that, when *hearing aids* are ordered for a patient and the patient does not return, the hearing aids may be returned for credit. But, keep in mind that the practice may lose the credit for shipping and handling and thus incur a small, but real, financial loss. In contrast, earmolds may not be returned for credit since they are custom made, so this would result in an even greater financial loss for the Division. To avoid this scenario, the Division decided to adopt a policy where patient's pay in full for the earmolds at the time the impressions are taken and the earmolds ordered.

When dispensing hearing aids, there are typically four patient visits. The first visit involves the audiometric and medical examination. A hearing aid evaluation (HAE) takes place during the second visit, where comprehensive counseling, additional measures, and impressions for earmolds or custom products are taken. The third visit is set aside for fitting the hearing aids, whereas the fourth visit is when the patient returns for fine-tuning (if necessary) and general follow-up procedures. This last visit typically is scheduled anywhere from 2 to 4 weeks after the fitting. Several years ago, our facility decided *not to charge* for the HAE, but instead bundled this charge into the dispensing fee. The reason for this decision is twofold. First, payment for the HAE was a stumbling block for many patients to pursue hearing aids because this was an expense whether or not the patient decided to proceed with ordering the hearing aids. Second, payment expectation for a visit that might not lead to pursuing hearing aids was confusing to many patients. To reduce the "fear" of an additional unnecessary expense and confusion, the Division decided to make this second visit a "no charge" visit, but instead added it to the cost of the dispensed hearing aids. We attribute some of our growth in our hearing aid practice directly to this decision, and would recommend the practitioner consider adopting a similar policy.

All earmolds, new hearing aids, repaired hearing aids, warranty extensions, hearing assistive technology, batteries, and hearing aid accessories require payment of 100% of the billable charge at the date of service. Several years ago our Division decided not to accept any third party reimbursement; our rationale is explained below.

Ability to Negotiate Hearing Aid Agreements

It is the strong opinion of the authors that no more than three manufacturers should serve as the primary source of hearing aids to be dispensed by the audiology staff. Certainly, there may be a need to order a hearing aid outside of these three major manufacturers, but for the most part, the practice should be limited to three manufacturers. There are several reasons for this recommendation. First, audiologists are in a better position to negotiate a higher level of discount because the hearing aids will be ordered from fewer sources. The author has always developed a long-term relationship with the manufacturers. Over time, the Director of Audiology negotiates greater and greater discounts because the Division has developed a history of "loyalty" to that product line. Second, the technology, and supporting software have gone through dramatic changes in a very short time. It is almost a full-time job trying to remain current with these changes. It becomes difficult to do this well with three manufacturers, and it becomes nearly impossible with more than three. Third, by keeping the options to three manufacturers, this provides a realistic opportunity for the staff to really know the software and specific aspects of the models from these manufacturers. This, in turn, provides better care to their patients. On occasion, it is inevitable that an audiologist will run into a situation requiring a special favor from a manufacturer. Granting of this favor becomes much more likely if the staff has a history of loyalty to a manufacturer than if this favor was asked of a less utilized and less familiar manufacturer.

Ability to Negotiate Contracts with Insurance Companies

The author has been directing the Audiology Division in a large medical school center for over 20 years. During many of those years, he has been involved in *direct* negotiations with representatives from a large number of insurance companies that wish to include hearing aids as a benefit for policy holders. In all the years the author has been involved in this aspect of his position, he has yet to find a single proposal that was financially feasible to accept for several reasons. First, the insurance company typically proposes to pay for hearing aids based on the invoice (discounted) cost of the hearing aids. This is obviously not going to advantage the profitability of the audiology practice. Second, negotiated payment for the *dispensing* component of the hearing aid related services typically is *extremely* low in comparison to the typical charge for patients who are not covered by insurance. Thus, audiologists are literally giving away their services for the promise that there will be an increase in patient referral volume from the insurance company. Therefore, the "promise" of the insurance company of greater patient volume will lead to a larger discount from hearing aid manufacturers. The insurers base this on the premise that the purchase of more hearing aids due to the greater patient volume will lead to greater discounts and that this will directly improve the bottom line. They will further argue that this increased discount will help defray the reduced income as a result of seeing patients referred from the insurance company. This will increase the "profit" when audiologists fit noninsured patients because the cost of the aids will be reduced due to decreases on the cost of goods of the hearing aids that have been negotiated by seeing the increased number of patients from the insurance company. The author has found the reality quite different: There were many cases where the amount to be paid by the insurer was less than the cost of purchasing the aid! The practitioner would be wise to recall that, if one loses money on every hearing aid, it cannot be made up by selling volume!

In addition, there also is the reality that insurance companies are infamous for informing billing and collection that:

1. "We never received the claim; can you send it again?"
2. "*That* patient isn't covered by our plan" in spite of the fact the staff have documentation (letter or E-mail) from the representative who stated the patient was covered, or
3. "We do not cover that aid" despite staff documentation that the insurance claims processor stated previously that the particular model *was* covered.
4. Finally, many insurance policies have a disclaimer in their contracts stating that the insurance company has the right to rescind the prior authorization!

When working with insurance companies, the audiology staff quickly may become billing/collection personnel, which then will evolve into an intolerable situation for obvious reasons. One must exercise extreme caution when getting involved in negotiations with insurance companies to cover hearing aids for their policy holders. In the 20 years that the author has been involved in these negotiations, there has not been a *single case* where the end result would have been in the financial best interest of the Division. Currently, our facility has no agreements with any insurance company to cover hearing aids under their plan. The author strongly urges the reader to review the fine print and recommend strong consideration against entering into an agreement to cover hearing aids. In addition to the financial considerations, it certainly is not positive for staff morale to spend large amounts of time verifying eligibility and subsequently pursuing payment. Finally, in a university setting, the author strongly suggests that it be the department policy that *all* negotiations to "carve out" hearing aids during insurance negotiations pass directly through the Director of Audiology and not through hospital/university personnel who negotiate other contracts. These fine professionals are simply not aware of the horrific outcome such agreements could have upon the financial well-being of the division and department. Negotiations must be made through experts in audiology and amplification who understand the nuances of negotiating bundled fees for goods and professional services.

Tracking Invoices and Credits

Every hearing aid invoice represents an expense. This figure can be very expensive because the invoice cost of one hearing aid can be over $1500. For this reason, it is strongly recommended to create a system where one person is assigned to track and associate each invoice to a patient and audiologist. Accurate records are crucial of documenting that each hearing aid is dispensed. It is not unreasonable to set a time line of within 60 days from receipt of the hearing aid from the manufacturer that it is expected to be dispensed. If the inventory record shows the aid has not been dispensed in this time line, then an E-mail should be forwarded to the audiologist to determine the status of the aid and reason for delay. Along the same line, the same individual must be in charge of keeping records of all hearing aids sent back for credit. This need to be tracked for a maximum time of 60 days from the time the aid is sent back for credit. If the credit has not been received within a reasonable period of time, then an E-mail is sent to the audiologist inquiring why the credit has not been received. Such a personnel tracking system of each aid (new and repaired) is important, by individuals who are familiar with audiology and division procedures. Computer technology and business office personnel are valuable resources, but errors can and do occur, which a tracking system can monitor.

Appropriate Charges for Services

A system to determine the appropriate charge for hearing aids must be established. At our facility, we take the single unit cost and add costs for accessory items that are dispensed with the aids (batteries, tubing blower, Dry and Store dehumidifier, ointment for easier insertion of earmolds or custom shells), sanitizer spray as well as the cost for the hearing aid evaluation (bundled into the dispensing fee) and dispensing fee. One fee is set for dispensing a monaural fit

and another is set for a bilateral fit. The monetary value of the price associated with the hearing aid evaluation and dispensing service is based on knowledge of all direct and indirect costs associated with providing this service. In addition, one must factor a set level of profitability. In our institution, all these data are placed into a spreadsheet developed by the author. The audiologist simply inputs the single unit cost of the aid to be dispensed and the spreadsheet calculates the cost to the patient. Values in the spreadsheet are updated annually to reflect changes in indirect and direct costs.

What was described above is known as bundling; there is a single charge for providing several layers of services and visits. That is, the patient pays one charge and the majority of subsequent services (reprogramming or minor repairs that can be completed in the office) are provided at no charge for the life of the hearing aid, unless the aid requires repair outside of the warranty period. Another way of charging for these services is called "unbundling" where a charge is applied to each visit depending upon the nature of the visit. In this scenario, the initial dollar amount paid by the patient is lower than the bundled model, but charges are added for each visit after the initial fit.

Finally, the audiologist must be constantly aware of current market trends. At the same time, we do not recommend undue influence by the current heavy marketing of very low-cost hearing aids from national chains. Our facility has not reduced our own charges in response to these marketing strategies. We did, however, negotiate with our hearing aid manufacturers to provide more low-cost, entry level digital hearing aids in order to be competitive with that segment of the outside market.

Marketing

Until recently, our Division did not engage in any external marketing. All marketing was targeted internally toward such areas as the medical school newsletters, community continuing education lectures, screenings, and similar avenues. A year ago, the Division decided to become more aggressive in spending money for marketing as well as some other innovative programs. Over the past year, some of the efforts have been successful, whereas others have not generated interest. The more successful efforts include:

1. Creating a trifold brochure that was delivered to every Washington University employee offering a 15% discount off the cost for hearing aids for the employee and members of his or her family
2. Sending this same brochure to every employee of the two hospitals directly affiliated with the medical school
3. Developing a Web site (http://audi ology.wustl.edu) that has attracted much attention
4. Creating another trifold brochure that provides mini-biographies of the staff that is handed out when completing community events, such as lectures or screenings
5. Developing a "call-back" postcard that is forwarded to patients to remind them that the warranty of their hearing aids will expire shortly. This is sent a month before the warranty expiration.

6. Developing another "call-back" post card that is forwarded to patients to remind them that it has been a year since their last hearing test and that they need to contact their physician to obtain a referral for an annual check if necessary. This is sent a month before the anniversary of the last audiologic evaluation.
7. Developing another "call-back" post card that is forwarded to patients to remind them that it has been a year since we last saw him or her for hearing aid related services. This is sent a month before the anniversary of the last visit for hearing aid repairs.
8. Forwarding a newsletter four times a year to all patients who have purchased hearing aids. Numerous patients receive the newsletter as an attached file to their E-mail addresses. The newsletter is also available on our Web site and in the waiting room of all three offices. We have received feedback that our patients enjoy hearing about the latest cutting-edge technology, new procedures and protocols, research activities of the Division, presentations and awards by the staff.
9. Developing a form that is sent to the Director for every patient who is referred by any physician. This form results in a timely personal letter to the referring physician or other referral source thanking him or her for the confidence he or she has in our staff. The physician is reminded that it is our pleasure to provide services to his or her patient. The physician is also provided contact information in the event our facility may be of further assistance.

Conclusion

This chapter provided the reader with some ideas of what is necessary for an audiology practice to be successful in a medical school and other medical environments. The recommendations here will fit in nicely with most private medical practice settings as well. With decreasing revenue for diagnostic procedures, the audiology program must develop and nurture an active hearing aid dispensing practice as part of the total services provided by the Division. It is essential that net income exceeds both direct and indirect expenses to allow the Division to remain profitable. This chapter has provided a "realistic" picture of steps that need to be taken to permit efficacious, cost-effective hearing aid dispensing.

17

The Future of Hearing Aid Research

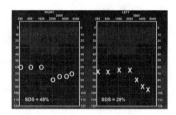

BRENT EDWARDS, PH.D.

Introduction

Hearing aid technology has progressed dramatically over the past decade. The introduction of digital signal processing (DSP) into hearing aids in 1996 allowed advanced signal processing algorithms to be introduced that increased benefit to hearing aid wearers. By 2007, 92% of the hearing aids sold in the United States had DSP in them (Kirkwood, 2007). Over half of the prescribed hearing aids today include directional microphones, providing verifiable improvements to speech understanding in noise. Open-canal products have increased in popularity because of improved comfort, the elimina-

tion of occlusion problems, and the lack of a requirement for custom shells or ear-molds. Finally, industrial design innovations in behind-the-ear case designs, make them look more like consumer electronics and less like prosthetic devices.

Few people would have predicted such advances in the hearing aid industry at the beginning of the 1990s. Multiband compression had been rejected as a valuable technology; directional microphones, noise reduction, and even open-canal fittings had been tried with hearing aids by 1990, none with much success.

So, what changed to make them successful today? Technology advanced enough to enable their application in a usable fashion: multiband compression could be implemented in a small form factor and with low noise; the directivity of directional microphones improved and they were designed to allow switching to omnidirectionality to avoid noise issues; feedback cancellation allowed greater gain in open-canal devices; and the acoustics were improved to increase the usable bandwidth.

New technologies are developed and are successful in the marketplace when they address the unmet needs of the consumers. Recent market data indicate that 71% of hearing aid users express overall satisfaction with their hearing aids, but there remain several well-defined areas that need improving (Kochkin, 2005). Table 17–1 shows customer satisfaction data from MarkeTrak VII that identifies current unmet needs that digital processing can address. As can be seen, there are many areas of opportunity for digital technology to provide improvement, such as improvements to the perception of wind noise and better loudness placement of sounds, which will drive new digital technology development.

Industry innovations occur in either incremental steps or radical changes. The incremental innovations are easier to predict because they involve natural progressions of existing technology. Radical innovations are difficult to predict because they involve new concepts with no current examples. Also, they often lead to disruptive technologies that completely change the marketplace of an industry (Christensen, 1997).

These types of innovation often involve bringing technology from one field into another, and the impact of these newly introduced technologies may be predicted by those knowledgeable in both fields. The introduction of DSPs and the appli-

Table 17–1. Customer Satisfaction Data from MarkeTrak VII

Signal Processing and Sound Quality	Percent Satisfied
Clearness tone/sound	74
Sound of voice	70
Natural sounding	69
Directionality	66
Able to hear soft sounds	64
Richness of sound fidelity	61
Comfort with loud sounds	60
Whistling/feedback/buzzing	55
Chewing/swallowing sound	54
Use in noisy situations	51
Wind noise	49

Note. The right-hand column indicates the percentage of hearing aid wearers who are satisfied with the aspect of hearing aid performance indicated in the left-hand column.
Source: From: Kochkin S. (2005). MarkeTrak VII: Customer satisfaction with hearing instruments in the digital age. *Hearing Journal, 58*(9), 30–42.

cation of feedback cancellation were radical innovations but could have been predicted by those who were aware of DSP use in nonhearing aid fields and who were able to see their potential benefit to hearing aid users.

Thus, although predictions about the future are often tenuous, estimates of where future potential benefits lie from new technology are not entirely ungrounded. This chapter attempts to outline where the hearing aid industry is heading and what new digital technologies and applications will be developed.

Digital Wireless Technology

Digital signal processing revolutionized the hearing aid industry 10 years ago and resulted in new applications that provided new benefit to the hearing impaired. Prior to its introduction, the possible benefit of digital technology to hearing aids was not well understood and many studies were conducted comparing digital hearing aids with analog hearing aids to determine if digital technology was providing benefit. Today, the benefit is clear, and what is also clear is that the use of DSP in a hearing aid was a revolutionary breakthrough that changed the hearing aid industry in unexpected ways. People have now started to wonder what the next revolutionary innovation will be. The most likely candidate—the one most likely to produce new applications and new patient benefits—is digital wireless technology.

Analog Wireless

Wireless technology has existed in the hearing aid industry for many years in the form of analog systems. These systems typically consist of a transmitter that is attached to a sound source, such as a lecturer's microphone or a movie theater's audio system, and a receiver that is connected to the hearing aid to receive the wirelessly transmitted signal. Examples of these systems are a microphone on a teacher that transmits an FM signal to an attachment on a BTE's direct audio input, or a loop system plugged into a lecturer's microphone in an auditorium whose electromagnetic signal is received by a telecoil inside of a hearing aid.

In the United States, neither FM systems nor loop systems have achieved significant success outside of specialized uses such as in a classroom. Their success has been limited by: (1) cost (a typical FM system costs thousands of dollars), (2) the requirement that other people use an accessory or that an establishment install a wireless system, (3) the requirement that accessories be carried around by the hearing aid wearer for use when they are needed, (4) the general incompatibility across systems (Beecher, 2000), (5) patient resistance to complicated technology, and (6) difficulties with electromagnetic interference and creating a homogeneous field strength with loop systems (Boothroyd et al., 2007; Ross, 2006). New digital wireless technology will improve on all of these limitations and add more functionality.

Technical Benefits

Digital wireless technology transmits a higher fidelity signal than do analog systems. With a typical wireless analog system, the signal quality decreases the farther the receiver is from the transmitter. Digital signals preserve their fidelity with greater consistency. The quality remains good up to some limiting distance, beyond which the quality drops dramatically. This becomes the usability distance, within which the user can be sure that the sound he or she hears will be uncorrupted by distortion and noise. This ability of digital wireless is in part due to error correction coding, a technique that detects when errors occur in the wireless data and corrects them. Digital coding schemes are also more resistant to interference from electromagnetic signals and to interference from other devices wirelessly transmitting in the area.

The large number of companies developing digital wireless technology (over 5000 companies have registered to create Bluetooth products per Yanz, Roberts, & Colburn, 2006) helps to advance the technology as well as drives down its cost and size. Digital wireless technology is lower in power and size than its analog counterparts, which improves its application to hearing aids

Connectivity

Digital wireless technology can enable hearing aids to be wirelessly connected to a wide array of audio products. This is possible because digital wireless technology is becoming ubiquitous in consumer electronics.

An increasing number of products are being produced with wireless capabilities. More importantly, audio products that hearing aid wearers want to listen to are being made with digital wireless technology embedded in the product, making them easier to connect to hearing aids wirelessly. If a television, for example, is transmitting its audio wirelessly, then a wireless receiver can be added to the hearing aid so that the hearing aid wearer can listen to TV audio that is not subject to room reverberation and not worry about bothering others in the room with a loud TV.

All of this wireless development would still not make connectivity easier for hearing aid wearers if every device transmitted its sound with different technology. Bluetooth, however, has become a standard that manufacturers have agreed to use when they digitally transmit their audio. This allows other products with a Bluetooth receiver to pick up the transmitted audio and play it without any spe-

cialized design requirements. A single Bluetooth receiver in or attached to a hearing aid can receive sound from all sorts of sound sources: televisions, radios, cellular phones, mp3 players. The use of Bluetooth for public broadcast systems as an alternative to loop systems has also been suggested (Myers, 2006).

Hearing aid companies are now creating Bluetooth accessories that plug into a BTE's direct audio input. They allow cell phone audio to be transmitted directly to the hearing aid and that will also pick up the wearer's voice and transmit it back to the cell phone. These accessories essentially convert the hearing aid into a hands-free cell phone earpiece. Microphones are also being manufactured that can be worn by the hearing aid wearer's companion so that their voice is wirelessly transmitted directly into the hearing aid. With this technology, the ratio of the speaker's voice to the background noise is improved well beyond the ratio improvement provided by a directional microphone on a hearing aid. As hearing aids become wirelessly connected to an increasing number of devices over the next several years, control of connectivity will become an important issue. User interface development and usability designs will become an increasingly important aspect of hearing aids.

This connectivity to audio products will be only the beginning of new benefits that digital wireless technology will provide.

The Bluetooth protocol provides connectivity not only for audio but also for nonaudio data such as control signals. When using Bluetooth to listen to a cell phone, for example, the wireless digital signal passes the sound back and forth between the phone to the earpiece and also transmits commands such as volume control, answer, mute, and hang up. This capability will allow hearing aids to control other products with user controls on the hearing aid.

In the consumer electronics field, wires that are currently used to transmit data and control signals between products will eventually be replaced by wireless technology: transmitting pictures from a digital camera to the PC, transmitting audio from a DVD player to speakers. Bluetooth is already being used to replace programming cables used to program hearing aids, and new applications will be developed that provide new benefits to hearing aid wearers and audiologists.

Yanz (2006) described a future where all audio sources communicate with a hearing aid wirelessly, and suggested that text-to-speech could be used in computers to relay E-mail wirelessly to hearing aids. Clearly, connectivity between the hearing aid and many devices will be the norm. Many more possibilities for interaction between hearing aids and audio products—or even non-audio products—are possible because of use of the Bluetooth standard for wireless connectivity.

Ear-to-Ear

Wireless ear-to-ear communication describes the situation where the left and right hearing aids of a bilaterally-fit wearer communicate wirelessly with each other. This functionality has been recently introduced into the industry and is becoming a common feature among the highest end devices. Current applications for this communication are synchronization of left and right volume controls and a few other basic functions.

As the wireless data rate increases, more functionality will become possible.

Eventually, a pair of hearing aids will be considered as a single system rather than as two separate hearing aids. With ear-to-ear connectivity, every function within the hearing aids can become synchronized. Processing could also be shared between the aids to overcome DSP chip limitations, where algorithms are computed in only one hearing aid and the results shared with the other rather than calculating the algorithm in both hearing aids independently. With this approach, computations are shared between the aids, overcoming computational limitations on any one hearing aid chip. The disadvantage of this, of course, would be that the two hearing aids are dependent on each other and do not function as well when the other is absent.

Once data rates for ear-to-ear communication increase enough to pass audio between them (requiring a rate of tens of thousands of bits per second rather than the current hundreds of bits per second), speech understanding in noise can be improved using beam forming techniques (van Veen & Buckley, 1988). At its most basic level, the signal from both hearing aids can be added together to increase the signal-to-noise ratio for a target signal in front of the wearer.

Figure 17–1 shows a directional pattern that can be achieved with this approach. Also shown with a dashed line is a directional pattern achieved by current directional microphones for comparison.

More complex algorithms such as adaptive beam forming and blind source separation will likely be applied when high data rate ear-to-ear audio transmission occurs, and the challenge in the application of these algorithms will be to ensure that speech understanding is improved without sacrificing sound quality.

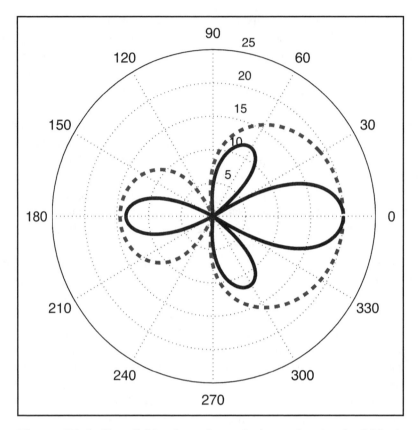

Figure 17–1. Free-field polar patterns for beam forming (*solid line*), and a first-order directional (*dashed line*).

Binaural perception will become an industry focus once ear-to-ear communication becomes mature. With multiband compression, noise reduction, and other adaptive algorithms operating independently at the two ears, there is the possibility that binaural cues are being distorted by hearing aids (Besing, Koehnke, Zurek, Kawakyu, & Lister, 1999; Desloge, Rabinowitz, & Zurek, 1997; Van den Bogaert, Klasen, Moonen, Van Deun, & Wouters, 2006). Wireless communication between hearing aids allows the possibility for algorithms that attempt to restore binaural perception to normal (Klasen, Moonen, Van den Bogaert, & Wouters, 2005). To date, little is known about the effect of independent hearing aids on such binaural phenomenon as localization and spatial release from masking. These effects are discussed later in this chapter, but ear-to-ear wireless communication could provide a mechanism for addressing any interactions between hearing aids and binaural perception by attempting to preserve binaural cues with processing synchronized between the ears.

Limitations

The reason that digital wireless technology isn't in every hearing aid today is because of power consumption. Currently, a Bluetooth chip requires over 30 mW to transmit and receive audio. Most hearing aids require less than 1 mw of power in total, so adding a Bluetooth chip would increase the power consumption dramatically and reduce the battery life of the hearing aid. Until this power problem is solved, Bluetooth chips likely will not be added as a component within a hearing aid. Yanz (2006) suggested an interim solution of a general-purpose relay device with a large battery that sits near the hearing aid, receives Bluetooth signals, and then relays them to the hearing aid using a wireless technology that requires less power than Bluetooth. This solution has been introduced in hearing aid systems from at least two manufacturers. Using a relay trades lower hearing aid power consumption for the need of an accessory, but has the potential to provide the widespread connectivity described earlier. Key aspects for the success of such relay devices with hearing aid wearers are reliability and usability: reliability because of wireless interference and the potential for lost wireless connectivity; usability because connectivity with multiple devices will require simple controls that are intuitive and easy for hearing aid users to use.

As digital wireless chips continue to be designed smaller in size and lower in power, these limitations will disappear and it is likely that the majority of hearing aids will have wireless receivers embedded in them in the same way that the majority of hearing aids today have DSPs. When this happens, hearing aids will contain new ear-to-ear algorithms and will be connected to most any audio source that the wearer wants to hear. The engineering challenge is to make connecting to these sources as easy as possible for the hearing aid wearer.

DSP Algorithms

Digital signal processing has reached a state of maturity in the hearing aid industry. Most hearing aids have a similar set of DSP algorithms that includes multiband compression, noise reduction, feedback cancellation, directional processing, and environment classification. Many thought-leaders in the industry have suggested that DSP chip development has outpaced the industry's ideas for its application, that is, that DSP chips in hearing aids now have more capabilities than companies know what to do with, and that we should not expect much future development in DSP functionality. In fact, the opposite is true.

Every major hearing aid company spends a considerable effort squeezing the signal processing that they want to provide into the restricted capabilities of hearing aid DSPs. In doing so, they often simplify the algorithms—making them less complex than what the engineer originally planned—in order for the algorithm code to fit within the restricted clock cycles and memory of the DSP chip. This is somewhat akin to scaling back the graphics on a computer game because the video card or CPU isn't powerful enough to handle all of the 3-D features that the software could provide—the basic functionality is there, but the experience is not nearly as good as it could be if the hardware were more powerful.

To keep their current drain well below 1 mA, DSP chips in hearing aids run their clock speeds at just a few MHz, as opposed to general purpose DSPs used in consumer electronics that can run at hundreds and thousands of MHz. The programming and data memory in hearing aid DSPs are also restricted to a few tens of thousands of words of RAM, rather than the hundreds of thousands or even millions of words of RAM in general purpose DSPs. Because of these hardware restrictions, algorithms currently found in hearing aids have been simplified so that they all can run on a single DSP chip and fit in its memory.

Current hearing aid DSP chip limitations also restrict the introduction of new types of algorithms that can run on more powerful commercial DSPs but not on hearing aid DSPs.

These facts mean two things for the future: (1) current hearing aid algorithms will improve over time, as hearing aid DSP chips become more powerful, and (2) algorithms not yet seen in the hearing aid industry will be introduced when hearing aid DSP chips become capable of running them.

The limitation with what hearing aids can do resides in the chip technology, not in the knowledge of what can be done with them. That being the case, what DSP algorithm innovations can we expect in the future?

Improved Algorithms

Algorithms that currently exist in hearing aids will be improved and refined as DSP capabilities increase and as we learn more about the benefit that current algorithms provide.

As a simple example, consider noise reduction. The telecommunication industry provides an example of how noise reduction and speech enhancements in hearing aids can be improved; cell phones have considerably more sophisticated noise reduction algorithms because of their more powerful DSP chips. Whereas current hearing aid noise reduction algorithms rely on envelope statistics and simple environment classifiers to function, similar algorithms in telecommunication use speech production models that attempt to simulate the acoustics of the vocal tract and resonances in the mouth and nasal cavity as a part of their speech detection and noise reduction systems.

As the speed and memory of hearing aid chips increase, the more sophisticated versions of current hearing aid algorithms will be developed by hearing aid companies, either through internal development or translation from universities and other industries, providing additional benefit to the hearing aid wearer.

New Algorithms

New computationally intensive algorithms will also be introduced as DSP chips increase in capability. Many of these new algorithms will also be borrowed from other industries that process audio, because they have had many years with more powerful chips to develop and optimize their processing schemes. For example, the music recording industry has sophisticated audio processing algorithms for compression, pitch shifting, and other effects that have been optimized by highly critical listeners. Most of these algorithms from other industries, however, will require considerable work to modify them for use in hearing aids. There are several reasons for this.

First, as already stated, hearing aids always have less powerful DSP capabilities than other products that do not have the same size and power constraints. This means that significant work will still exist to simplify algorithms and to integrate them with existing hearing aid algorithms. Many algorithms from other industries will have to be translated from 32-bit floating point implementations into more difficult 16-bit fixed point implementations.

Second, most audio industries process very specific types of sound. The telecommunication industry usually processes speech at high signal-to-noise ratios; the music industry only processes voice and musical instruments, often separated into individual tracks; the teleconference industry only processes sounds that exist in conference rooms such as speech and HVAC noise.

Hearing aids, however, have to be able to process all possible sounds with imperceptible distortion and good perceived quality for someone listening all day long. In other words, they have to be able to handle every sound and any sound in all possible combinations. Algorithms that are designed to only work with headsets in an office cannot simply be ported to a hearing aid without serious alteration to ensure that they work in all of the conditions that a hearing aid wearer might experience. Customers do not return their cell phones because the sound of a fork on a plate wasn't processed properly.

Third, algorithms in other industries were designed for normally hearing listeners. If and how they would have to be modified for listening by those with hearing impairment is unknown. Wider auditory filters, loudness recruitment, and changes to forward masking functions may cause hearing impaired listeners to prefer different processing designs than those optimized for normally hearing listeners. The interaction of new algorithms with other hearing aid algorithms such as multiband compression will also have to be carefully investigated to ensure that algorithms work together gracefully.

Intelligent Systems

Hearing aids today have many automatic features: turning directionality and noise reduction on and off, classifying the environment that the user is in (e.g., car, noisy restaurant, quiet office, etc.), and making adjustments to the hearing aid settings. This automation will continue to evolve, but learning also will be added to hearing aids, making them "intelligent."

Current adaptive algorithms in hearing aids should not be classified as intelligent because they lack learning, which is the ability to improve behavior over time in response to sensor information. Techniques such as neural networks, fuzzy logic, and genetic algorithms have been researched extensively in academia for use in systems that learn behavior and alter how they work in an optimal way, and we should expect their emergence into the hearing aid industry.

One application for intelligent systems is to assist with individualized fittings. The proper fitting of the parameters of a hearing aid by the audiologist or hearing instrument specialist to the needs of the hearing aid wearer is critical to the success of the hearing aid. Unfortunately, not all dispensers are skilled at providing the best hearing aid setting for their patient needs, and often getting the proper fit requires several office visits. A hearing aid that can automatically alter how it works over time to better fit the needs of the hearing aid wearer would benefit patients who were not fit by an expert fitter. The dispenser also would benefit by not having to spend as much office time fine-tuning the hearing aid parameters. The challenge with implementing intelligent systems in hearing aids is to ensure that the system is able to adapt over time so that the sound processing is improved for the hearing aid wearer.

Durant et al. (2004) implemented a genetic algorithm that adjusted the parameters of a feedback canceller in a hearing aid such that the feedback canceller improved its performance over time. The genetic algorithm required the wearer to assess the sound quality of the hearing aid with different parameter settings, and the algorithm used the listener's responses to continually adjust and improve the feedback canceller and the resulting sound quality. One can imagine that this approach could be applied to many aspects of hearing aid use. Such a system would need to be to designed to be easy to use and to ensure that the hearing aid continues to improve as it adapts rather than mistakenly get worse.

Hearing Science

The science of auditory perception is a mature field, as is our understanding of the psychoacoustics of hearing impairment. Surprisingly little of the research in these areas has contributed to hearing aid design and hearing aid fitting. The articulation index has been used to optimize the audibility of speech, and loudness recruitment data has led to the design and fitting of multiband compression. Attempts to design other hearing aid algorithms based on the psychoacoustics of hearing impairment, such as the application of spectral contrast enhancement to compensate for the broader auditory filters of the hearing impaired (Baer, Moore, & Gatehouse, 1993), have not been successful.

The future will see the successful application of hearing science to DSP technol-

ogy innovations, but most of the advances will require an integrated development of new diagnostics, signal processing, and validation measures as discussed later. The most direct application of hearing science to new digital technology in the future will be the application of auditory models to hearing aid signal processing.

Auditory Models

Auditory models have been used successfully in a variety of audio processing applications (e.g., in perceptual vocoders such as MP3 and as front-ends to automatic speech recognition systems). Multiband compression might even be considered a simplistic model of cochlear function. The application of auditory models to hearing aid processing seems logical given that hearing aids attempt to compensate for changes to auditory function. Auditory models are one way to understand normal and impaired auditory function, and certainly illuminate how processing might compensate for the difference.

Auditory models may also help with non-hearing-loss related algorithms such as environment classification. Humans can recognize sound sources and environments with much greater accuracy than computer-based systems; modeling the way that the human auditory system processes sound may provide insight into the best approach for designing DSP-based sound-source identification and environment classification.

The application of sophisticated auditory models to hearing aids has been prevented thus far by the computational limitations of hearing aid DSPs. As these DSPs become more powerful, however, the possibility of applying auditory models becomes more realistic.

Models that could prove to be beneficial when implemented in hearing aids include cochlear models that simulate level-dependent filter bandwidths and suppression with resolution equivalent to cochlear filters (Zhang, Heinz, Bruce, & Carney, 2001), modulation filterbank models that represent the perception of envelopes in different frequency regions (Dau, Kollmeier, & Kohlrausch, 1997a, 1997b), and temporal-spectral models that represent how we perceive complex features (Chi, Ru, & Shamma, 2005). Such auditory models have been derived from perceptual and physiologic data on how sound is perceived. To the extent that these models can be modified to reflect auditory perception by the hearing impaired, they could improve hearing aid design by modeling the changes to perception from an individual's specific loss.

Bondy et al. (2004) applied this approach to derive the optimal linear gain prescription for a given audiogram. A model of the cochlea and auditory nerve was used to determine the auditory nerve's response to speech for a normal auditory system and for impaired auditory systems with varying amounts of hearing loss. Bondy et al. calculated linear gain fitting algorithm parameters that brought the model of the impaired systems' auditory nerve response as close to normal as possible. The fitting prescription that resulted from this model-based approach was similar to the NAL-R fitting prescription (Byrne & Dillon, 1986) that was derived using a combination of theory and empirical data. Bondy et al.'s results demonstrate that auditory models can be used to optimize hearing aid function that had previously required empirical data to derive. The use of an auditory model also provides an explanation for why the NAL-R fitting algorithm has been

successful: the optimal gain was that which brought the auditory nerve response of the damaged auditory system closest to the response of an undamaged auditory system. Although this application did not require the model to function on the hearing aid DSP chip because the application was a fitting algorithm, one can imagine using the same model to determine proper hearing aid processing instantaneously within the hearing aid itself.

As another example, Shi et al. (2006) designed a signal processing strategy that compensated for the change to cochlear phase response caused by hearing impairment. The instantaneous phase responses of both a healthy cochlea and a damaged cochlea were modeled, and then the difference in phase was applied to the signal in order to restore the normal phase response to the hearing impaired listener. Limited results indicated an improvement to speech understanding and sound quality in some subjects.

Both of these approaches are similar to the general strategy described by Edwards (2002), who proposed that hearing aid processing should restore the psychoacoustic and physiologic measures of a damaged auditory system to normal. Accurate models of normal and impaired auditory function can be used to facilitate this approach.

Individualization

Hearing aid technology will change as the industry alters how it approaches the pathologies and needs of individual hearing impaired patients. The biotech industry is in a similar transition in its approach to disease, diagnoses, and treatment, and Table 17–2 has been adapted from a table

Table 17–2. How Hearing Loss Has Been Treated in the Past (*left column*) and in the Future (*right column*)

Past	Future
Loss defined by *audiogram*	Loss defined by *mechanism*
Uniformity of patients	Individuality of patients
Universal treatment	Individual therapy

Source: Adapted from S. Burrill (2005, April). *Biotech state of the industry.* Presented at: BayBio2005: Returns on Innovation, San Mateo, CA.

created by a biotech industry analyst (Burrill, 2005). The left column in Table 17-2 identifies how hearing aid patients have been addressed up until now, and the right column identifies how this will change in the future.

As the first entry in Table 17-2 indicates; hearing loss will become less defined by diagnostic measures, such as the audiogram, and more defined by the mechanism of the loss. Today, hearing aids are primarily fit to the audiogram of the hearing aid wearer, yet the nature of an individual's hearing loss is more complex than that simple description.

Pure-tone thresholds do not identify whether a sensorineural hearing loss is caused by damage to the outer hair cells, the inner hair cells, or a mixture of both. A rule of thumb typically has been that hearing loss up to approximately 60 dB HL is from outer hair cell loss and greater levels of loss are a result of additional damage to inner hair cells. In all likelihood, even losses below 60 dB HL contain a mixture of inner and outer hair cell damage.

Additional mechanisms of hearing loss include changes to the endocochlear potential. Schmiedt et al. (2002) has suggested that presbycusis may result from damage to the cochlear lateral wall, reduc-

ing the voltage within the cochlea and altering the function of the hair cells. In this case, the hair cells are not damaged, just altered in function, and amplification will not cause auditory nerves to respond at the same level as they would with a healthy cochlea.

Clearly, in order to best treat the hearing loss of a patient, the physiology of his or her hearing loss must be understood. To do so, additional diagnostic procedures are needed from which the mechanism of hearing loss can be estimated. For example, the amount of compression at a specific frequency region can be estimated using a masked-threshold technique (Oxenham & Plack, 1998), which may provide information on the health of outer hair cells in that frequency region. Otoacoustic emissions have been demonstrated to be correlated with compression as well (Epstein & Florentine, 2005), where the growth of OAEs with increasing stimulus level matched the growth of loudness with stimulus level. As the slope of the loudness growth function has been assumed to be related to the state of outer hair cell health, this measure of OAE response also may be useful in estimating the residual compression. Such information could be used to alter hearing aid signal processing or to design new algorithms based on a better understanding of the mechanism of someone's hearing loss.

The second entry in Table 17–2 indicates that patients with the same diagnostic characteristics of hearing loss, and maybe even the same mechanism of loss, no longer will be treated as having the same needs. Although the general approach of the industry is to treat hearing aid wearers as the same if they have identical loss, the reality is that they respond differently to the same treatment. In part, this may be because they have different mechanisms of hearing loss, but also may be because they have other differences as well.

These other differences between patients include dexterity, lifestyle, speech understanding ability, and cognitive ability. Each of these differences may result in one patient requiring different technology than another patient who has similar levels of hearing loss.

These individual differences will require different treatments to hearing impairment, as indicated by the third entry in Table 17–2. Different hearing aid technologies and feature settings will be applied as we understand the individual differences of the patients better and what their corresponding needs are. For example, the finding that IQ test scores have been positively correlated with speech understanding benefit from fast-acting compression (Gatehouse, Naylor, & Elberling, 2003) suggests that different compressor time constants might be prescribed for patients with different cognitive ability.

The increased use of mobile and home computing will allow those individual needs to be met with innovative therapies integrated with hearing aid solutions. Some patients will require more assistance in adapting to their hearing aids than others, and home-administered therapies such as LACE (Sweetow & Henderson-Sabes, 2004) could become a common method to assist patients in optimizing their use of their hearing aid technology. LACE trains users to improve their hearing with their hearing aids and adapts itself to the performance of the user. If the patient improves quickly, then LACE adjusts its difficulty quickly; if the patient has more difficulty adapting to the hearing aid and has difficulty with the tasks in LACE, then the program adjusts its difficulty slowly. One can imagine that hearing aids will adapt over time as patients adapt to their new technology in the same way that LACE training adapts the difficulty of its tests to the subject's performance. Combined with the intelligent algorithms in hearing aids discussed earlier, hearing aids become systems that are designed to refine their treatment to the individual needs of the user.

Assessment Procedures

Standard assessment procedures for measuring hearing aid benefit have focused on audibility-related performance with speech understanding measured in the presence of speech-shaped noise. Audibility is one aspect of auditory perception that is now well understood and essentially is a solved problem for hearing aids for mild and moderate levels of impairment.

Auditory perception is defined by much more than audibility, however. Suprathreshold processing can affect not only speech intelligibility, but also sound quality and factors that affect our ability to extract information about the world through what we hear. To determine how digital signal processing is affecting these factors, we need assessment procedures that are sensitive to more than audibility effects.

How does the perception of noise reduction artifacts vary with hearing loss configuration? What is the impact of multiband compression on the perception of echoes? These more complex aspects of auditory perception must now be addressed. Additional areas of investigation include the perception of amplitude and frequency modulation, cross-frequency coherence, binaural perception, and timbre. A more sophisticated understanding of how hearing impairment and hearing aid processing affects complex auditory processing such as source segregation, auditory streaming, feature extraction, and auditory-visual integration also need to be better understood in order to better design the signal processing within hearing aids. Some of these issues are addressed in the next section.

Cognition

In general, the hearing aid research community and the hearing aid industry take a bottom-up approach to hearing impairment research and hearing aid design. They are concerned with how the impairment in the auditory periphery alters the auditory signal, and how hearing aids change this peripheral representation. Diagnostics assess the function of the auditory periphery, hearing aids are designed to account for changes to auditory processing in the cochlea, and validation procedures assess speech understanding ability that primarily is affected by audibility.

A significant amount of auditory perception, however, is top-down, involving the cognitive system. Hearing impairment

and hearing aids likely have an impact on this higher-level function. Cognitive function and its interaction with both hearing impairment and hearing aids have not received much clinical or research effort. The interaction between hearing aids and cognitive function is also not considered in the design of hearing aids.

In the future, hearing aids will be designed not only to take into account the effect of processing on signal representation in the auditory periphery, but also to take into account the impact of processing on cognitive function.

Attention and Effort

A common complaint of the hearing impaired is that listening in noisy situations is an exhausting experience, and a hearing-impaired person is far more tired after an hour of conversing in a noisy situation than someone with normal hearing. This likely is due to the increased listening effort necessary to understand speech through the distorted auditory system.

Communication is a complex process that embodies far more than audibility-related auditory function. When listening to speech in a noisy situation, linguistics and context information are used to assist in the speech understanding process. Sentences with inaudible words, such as in the sentence "The hungry cat chased a small gray _____," can still be accurately understood with above chance probability because of context and linguistics. The missing word in the example can be anticipated to be "mouse" because of the topic, because of the modifiers "small" and "gray," because it must be a noun, and perhaps because the person listening was able to determine that the word was a single syllable even though the phonemes were unidentifiable. If the missing word occurs earlier in the sentence, such as "a _____, small and gray, was being chased by a hungry cat," the listener can hold the sentence in memory, then go back and fill in the missing word after hearing the whole sentence.

These are cognitive aspects of speech understanding that affect the amount of attention and effort that the cognitive system expends during communication. In actual conversation (as opposed to standard speech-in-noise tests), the listener also is generating thoughts that are produced by what they are hearing, creating relationships between different sentences while drawing higher level contexts, storing information in memory, and thinking about what he or she is going to say during the conversation in response to what they are hearing. In other words, far more cognitive activity is involved in conversation than is tested with phoneme recognition tests or simple speech in noise tests. Figure 17–1, adapted from Sweetow and Henderson-Sabes (2004), graphically illustrates this complex situation. Of course, listeners may be taxing their attentional system even more by performing secondary tasks during conversation, such as reading a menu or driving.

If speech information is being missed due to poorer audibility from hearing loss in the auditory periphery, the cognitive system will have to work harder to maintain an acceptable level of understanding. Situations may exist where a hearing impaired person understands speech as well as a normal hearing person but is relying more on processing of context and linguistic information to help interpret parts of speech that are inaudible. Pichora-Fuller et al. (1995) have demonstrated that older hearing-impaired listeners benefit more from context in speech than normally hearing older listeners, possibly due to the hearing impaired listeners' more frequent use of their cognitive system to assist in speech understanding. In the same study, they also demonstrated that background noise babble affects word memory in the same way that hearing impairment does, suggesting that distortion to the speech signal either by hearing impairment or by additive noise causes the cognitive system to function poorer. The possibility also exists that the combination of hearing impairment and background noise may cause an even greater impairment to the cognitive system.

A fundamental concept in attention and effort is that the cognitive system has limited resources available at any given time, and as one system is tasked more, other systems have their capabilities negatively impacted (Kahneman, 1973). Several researchers have demonstrated that poorer speech understanding and memory function in the aging population that is normally attributed to a decline in brain function are in part caused by a deterioration of the auditory periphery (Lindenberger & Baltes, 1994; Schneider, Daneman, & Murphy, 2005; Schneider, Daneman, Murphy, & See, 2000). Deterioration to the perceptual system (bottom-up) can impair the cognitive system (top-down) by increasing the cognitive load necessary for auditory processing and limiting the cognitive ability left for other functions.

When more cognitive resources are needed to process speech in noise, fewer resources are available for other cognitive tasks. McCoy et al. (2005) found that older subjects with hearing impairment performed worse in a word recall task than a similar age group with normal hearing. Their conclusion was that the additional cognitive resources required by the hearing impaired group to understand words in sentences impaired their ability to remember the words because fewer cognitive resources were available. Schneider et al. (2000) found a similar interaction between hearing ability and speech comprehension.

These results and others indicate that hearing impaired listeners expend greater effort than normally hearing listeners even when the two groups are understanding speech at the same level of performance. This greater effort not only denies cognitive resources for other activities, but could account for their self-reported increased level of stress and exhaustion when having a conversation in a noisy environment.

Whether or not current hearing aid processing reduces or increases listening effort is unknown. Evidence using a dual-attention task (Sarampalis, Kalluri, Edwards, & Hafter, 2008) suggests that signal-to-noise ratio improvement resulting from directional microphones and from noise reduction can reduce listening effort. Reaction times for a dual-attention task were measured in which the primary task was to understand speech in noise and the secondary simultaneous task was to monitor a computer monitor and respond with a keyboard stroke according to what was seen. In this paradigm, a decrease in the reaction time indicates a reduction in the effort applied to the primary task: understanding speech in noise. Their results are strongly suggestive of both directional microphones and noise reduction technology reducing the amount of effort necessary to understand speech in noise.

If this continued line of research proves successful, a new dimension of hearing aid benefit will be associated with hearing aid technology. Figure 17–2 shows possible future specifications for noise reduction and directional microphone benefit. The left figure represents the current state of characterizing hearing aid benefit, in which an increase in directional strength increases speech understanding whereas an increase in noise reduction strength has no impact on speech understanding. The figure on the right hypothesizes one possible future outcome, in which both algorithms are shown to provide cognitive benefit by reducing the listening effort required for speech understanding. If such interactions between hearing aid processing and cognitive function are discovered, cognitive function metrics such as listening effort could be used by hearing aid companies to select between different signal processing designs and to improve current ones. Both patients and dispensers also will appreciate the greater extent to which signal processing provides benefit to the hearing aid wearer, and increased user satisfaction is possible.

Auditory Scene Analysis

Auditory scene analysis is "the organization of sound scenes according to their inferred sources" (Bregman, 1990). It is the ability to make sense of the world around us from what we hear, to take a complex auditory signal that consists of sound from multiple sources and be able to separate the individual auditory components and "hear" the individual sound sources. The ability to pay attention to one person speaking while several other speakers are also heard, or to perceive music from a band as consisting of individual instruments playing rather than

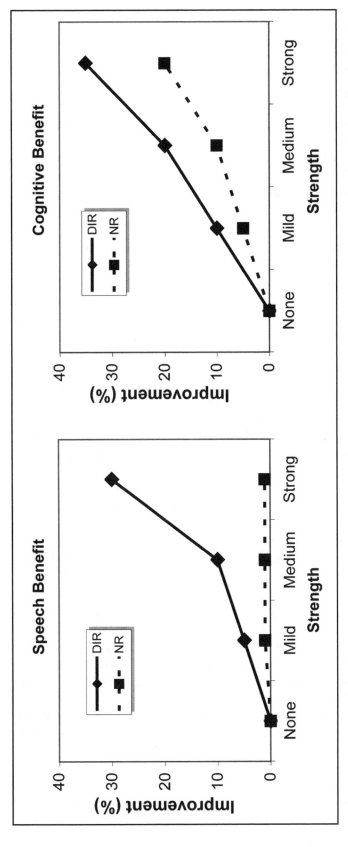

Figure 17–2. Future measures of hearing aid benefit. The left panel shows theoretical improvements to speech understanding from noise reduction and directionality. The right panel shows theoretical improvements to listening effort from noise reduction and directionality.

one jumbled cacophony, is a result of our cognitive ability performing auditory scene analysis.

Research in this field has determined that listeners are able to easily combine acoustic components across frequency and time into individual sources by identifying certain features that bind acoustic components together. These features include:

- common harmonicity
- common onsets and offsets
- common amplitude and frequency modulation
- common spatial location
- common timbre.

Listeners pre-attentively group together sound using these auditory features into auditory objects, which then allows them to focus their attention on a specific sound source (e.g., a conversation to their left or a trumpet in a jazz ensemble. An example of this ability was demonstrated by Summerfield and Assman (1991), where subjects' ability to identify two simultaneously spoken vowels was improved when the fundamental frequency of the two vowels differed. Harmonicity was used as a cue to separate temporally and spectrally overlapping speech components into two separate auditory objects (i.e., two vowels).

The difficulty that hearing impaired listeners have understanding speech in noisy environments, such as a loud restaurant, even when all sounds are audible, may be related to a dysfunction in their auditory scene analysis process. A room full of people speaking often is described by people with significant hearing impairment as sounding like a jumble akin to a bee hive, where they can hear but cannot understand speech. This deficit

could result from an inability to separate sound components into auditory objects, preventing the listener from focusing attention on and listening to a single talker.

The effect of hearing impairment and hearing aid processing on auditory scene analysis will become a significant research effort in the near future. The possibility exists that current hearing aids may interfere with auditory scene analysis ability (Edwards, 2003). If interactions are found, hearing aids could be developed with the specific goal of improving a listener's auditory scene analysis ability.

Algorithms such as multiband compression and noise reduction can alter the amplitude modulations, onsets, offsets, and perceived locations of sounds—cures necessary for the creation of auditory objects—and therefore could impact auditory scene analysis ability. If this occurred, listeners would have difficulty focusing their attention on specific sound sources, and their ability to understand speech in the presence of other talkers would be affected along with other auditory activities such as listening to music. Freyman et al. (2001) have demonstrated that informational masking, a phenomenon associated with auditory scene analysis, affects a listener's ability to understand speech in the presence of other talkers, and that perceived spatial separation between the talkers improves a person's ability to understand the target speaker. Any interference on sound source localization by hearing aids may affect improvements to speech understanding caused by spatial separation (Kalluri, Shinn-Cunningham, & Edwards, 2006).

Other high level functions that occur in the midbrain also could affected by hearing impairment and hearing aids. Hearing-impaired listeners have a more difficult time understanding speech in reverberation than normally hearing listeners. The binaural auditory system is designed to suppress echoes, a phenomenon known as the precedence effect or the law of the first wavefront whereby the auditory system attends to the first instance of a sound and suppresses the perception of subsequent echoes. The impact of hearing impairment and hearing aid processing is not well understood, but research in this area could suggest hearing aid designs that help hearing impaired listeners understand speech in noise by allowing normal auditory function such as the precedence effect to operate effectively.

Finally, auditory scene analysis may have other applications to hearing aids. Edwards (2003) noted that models of auditory scene analysis have been applied to computer speech recognition systems, and he suggested that similar models could be implemented in hearing aids as a way of preprocessing speech to improve speech understanding by the hearing impaired. Clearly, significant work in the combined fields of auditory scene analysis and perception with hearing aids needs to be conducted to better understand how these two fields can be combined to produce better hearing aids.

In general, the assessment of hearing aid benefit needs to be applied to auditory function that is mitigated by more than audibility. The functioning of the complete auditory and cognitive systems need to be assessed when determining the benefit from hearing aids. This will lead to a better understanding of the needs of the hearing impaired, and will provide additional metrics from which to compare different hearing aid technologies. Basing hearing aid designs on simple measures of speech understanding ability in speech-shaped noise do not capture the complexities of auditory perception and cannot determine whether hearing aid technology is improving or making worse complex auditory and cognitive function. With the introduction of new performance measurement procedures, hearing aid technology will be improved in ways that cannot be assessed today, and hearing aid wearers will better appreciate the benefit provided to them by hearing aids, which will possibly produce more satisfied hearing aid users.

Summary

As digital hearing aid technology matures, new innovations become more difficulty to develop. Straightforward engineering approaches have driven applications up until now, but future advances will require collaboration across many fields including psychoacoustics, signal processing, and clinical audiology.

The methods by which new digital hearing aid technology is developed are about to change. Concepts of connectivity and individuality will drive much of the new applications. As the interaction between hearing aid processing and complex auditory and cognitive function becomes better understood, new concepts in digital hearing aid technology will be developed to account for these interactions. As DSP chips become more advanced in capability, improvements to current algorithms will be made and new algorithms will be created with inspiration from such sources as auditory models and other audio industries.

Patient benefit should drive all of this development, and producing evidence of this benefit when new technology is introduced will become more commonplace as evidence-based practice becomes more popular. This alone will cause engineering development to work closely with audiologic and auditory science to see that new diagnostic measures and validation procedures are developed in conjunction with new digital technology (Cox, 2005; Edwards, 2006).

References

Baer, T., Moore, B. C., & Gatehouse, S. (1993). Spectral contrast enhancement of speech in noise for listeners with sensorineural hearing impairment: Effects on intelligibility, quality, and response times. *Journal of Rehabilitation and Research Development*, *30*(1), 49-72.

Beecher, F. (2000). A vision of the future: A 'concept hearing aid' with Bluetooth wireless technology. *Hearing Journal*, *53*(10), 40-44.

Besing, J., Koehnke, J., Zurek, P., Kawakyu, K., & Lister, J. (1999). Aided and unaided performance on a clinical test of sound localization. *Journal of the Acoustical Society of America*, *105*, 1025.

Bondy, J., Becker, S., Bruce, I., Trainer, L., & Haykin, S. (2004). A novel signal processing strategy for hearing aid design: neurocomputation. *Signal Processing*, *84*(7), 1239-1253.

Boothroyd, A., Fitz, K., Kindred, J., Kochkin, S., Levitt, H., Moore, B. C. J., et al. (2007). Hearing aids and wireless technology. *Hearing Review*, *14*(6), 44-48.

Bregman, A. (1990). *Auditory scene analysis.* Cambridge, MA: MIT Press.

Burrill, S. (2005, April). *Biotech state of the industry.* Paper presented at the BayBio-2005: Returns on Innovation, San Mateo, CA.

Byrne, D., & Dillon, H. (1986). The National Acoustic Laboratories' (NAL) new procedure for selecting the gain and frequency response of a hearing aid. *Ear and Hearing*, *7*(4), 257-265.

Chi, T., Ru, P., & Shamma, S. A. (2005). Multiresolution spectrotemporal analysis of complex sounds. *Journal of the Acoustical Society of America*, *118*(2), 887-906.

Christensen, C. M. (1997). *The innovator's dilemma.* Cambridge, MA: Harvard Business School Press.

Cox, R. M. (2005). Evidence-based practice in provision of amplification. *Journal of the American Academy of Audiology*, *16*, 419-438.

Dau, T., Kollmeier, B., & Kohlrausch, A. (1997a). Modeling auditory processing of amplitude modulation. I. Detection and masking with narrow-band carriers. *Journal of the Acoustical Society of America*, *102*(5, Pt. 1), 2892-2905.

Dau, T., Kollmeier, B., & Kohlrausch, A. (1997b). Modeling auditory processing of amplitude modulation. II. Spectral and temporal integration. *Journal of the Acoustical Society of America*, *102*(5, Pt. 1), 2906-2919.

Desloge, J., Rabinowitz, W., & Zurek, P. (1997). Microphone-array hearing aids with binaural output Part I: Fixed-processing systems. *IEEE Transactions on Speech, Audio, and Language Processing*, *5*, 529-542.

Durant, E. A., Wakefield, G. H., Van Tasell, D. J., & Rickert, M. E. (2004). Efficient perceptual tuning of hearing aids with genetic algorithms. *IEEE Transactions on Speech, Audio, and Language Processing*, *12*(2), 144-155.

Edwards, B. (2002). *Signal processing, hearing aid design, and the psychoacoustic Turing test.* Paper presented at the IEEE International Conference on Acoustics, Speech, and Signal Processing, Orlando, FL.

Edwards, B. (2003). Hearing aids and hearing impairment. In A. Greenberg, A. Popper, & R. Fay (Eds.), *Speech processing in the auditory system.* New York: Springer.

Edwards, B. (2006). What outsiders tell us about the hearing industry. *Hearing Review*, *13*(3), 88-92.

Epstein, M., & Florentine, M. (2005). Inferring basilar-membrane motion from tone-burst otoacoustic emissions and psychoacoustic measurements. *Journal of the Acoustical Society of America, 117*(1), 263–274.

Freyman, R. L., Balakrishnan, U., & Helfer, K. S. (2001). Spatial release from informational masking in speech recognition. *Journal of the Acoustical Society of America, 109*(5, Pt. 1), 2112–2122.

Gatehouse, S., Naylor, G., & Elberling, C. (2003). Benefits from hearing aids in relation to the interaction between the user and the environment. *International Journal of Audiology, 42*(Suppl. 1), S77–S85.

Kahneman, D. (1973). *Attention and effort.* Englewood Cliffs, NJ: Prentice-Hall.

Kalluri, S., Shinn-Cunningham, B., & Edwards, B. (2006, April 6–8). *Effect of hearing-aid compression on spatial unmasking.* Paper presented at the American Academy of Audiology, Minneapolis, MN.

Kirkwood, D. H. (2007). Bucking bad economic news, hearing aid sales rise by 5.4% on way to record year. *Hearing Journal, 60*(12), 11–16.

Klasen, T. J., Moonen, M., Van den Bogaert, T., & Wouters, J. (2005). *Preservation of interaural time delay for binaural hearing aids through multi-channel wiener filtering based noise reduction.* Paper presented at the Proc. IEEE-ICASSP.

Kochkin, S. (2005). MarkeTrak VII: Customer satisfaction with hearing instruments in the digital age. *Hearing Journal, 58*(9), 30–42.

Lindenberger, U., & Baltes, P. B. (1994). Sensory functioning and intelligence in old age: A strong connection. *Psychology and Aging, 9*(3), 339–355.

McCoy, S. L., Tun, P. A., Cox, L. C., Colangelo, M., Stewart, R. A., & Wingfield, A. (2005). Hearing loss and perceptual effort: Downstream effects on older adults' memory for speech. *Quarterly Journal of Experimental Psychology, A, 58*(1), 22–33.

Myers, D. G. (2006). In a looped America, hearing aids would be twice as valuable. *Hearing Journal, 59*(5), 17–23.

Oxenham, A. J., & Plack, C. J. (1998). Suppression and the upward spread of masking. *Journal of the Acoustical Society of America, 104*(6), 3500–3510.

Pichora-Fuller, M. K., Schneider, B. A., & Daneman, M. (1995). How young and old adults listen to and remember speech in noise. *Journal of the Acoustical Society of America, 97*(1), 593–608.

Ross, M. (2006). Telecoils are about more than telephones. *Hearing Journal, 59*(5), 24–28.

Sarampalis, A., Kalluri, S., Edwards, B., & Hafter, E. (2008). *Objective measures of listening effort: Effects of background noise and noise reduction.* Manuscript submitted for publication.

Schmiedt, R. A., Lang, H., Okamura, H. O., & Schulte, B. A. (2002). Effects of furosemide applied chronically to the round window: A model of metabolic presbyacusis. *Journal of Neuroscience, 22*(21), 9643–9650.

Schneider, B. A., Daneman, M., & Murphy, D. R. (2005). Speech comprehension difficulties in older adults: Cognitive slowing or age-related changes in hearing? *Psychology and Aging, 20*(2), 261–271.

Schneider, B. A., Daneman, M., Murphy, D. R., & See, S. K. (2000). Listening to discourse in distracting settings: the effects of aging. *Psychology and Aging, 15*(1), 110–125.

Shi, L., Carney, L. H., & Doherty, K. A. (2006). Correction of the peripheral spatiotemporal response pattern: A potential new signal-processing strategy. *Journal of Speech, Language, and Hearing Research, 49*(4), 848–855.

Summerfield, Q., & Assmann, P. F. (1991). Perception of concurrent vowels: Effects of harmonic misalignment and pitch-period asynchrony. *Journal of the Acoustical Society of America, 89*(3), 1364–1377.

Sweetow, R., & Henderson-Sabes, J. (2004). The case for LACE (Listening and Communication Enhancement). *Hearing Journal, 57*(3), 32–38.

Van den Bogaert, T., Klasen, T. J., Moonen, M., Van Deun, L., & Wouters, J. (2006). Horizontal localization with bilateral hearing aids: Without is better than with. *Journal of the Acoustical Society of America*, *119*(1), 515–526.

van Veen, B. D., & Buckley, K. M. (1988). Beamforming: A versatile approach to spatial filtering. *IEEE ASSP Magazine*, *5*, 4–24.

Yanz, J. L. (2006). The future of wireless devices in hearing care: A technology that promises to transform the hearing industry. *Hearing Review*, *13*(1), 18–20.

Yanz, J. L., Roberts, R., & Colburn, T. (2006). The ongoing evolution of Bluetooth in hearing care. *Hearing Review*, *13*(1), 18–20, 93.

Zhang, X., Heinz, M. G., Bruce, I. C., & Carney, L. H. (2001). A phenomenological model for the responses of auditory-nerve fibers: I. Nonlinear tuning with compression and suppression. *Journal of the Acoustical Society of America*, *109*(2), 648–670.

Index